Mass Action in the Nervous System

MASS ACTION IN THE NERVOUS SYSTEM

Examination of the Neurophysiological Basis
of Adaptive Behavior through the EEG

WALTER J. FREEMAN

Department of Physiology–Anatomy
University of California
Berkeley, California

ACADEMIC PRESS   New York   San Francisco   London   1975

A Subsidiary of Harcourt Brace Jovanovich, Publishers

ACADEMIC PRESS, INC.
111 Fifth Avenue, New York, New York 10003

United Kingdom Edition published by
ACADEMIC PRESS, INC. (LONDON) LTD.
24/28 Oval Road, London NW1

Library of Congress Cataloging in Publication Data

Freeman, Walter J.
    Mass action in the nervous system.

    Bibliography: p.
    Includes indexes.
    1.   Neurophysiology—Mathematical models.
    2.   Adaptation (Physiology)—Mathematical models.
    3.   Electroencephalography.   I.   Title.
    [DNLM: 1.   Electroencephalography.   2.   Neurophysiology.
    WL150 F855m]
    QP356;F72   612'.822   74-27781
    ISBN 0–12–267150–3

To my father

Contents

PREFACE   xi
ACKNOWLEDGMENTS   xiii
NOTATION   xv

Chapter 1 Topological Properties

1.1.   The Approach to Neural Masses   1
       1.1.1.   Direct and Indirect Observations   1
       1.1.2.   The Use of Models in a Hierarchy   3
       1.1.3.   Macroscopic Forms of Cooperative Neural Activity   5
1.2.   Single Neurons   10
       1.2.1.   The Structures of Neurons   10
       1.2.2.   The Operations of Neurons   11
       1.2.3.   The State Variables of Neurons   13
       1.2.4.   Specification of the Active States and Operations   16
       1.2.5.   Input–Output Relations of Single Neurons   19
       1.2.6.   Multiple Stable States of Neurons   22
       1.2.7.   Basic Topologies of Networks of Neurons   24
1.3.   Neural Masses   25
       1.3.1.   A Topological Hierarchy of Interactive Sets   25
       1.3.2.   The State Variables of KO and KI Sets   34
       1.3.3.   The Operations of Neural Sets   37
       1.3.4.   Feedback Gain as a Parameter for Interaction   39
       1.3.5.   Multiple Stable States and the Levels of Interaction   42
       1.3.6.   The Relation of Multiple Stabilities to Neural Signals   46
       1.3.7.   The Conditions for Realizability   47
       1.3.8.   The Use of Differential Equations   49

vii

Chapter 2   Time-Dependent Properties

2.1. Measurement of Neural Events   51
    2.1.1. Representation of Events by Functions   51
    2.1.2. Input–Output Functions   55
    2.1.3. Linear Input–Output Functions   57
    2.1.4. The Impulse and the Impulse Response   60
2.2. Linear Models for Neural Membrane   61
    2.2.1. The Topology of the Membrane   61
    2.2.2. Differential Equations   64
    2.2.3. The Laplace Transform   67
    2.2.4. Application of the Laplace Transform to the Membrane   70
2.3. Linear Models for Parts of Neurons   72
    2.3.1. Convolution   72
    2.3.2. The Convolution Theorem   76
    2.3.3. Transfer Functions for Pulse Transmission   80
    2.3.4. The Core Conductor Model   86
    2.3.5. Synaptic Delay   91
2.4. Linear Models for Neurons   94
    2.4.1. Formulation of the Topology   94
    2.4.2. Input–Output Pairs and the Differential Equation   96
    2.4.3. Interpretation of the Parameters   99
    2.4.4. Linear Function for Wave to Pulse Conversion   101
2.5. Linear Models for Neural Masses   103
    2.5.1. Use of Nonlinear Regression   103
    2.5.2. The KO Neural Set   106
    2.5.3. Oscillatory Responses from a KII Set   110

Chapter 3   Amplitude-Dependent Properties

3.1. Nonlinear Models for Neural Membranes   121
    3.1.1. The Ionic Hypothesis   121
    3.1.2. Metabolic Forces   125
    3.1.3. The Concept of Equilibrium Potential   126
    3.1.4. The Sodium Permeability Model   129
3.2. Nonlinear Models for Neurons and Parts of Neurons   134
    3.2.1. Action Potentials in Axons   134
    3.2.2. Threshold Uncertainty in Axons   138
    3.2.3. Postsynaptic Potentials in Dendrites   140
    3.2.4. Amplitude-Dependent Input–Output Relations   144
3.3. Nonlinear Models for Neural Masses   146
    3.3.1. Background Activity in the Wave Mode   146
    3.3.2. Background Activity in the Pulse Mode   150
    3.3.3. Relations of Waves and Pulses   154
    3.3.4. Wave to Pulse Conversion in the KI Set   159
    3.3.5. Pulse to Wave Conversion in the KI Set   163
    3.3.6. The Forward Gain of the KI Set   165

Chapter 4   Space-Dependent Properties

4.1. Potential Fields of Single Neurons   172
      4.1.1. Basis Functions for Measurement of Potential in Space   173
      4.1.2. Basis Functions for Potential in Current Fields   177
      4.1.3. Potential Functions for the Core Conductor   180
      4.1.4. Potential Fields of Axons   185
      4.1.5. Nodes and Branched Fibers   188
4.2. Potential Fields of Neural Masses   193
      4.2.1. Measurement of Observed Fields   193
      4.2.2. Basis Functions for Potential Fields of Neural Masses   196
      4.2.3. Compound Potential Fields: Modular Analysis   202
4.3. Potential Fields in the Olfactory Bulb   211
      4.3.1. Bulbar Geometry and Topology   212
      4.3.2. Analysis of the Spatial Function of Potential   219
      4.3.3. Time-Dependent Activity   228
4.4. Potential Fields in the Prepyriform Cortex   234
      4.4.1. Cortical Geometry and Topology   234
      4.4.2. Observed Fields of Cortical Potential   238
      4.4.3. Relation of Potential Fields to Active States   245
4.5. Divergence and Convergence in Neural Masses   249
      4.5.1. The Operation of Divergence   249
      4.5.2. Evaluation of Spatial Distributions of Active States   253
      4.5.3. Evaluation of Synaptic Divergence   260
      4.5.4. Evaluation of Tractile Divergence   264

Chapter 5   Interaction: Single Feedback Loops with Fixed Gain

5.1. General Properties of Single Feedback Loops   270
      5.1.1. Types of Neural Feedback   271
      5.1.2. Derivation of the Lumped Piecewise Linear Approximation   273
      5.1.3. Root Locus as a Function of Feedback Gain   278
      5.1.4. Amplitude-Dependent Gain and Stability   284
5.2. Reduction from the KI Level   285
      5.2.1. Topological Analysis of the Glomerular Layer   285
      5.2.2. Differential Equations for the KI_e Set   291
      5.2.3. Self-Stabilization of the KI_e Set   299
5.3. Reduction from the KII Level   305
      5.3.1. Topological Analysis of the Olfactory Bulb   305
      5.3.2. Differential Equations for the Open Loop Cases   309
      5.3.3. Differential Equations for the Closed Loop Cases   314
5.4. Reduction from the KIII Level   321
      5.4.1. Topological Analysis of the Prepyriform Cortex   321
      5.4.2. Differential Equations for the Cortex   326
      5.4.3. Transfer Function of the LOT Input Channel   330
      5.4.4. Pulse–Wave Relations in Cortex and Bulb   334
      5.4.5. Channels for Centrifugal Input   338

Chapter 6   Multiple Feedback Loops with Variable Gain

6.1. Equilibrium States: Characteristic Frequency   342
    6.1.1. Definition of the Three Types of Feedback Gain   342
    6.1.2. Solution of the Differential Equations   349
    6.1.3. Experimental and Theoretical Root Loci   355
    6.1.4. Bias Control of Characteristic Frequency   366
    6.1.5. Root Loci Dependent on EEG Amplitudes   370
6.2. Limit Cycle States: Mechanisms of the EEG   378
    6.2.1. Stability Properties of KII Sets   378
    6.2.2. Limit Cycle States in the First Mode   381
    6.2.3. Limit Cycle States in the Second Mode   386
    6.2.4. Sources of Error and Limitation   390
    6.2.5. Comparisons with Related Mathematical Models   396

Chapter 7   Signal Processing by Neural Mass Actions

7.1. Behavioral Correlates of Wave Activity in KII Sets   402
    7.1.1. The Operational Basis for Correlation   402
    7.1.2. Factor Analysis of AEPs   407
    7.1.3. Patterns of Change in AEPS with Attention   414
    7.1.4. A Proposed Cortical Mechanism of Attention   422
7.2. Transformations of Neural Signals by KII Sets   427
    7.2.1. Neural Coding in the Olfactory Bulb   429
    7.2.2. Bulbar Mechanisms for Phase Modulation   434
    7.2.3. Attention and the Cortical Expectation Function   440
    7.2.4. Possible Mechanisms of Cortical Output   446
7.3. Comments concerning Neocortical Mass Actions   448
    7.3.1. Rhythmic Potentials and Rhythmic Stimulation   449
    7.3.2. DC Polarization and Steady Potentials   452
    7.3.3. Unit Activity Correlated with Sensory and Motor Events   455

References   462

AUTHOR INDEX   473
SUBJECT INDEX   477

Preface

This book was written to answer the questions: What are the neural mechanisms, and what is the behavioral significance of the electroencephalogram (EEG)? The answers are partial, tentative, and predictably complex. Emphasis is given to observations made on the mammalian olfactory system for reasons stated below. Citations to the literature are restricted to reports exemplifying particular points. Extensive bibliographies can be found in several recent reviews of the olfactory system (LeGros Clark, 1957; Ottoson, 1963; Moulton & Tucker, 1964; Wenzel & Sieck, 1967; Shepherd, 1972). Some appropriate introductory textbooks in relevant fields of study are also suggested.

The book is organized as follows. Chapter 1 consists of a brief nonmathematical review of the concept of the neuron and the interrelations among neurons that lead to the formation of interactive masses. New terms are defined and the central argument is presented.

In Chapter 2 the linear properties of neurons and their parts are reviewed. This provides an opportunity to introduce the use of linear differential equations and the Laplace transform method for solution. Mathematical description is not a prerequisite for understanding single neurons and is usually deemphasized. Description and prediction of the properties of masses of neurons cannot, however, be undertaken without the use of mathematics, and the review provides both some experience in describing the lower level models and some equations to be used as elements in constructing models at a higher level.

In Chapter 3 the ionic hypothesis is reviewed, and the nonlinear input–output relations of neurons in masses are expressed in terms of amplitude-dependent coefficients in linear differential equations. Chapter 4 deals with the relations between the states of activity of neurons, both singly and in

xi

masses, and the electrical fields of potential which are the principle means for indirect observation of the activity. Chapter 5 describes the properties resulting from feedback within neural masses. Chapter 6 analyzes the effects of the nonlinearities in the input–output relations of neurons on the behavior of masses. Chapter 7 contains some inferences concerning the mechanisms of neural signal processing at the level of neural masses.

The book is intended as a model for an advanced text in neurophysiology, and some understanding is assumed of the elements of the fields of linear analysis (DiStefano *et al.*, 1967), probability (Parzen, 1960), statistics Anderson, 1958), theory of potential (Rogers, 1954), neuroanatomy (Gardner, 1968), electrophysiology (Katz, 1966), neuropharmacology (Goodman & Gilman, 1970), and experimental psychology (Hebb, 1958). Introductory courses in neurobiology and calculus should suffice for understanding the basic approach, with the help of a textbook on linear systems analysis. Introductory materials have been included to provide a coherent argument from first principles, and to provide guidelines for extraction of essential background from standard textbooks in neurophysiology and linear analysis, but not as a substitute for the textbooks.

The greater part of the experimental detail in this book is drawn from the mammalian olfactory system. There are two reasons for this. The primary reason is that neural mass actions reflected in the EEG are mainly identified with the mechanisms of adaptive behavior in vertebrates. The neural machinery of the spinal cord, brainstem, and cerebellum has the property of modifiability, but only the forebrain is capable of elaborating adaptive, goal-oriented, purposive, learned, teleological behavior. The neural masses in the forebrain are also the only brain structures that generate well-developed EEG waves in the range of 1 to 100 Hz. When the EEG is present and orderly, adaptive behavior is generally found. When the EEG is absent, or is disorganized as in deep sleep, epilepsy, or general anesthesia, there is no adaptive behavior. By inference, the EEG is like a Rosetta Stone for deciphering the neural coding of adaptive behavior. The olfactory system is the simplest part of the brain to elaborate both.

The more obvious reason for emphasizing the olfactory system is that a particular point of view is being presented which has evolved from the study of the properties of this system. The application of the theory and methods described here to other systems must be based on detailed reexamination of the anatomy, electrophysiology, and behavioral correlates of those systems and not on casual generalizations. The intention in giving examples is to illustrate what kinds of data are needed and how they are obtained, as much as to construct a general theory. Students of spinal, cerebellar, and brainstem machinery may find the means to break some intellectual log-jams with the methods and concepts described here, but the message is mainly directed to students of the cortex and basal ganglia.

Acknowledgments

The work described here has been financially supported by grants from the National Institute of Mental Health, MH 06686, the Foundations' Fund for Research in Psychiatry, 59–204, and the Guggenheim Foundation. Many of the illustrations in this book were prepared with the help of Brian Burke, Charmane Thomson, The Scientific Photographic Laboratory, and the Computer Center on the Berkeley Campus. Computer programming was by Brian Burke. The manuscript was typed by Barbara Kitashima. Permission is achnowledged for reproduction of figures from *Biophysical Journal*, The Rockefeller Institute; *Journal of Comparative Neurology*, The Wistar Institute of Anatomy and Biology; *Experimental Neurology*, Academic Press, Inc.; *The Conduction of the Nervous Impulse*, Liverpool University Press; *American Journal of Physiology*, American Physiological Society; *Brain Mechanisms, Progress in Brain Research*, American Elsevier Publishing Co., Inc.; *Studies from the Rockefeller Institute*, Rockefeller Institute for Medical Research; *Journal of Cellular and Comparative Physiology*, Wistar Institute of Anatomy and Biology; *Journal of Physiology*, Cambridge University Press; *Physiology of Nerve Cells*, The Johns Hopkins Press; *Transactions of Biomedical Engineering*; Institute of Electronics and Electronic Engineers.

The author wishes to express appreciation to the students, former students, and colleagues on the Berkeley faculty, particularly Professor O. J. M. Smith for introducing us to systems analysis, Dr. Heinrich Bantli and Dr. Soo-Myung Ahn for advice and comment on the manuscript, and Professor I. Prigogine whose invitation to lecture as Titulaire de la Chaire Solvay 1974 at the Université Libre de Bruxelles provided an impetus for writing this book.

Notation

A. *Individual Neurons and Neural Sets*

A1. Coordinate Variables

t	real time	14, 52
T	lag time (e.g., from stimulus)	55
T_a	conduction (propagation) delay	83
s	Laplace complex frequency	41, 68
ΔT	duration of an observation or time window	55
x, y, z	Cartesian spatial coordinates	34
X	vector denoting x, y, z	37

A2. Time-Dependent Functions and Operations

$\delta(t)$	Dirac delta function	60, 77
$\mu(t)$	step function	65, 77
$o(t)$	time function for active state	17
$f(t), v(t), p(t)$	time functions for observable events	52
$\mathscr{L}, \mathscr{L}^{-1}$	Laplace transform and its inverse	69
$F(s), V(s), P(s)$	linear operations in the frequency domain	68, 272
$v'(t)$	measured (digitized) time function in the wave mode	53
$p'(t)$	measured (digitized) time function in the pulse mode	53
$\mathscr{E}[v'(t)] = \hat{v}(T)$	wave mode ensemble averages for fixed T	55
$\mathscr{E}[p'(t)] = \hat{p}(T)$	pulse mode ensemble averages for fixed T	55
$\bar{v}, \bar{p}$	average of $v'(t), p'(t)$ over time t	207, 303
$\varepsilon(t), \varepsilon(T, X)$	random error, noise, or least mean square deviation, e.g., $[\hat{v}(T) - v(T)] = \varepsilon(T)$	53

A3. Equivalence Statements

$=$	equals
$\triangleq$	is defined by
$\approx$	is approximated by
$\propto$	is equivalent to or replaced by

B. *Individual Neurons*

B1. Subscripts Denoting Structure

a	axonal	95
d	dendritic	95
s	soma	95
m	membrane	64, 87
l	longitudinal	65, 87
e	external	64, 87
i	internal	64, 87

B2. State Variables

o	active state	14
i	current	52
v	potential difference	52
p	pulse rate	52
$\mathbf{j}$	current density (vector)	177
j	current source–sink density	179
q	fixed charge equivalent to j	173
ξ	fixed charge density	173
$\mathbf{E}$	electrical field intensity (vector)	173

B3. Amplitude-Dependent Functions

$G_d(p, t)$ nonlinear time-varying function for pulse to wave conversion   17, 144

$G_s(v, t)$ nonlinear time-varying function for wave to pulse conversion   17,101

B4. Functional Parameters and Acronyms

τ	passive membrane time coefficient (fixed number)	88
a	passive membrane rate coefficient (fixed number)	99
T_b	distributed delay time coefficient (fixed number)	92
b	lumped cable delay rate coefficient (fixed number)	98
$T_c, 2/c$	lumped synaptic delay time coefficient (fixed number)	93

λ	membrane length coefficient (fixed number) 88
θ	axonal conduction velocity 82
EPSP	excitatory postsynaptic potential 20
IPSP	inhibitory postsynaptic potential 20
v_{EPSP}	equilibrium potential for EPSP 141
v_{IPSP}	equilibrium potential for IPSP 141

B5. Structural Parameters (capital letter = total; lower case = specific)

c_m, C_m	transmembrane capacitance 63
r_m, R_m	transmembrane resistance 63
g_m, G_m	transmembrane conductance 122
r_l, R_l	longitudinal resistance 87
r_e, R_e	external resistance 87
r_i, R_i	internal resistance 87
ρ	volume specific resistance 178
μ_y	mobility of the yth ion species 123
$\mathbf{p}_y$	membrane permeability to yth species 128

C. Neural Sets

C1. Topological Hierarchy Based on Interconnectivity

KO_e	noninteractive excitatory set 26
KO_i	noninteractive inhibitory set 26
KI_e	interactive excitatory set 29
KI_i	interactive inhibitory set 29
KII	KI_e set interactive with KI_i set 31
KIII	interactive KII sets 34

C2. State Variables

o, O	active density in any form 34
o_p, O_p	pulse density (o, O in pulse mode) 35
o_v, O_v	wave amplitude (o, O in wave mode) 35
f, F	lumped piecewise linear activity density 43
p, P	pulse rate of neuron or of unit cluster 193
v, V	potential difference in a neural mass 194
u, U	o, O in wave and/or pulse mode 37
j	current source–sink density at a point in space 179
q	fixed charge at a point in space, equivalent to j 180
ψ, Ψ	pulse density at a point in space, homologous to q 86, 250

C3. Time-Dependent Functions and Operations

AEP   average evoked potential, a form of $\hat{v}(T)$ 37
PSTH   poststimulus time histogram, a form of $\hat{p}(T)$ 37
EEG   electroencephalogram, a form of $v'(t)$ 45, 49
See also A2.

C4. Amplitude-Dependent Functions and Operations

$G(v) \triangleq G[v(t)]$ nonlinear function for wave to pulse conversion   38, 161
$G(p) \triangleq G[p(t)]$ nonlinear function for pulse to wave conversion   38, 165
$g(v)$ nonlinear gain function for wave to pulse conversion   39, 168
$g(p)$ nonlinear gain function for pulse to wave conversion   39, 167

C5. Probability Functions in Pulse and Wave Modes

$P(v)$ wave amplitude probability density   148
$P(p \cap v)$ joint pulse and wave amplitude probability density   155
$P(p \mid v)$ conditional pulse probability on wave amplitude   155
$P(p \mid T \cap v)$ conditional pulse probability on wave time and amplitude   156
$P(p \mid T \cap v \cap \omega)$ predicted pulse probability conditional on wave time, amplitude and frequency   162
$\hat{P}(p \mid T \cap v \cap \omega)$ observed pulse probability conditional on EEG time, amplitude and frequency   162
$P(T), \hat{P}(T)$ predicted observed normalized pulse probability wave   159
$P(v), \hat{P}(v)$ predicted observed normalized pulse probability sigmoid curve   159

C6. Space-dependent functions and operations

$h(x, y)$ spatial component of a neural activity distribution   194
$H(X) \triangleq H[h(x, y), z]$ linear divergence operation in the spatial domain   250
$H^{-1}(X) \triangleq H^{-1}[h(x, y), z]$ linear convergence operation in the spatial domain   252
$p(t, x, y, z), p(T, X)$ space–time distribution of action potentials   194
$v(t, x, y, z), v(T, X)$ extracellular potential field   194
$f_X(T), p_X(T)$ basis function in time for potential field   196
$v_T(X), p_T(X)$ basis function in space for potential field   198
$q(X)$ equivalent charge distribution for potential field   197
$\psi(X)$ spatial distribution of activity in pulse mode   250
x, y coordinates of a neural surface   34

x coordinate parallel to direction of propagated input over surface   219, 254

y coordinate orthogonal to direction of propagated input over surface   220, 254

z coordinate orthogonal to a neural surface   223, 254

x_0, y_0, z_0 center of a response domain   223

$x_0, y_0, z = 0$ epicenter of a response domain   220

$x = 0, y = 0, z = 0$ stimulus site   219

C7. Generalized Functions and Operations

$o(t, x, y, u)$ activity density function   41, 249

$o_v(t, x, y, u)$ activity density function in the wave mode   41, 249

$o_p(t, x, y, u)$ activity density function in the pulse mode   41, 250

$O(s, X, U)$ operation in the domains of frequency, amplitude, and space; if separable, equivalent to $G(U)H(X)F(s)$ 41, 275

Ω time and space operator denoting the form of neural signals transmitted by KII sets   434

$o(\Omega)$ wave packet carrying signal of a KII set and constituting a form of $o(t, x, y, u)$ of a component KI set   434

$\varphi(X)$ phase of $P(T)$ as a function of X in $P(p \mid T \cap v \cap \omega)$ in a KI component of a KII set   432

$\tilde{p}(X)$ modulation amplitude of $P(T)$ as a function of X in $P(p \mid T \cap v \cap \omega)$ in a KI component of a KII set   159, 433

C8. Parameters Relating to Interaction

$e, +$ excitation   19, 26

$i, -$ inhibition   19, 26

K_f, K', K_μ forward gains of input channels   293

g_e, g_i, g_o forward gains of transmitting to receiving subsets in KI sets   39, 166

K_e excitatory positive feedback gain   40, 277

K_i inhibitory positive feedback gain   41, 343

K_n negative feedback gain   42, 280

K_o reference feedback gain in steady state   44, 299

K_2 lumped feedback gain—KII feedback modeled by a diffusion process   327

T_2 lumped feedback delay—KII feedback modeled by a diffusion process   328

δ_e, δ_i operating bias coefficients of KI_e, KI_i, and KII sets   348

γ_e, γ_i rate constants for wave to pulse conversion   160

ζ_e, ζ_i rate constants for pulse to wave conversion   165

v_o, p_o mean wave amplitude and pulse density   160

$\tilde{v}_e, \tilde{v}_i$ difference between v_0 and v_{EPSP}, v_o and v_{IPSP} 164

r ratio of v_e/v_i or ζ_i/ζ_e 165

v_e^*, v_i^* effective operating amplitudes of KI_e and KI_i sets   170, 348

C9. Parameters Relating to Time and Space

$a, b, c, d, \ldots$ open loop rate coefficients (fixed numbers)   108

$\alpha, \beta, \gamma, \ldots, \omega$ closed loop rate coefficients (gain-dependent variables) 61, 110

φ_j phase of the jth sinusoidal time function   61, 111

$A_j, B_j, \ldots, P_j, V_j$ amplitude coefficients of the jth time function   110

d_j the jth pole of a transfer function   69, 108

z_j the jth zero of a transfer function   69, 108

$\times, *$ open loop single pole, double pole   278

$\bigcirc$ open loop zero   278

$\triangle$ closed loop pole   278

$\square$ closed loop zero   278

η distance (fixed number)   82

σ_x, σ_y standard deviations of a spatial Gaussian (normal) distribution $h(x, y)$ 253, 255

$\sigma_{\mu \cdot \mu + 1}$ standard deviation of a Gaussian divergence (spatial) operation $H(X)$ 260

σ_t standard deviation of a Gaussian dispersion (time) operation $F(s)$ 83

C10. Subscripts and Acronyms Referring to Structure

A   Type A prepyriform neurons (excitatory), KI_A set   47

B   Type B prepyriform neurons (inhibitory), KI_B set   47

C   Type C prepyriform neurons (excitatory), KO_C or KI_C set 47

G   bulbar granule cells (inhibitory), KI_G set   32

M   bulbar mitral–tufted cells (excitatory), KI_M set   32

N   anterior olfactory nucleus (unclassified)   47

P   bulbar periglomerular neurons (excitatory), KI_P set   33

R   olfactory receptors (excitatory), KO_R set   32

LOT   lateral olfactory tract   215, 234

PON   primary olfactory nerve   32, 212

$A_m(s)$ transfer function for PON, orthodromic to bulb   308

$A_k(s)$ transfer function for LOT, antidromic to bulb   308

$A_t(s)$ transfer function for LOT, orthodromic to cortex   325

CHAPTER 1

Topological Properties

1.1. The Approach to Neural Masses

1.1.1. DIRECT AND INDIRECT OBSERVATIONS

The basis for our curiosity about the brain is the fact that we observe interesting and purposive behavior in ourselves and in animals with intact brains, and that this behavior is disorganized or absent when the brain is damaged or destroyed. We infer that the brain is a kind of biological machine that is susceptible to manipulation through specialized receptors on and in the body, that can store and modify past input, and that can organize complex sequences of muscular contraction and glandular secretion. For 2000 years we have been interested in the physicochemical properties of this machine, and new developments in our understanding have seldom lagged more than a generation behind the major advances in physical theory and technology.

Direct examination of the living brain is not very rewarding. When deprived of its protective coverings, the brain surface appears smoothly folded, pinkish grey, and faintly translucent with a web of pulsating red and purple blood vessels on its surface. It is yielding and moist to the touch. When removed from the cranium and cut, it has the texture and faint aroma of soft cheese. The cut surface is marbled pink and white. (The "grey matter" of the outer shell or cortex and the nuclei becomes grey only when it is hardened by formaldehyde.) Its features are so incongruous that artists notoriously have difficulty in drawing the brain, unless helped by a skilled anatomist. The point is instructive, because for no other organ is what

1

we see so strongly dependent on what we expect or are told to see (Section 7.2.3).

Most of what we know and believe about the brain has come from indirect observations. These include stimulus–response relationships with or without brain lesions or the prior administration of drugs, recordings of amplified electrical potentials found or induced in the brain, and the structural residues seen under microscopes following exsanguination, chemical impregnation, and thin-sectioning of brain tissues. But the technologies of indirect observation are so complex, and the results are so dependent on variations of factors too numerous to explore systematically, that we cannot collect "facts" in the way a naturalist collects specimens for classification. Instead we maintain a dialectical process in which our expectations largely determine the techniques, and the results modify the expectations or are rejected.

This dialectic cannot be avoided, because fundamentally we have no conception of how the brain functions as a physicochemical machine. That is one of the main objectives of our search. Most new developments in understanding arise unexpectedly from the availability of new techniques for indirect observation and not from a basis in theory. They give limited insight into narrow aspects of brain function, falling far short of our ultimate aim. Often in our impatience to bridge this gap we apply to brain function certain broad concepts which accompany a new technology, but which hold for the brain only by analogy or metaphor. Familiar examples are the Cartesian pump, the Helmoltz telegraph system, and more recently the servomechanism, the digital computer, and the holograph. The use of analogies to guide experimentation is at best merely suggestive and at worst can be highly misleading.

Despite this and other pitfalls the circuitous and tentative dialectical process over the past 300 years has enabled us to accumulate a solid core of data on some elementary physicochemical properties of the brain and its parts. In order for us to interrelate and understand these data, we have evolved a series of symbolic (verbal and mathematical) representations or concepts, which are commonly called *models*. Some classic examples are the passive membrane, ionic permeability, the core conductor, the volume conductor, the synapse, the neuron, the neuron pool, and the neuron chain or reflex arc. These and related models constitute our best approximation to date of a systematic understanding of brain function on its own terms without recourse to metaphorical generalizations. They are characterized by flexibility and adaptiveness; they may be presented in very simple form or made as elaborate as the needs of the user require. They are always abstractions; the only complete description of a system is the system itself. Because models are made to interrelate facts, they are used to predict facts. Their hallmark is immediate testability by means of comparison of prediction with experimental observation, and it is conformance to the predictions of a model that makes a "fact" significant and not trivial. They are the foundation for future developments in our understanding, and, as successful models, they provide us with some insights into what the epistemological characteristics of future models will be.

1.1.2. THE USE OF MODELS IN A HIERARCHY

Each of our models has four essential aspects. The first is a structure corresponding to an anatomical or material element in the brain, such as a membrane or a neuron, which has an inside, an outside, and some sort of boundary. Specification of structure includes also a list of connections and interconnections, which is the topology of the model. The second is an abbreviated list of input–output relations that summarizes the experimental observations on the element being modeled, including specification of the conditions and their limits within which the model is thought to be valid. The third is a set of statements describing the flow or transfer within or across the structure, the nature of what is being transferred, i.e., whether it is a form of energy, a substance, a signal, or a state of activity, and the magnitude of that entity in each part of the model. The fourth is a description of the relations of the model to its parts, which are models of a lower order, and to other models, which together comprise a model of a higher order. For example, the membrane model can be interpreted in terms of the properties of the bimolecular lipid layer, which is a model for a component of the membrane, or in terms of the model of a neuron of which it is a part.

The fourth aspect is by far the most difficult for comprehension and yet the most important for understanding the physicochemical properties of the brain. As a tissue, the brain consists of molecules, organelles, neurons, and masses of neurons. In parallel to this hierarchy of structure, we have a hierarchy of models at each of these levels as well as some in between. The power of these models for understanding lies in their use in predicting relations between data taken at different levels in the hierarchy. An example is the prediction by Hodgkin & Huxley (1952) of the amounts of sodium and potassium transferred across the axon membrane for each nerve impulse at the ionic level from measurements on the transmembrane potential and conductance at the cellular level. The difficulty lies in establishing correspondences between a part of a model at one level and the part conceived as a model in its own right. Strong models minimize the difficulty by achieving conceptual proximity, so that, for example, ionic conductance can plausibly be interpreted in terms of a diffusion channel through a membrane or a carrier molecule. Weak models are characterized by too great a jump between the parts and the whole, as when attempts are made to link ionic conductance changes to the process of memory as defined, for example, in relation to conditioned reflexes. It is not illogical to try this, but the interpretations are vague, ambiguous, and uncertain.

Yet in studies of the brain it is necessary to establish relations between physicochemical measurements and on-going behavior, because the brain is infinitely complex, and we wish to identify and emphasize those of its properties related to behavior, not merely those related to our choice of instruments. We establish these relations by means of hierarchical sets of models that form traditional views of the brain.

This book is based on the idea that two of the main traditions in neurophysiology are ripe for fusion. In each tradition it is held that the brain is composed of neurons, and that the behavior of animals depends both on the properties of neurons and on the ways in which they are functionally connected and interconnected. This is their topology. The older tradition emerged from 19th century studies of the reflex properties of the brain and spinal cord and was brought to fruition principally by Sherrington (1906). Owing to the limitations of his techniques consisting of surgical ablation, the inductorium, the focal electrode, and the muscle lever, the central nervous system in this tradition is conceived as a mosaic of centers. Each center is a pool of neurons acting in parallel with each other, and the action of each center is considered to be the sum of the actions of its neurons. Interconnections are between centers rather than within centers. There are centers for receiving each modality of input and for initiating each type of motor response. The main tasks of neurophysiologists for brain analysis are to locate the centers and chart the fixed and temporary connections between them. Fine structure of neural activity is not denied, but it is considered to be inaccessible to observation.

The introduction of the oscilloscope, the electronic amplifier, and the microelectrode has brought a new tradition in the second quarter of this century. The neural action potential has come to be viewed as the universal currency of the nervous system. Theorists such as McCulloch & Pitts (1943), Hebb (1949), and Walter (1953) have shown that *networks* of individual neurons might perform virtually all of the operations seen or inferred in animal behavior, and experimentalists such as Sperry (1951), Barlow (1953), Mountcastle (1957), Lettvin, Maturana, McCulloch & Pitts (1959), and others have demonstrated remarkable specificities in the topographical arrangements and behavioral correlates of single neurons. The traditional Sherringtonian central excitatory and inhibitory states are entirely too gross to account for these fine structures. The concept of the center is replaced in this tradition by the concept of the neuron as the bearer of behaviorally significant information. The telegraphic network of centers is replaced by the telegraphic network of individual neurons.

In this book it is proposed that both concepts are partially correct. The center is redefined as a domain of cooperative activity rather than as an anatomical pool of neurons. Activity sustained by a mass of neurons comprising a center is cooperative by virtue of synaptic interconnections among the neurons. Within the cooperative domain each neuron generates a pulse train, which has a different but related time sequence compared with those of its neighbors. The nature of the transmitted information can only be found by examining the pulse trains of many neurons recorded over the same period of time, because it is the interrelation of the output of all the neurons in the domain that defines the signals, and not the averaged activity across the domain or the activity of one or a few neurons.

The models for interactive neural masses are designated as *neural sets*. These models of masses differ as much from the model of the neuron as that does from the model of the membrane. The basis of the difference is the existence of locally dense synaptic *interaction*. When a large number of such highly nonlinear elements as neurons mutually influence each other diffusely over an extended range in time and space, a *macroscopic entity* emerges in the mass that requires a new model for description. If the flow of influence within the mass is sufficiently strong and over a sufficient number of channels, then sudden transitions occur in which completely new macroscopic properties emerge and define a new state or a new set of states for the mass. Such states are called *macrostates* and are characterized by widespread cooperative activity of neurons. Neither the macroscopic properties nor the cooperative activity can be explained or understood at the level of the individual neuron, any more than the properties of ice can be explained in terms of a molecule of water.

1.1.3. MACROSCOPIC FORMS OF COOPERATIVE NEURAL ACTIVITY

Models of cooperative activity have been advanced in numerous forms during the past 20 years by physiologists (Lilly & Cherry, 1954; Cragg & Temperley, 1954; Gerard, 1960) psychologists (Lashley, 1929; Köhler, 1940; Tolman, 1948; John, 1967; Pribram, 1971; Grossberg, 1974b), and theorists (von Neumann, 1958; Beurle, 1956; Griffith, 1963; Wilson & Cowan, 1972) among others. Until recently there have not been sufficient experimental data with which to test, elaborate, and adapt these concepts, nor an adequate language to describe them.

In relation to specific brain systems two developments have changed this situation. One is the availability of a new technology. It is based on the integrated circuit that permits construction of large numbers of reliable amplifiers, so that observations can be made simultaneously on many electrodes, and on the digital computer that permits the acquisition, storage, and processing of measurements in quantities that only 10 years ago were almost inconceivable. This technology will be as revolutionary in its impact as the Faradic stimulator and the cathode ray oscilloscope were in their times. We have only begun to learn how to use it.

The other development, which is more a promise than an actuality, comes from theoretical chemistry. When several chemical reactions in a distributed system are coupled by diffusion, so that the products of each reaction become the reactants of another, steady state inhomogeneities in the distribution of the reactants and products may occur. The inhomogeneities arise in a previously homogeneous system. At any instant the inhomogeneous concentrations conform to a geometric pattern in the space of the reaction system, so it is said to have a *dynamic pattern*. The pattern may or may not vary with time, and if it does, the variation may be periodic.

Four conditions are required for the formation of such dynamic patterns. There must be two or more nonlinear transformations of substance or energy in the system. The transformations must be coupled, so that the reactions occur topologically in one or more closed loops. There must be delays in either the transformations or in the diffusional flows or both. Finally, the system must have a continuing source of energy. The patterns are in fact dynamic structures, which feed on energy and dissipate it as heat. For this reason Prigogine (1969) used the term *dissipative structures* to distinguish them from equilibrium structures, such as crystals.

Because such reaction systems are open, the theory of equilibrium thermodynamics does not hold. Over the past 20 years the theory of irreversible thermodynamics has been further developed and applied by Turing (1952), Glansdorff & Prigogine (1971), Katchalsky, Rowland & Blumenthal (1974), and others, as a means for the mathematical description of diffusion-coupled chemical reactions leading to spatial forms.

Katchalsky (1971) and Katchalsky et al. (1974) were quick to leap beyond Liesegang rings and the Zhabotinsky reaction and to see an equivalence between diffusion-coupled reactions and the interactions within masses of neurons. Each neuron continually performs nonlinear transformations at synapses and trigger zones. Feedback connections exist between neurons at high densities, and neurons in masses are coupled with sufficient density to simulate the continuum of chemical reactions and thus to create neural macrostates. The flow of neural activity along axons and across synapses in masses is analogous to the diffusion of chemical reactants. Also self-sustaining levels of activity in excitatory neural masses with internal feedback provide the analog of varying levels of energy input to other masses.

Katchalsky and co-workers reasoned that in any system containing a large number of nonlinear elements, which are diffusely coupled and there-fore interactive in a continuum, the properties of the whole depend on the rates of energy inflow. If there is no inflow, the system stabilizes in a zero equilibrium state. If energy is fed in, the system is driven progressively away from equilibrium until a critical level is reached at which a sudden change in state occurs. A new macroscopic entity emerges that is character-ized by a dynamic pattern or dissipative structure. With further increase in energy inflow, the system changes within this state and may then jump to yet another state, or through a series of new states, each with a dynamic pattern uniquely different from the others. Each new state may be a stable state and yet none is at zero equilibrium.[†]

The postulate that macroscopic forms of cooperative neural activity exist in the cortex, which transcend action potentials and synaptic potentials and which are analogous to diffusion-coupled chemical reaction rates, depends on several *assumptions* regarding the conditions of central neural activity.

(1) The global connections among neurons can be determined, in the sense of topographically organized tracts connecting areas of cortex and nuclei, but the precise local connections cannot be known, except for a small sample of representative neurons, and in any case need not be known with respect to most forms of animal behavior. That is, the precise trajectories of all pulse or wave transmissions in the cortex during a behavioral event are not knowable and need not be known, but only an average or instances representing the average (see Griffith, 1971, Chapter 8, for an equivalent statement regarding statistical mechanics) need be known (see also Goodwin, 1963).

(2) Macroscopic activity is continuously distributed in space in certain masses of the brain (Freeman, 1972f). We may then define a volume or surface element, which is sufficiently large that the level of activity of the element is an average over the ensemble of neurons in the element and which is sufficiently small with respect to the entire mass that the average is valid over the element, though the activity level over the mass is not homogeneous. This assumption is analogous to the assumption for an inhomogeneous chemical reaction system that a volume element exists around each point large enough to define a concentration for each ion

---

[†] Katchalsky was enormously enthusiastic over the latent possibilities in further exploration of these concepts, both in mathematical and experimental analysis. His participation was cut short by his tragic death. Nevertheless he contributed some remarkable insights into the nature of neural activity, which stemmed from his deep knowledge of polymer chemistry. For purposes of analyzing different kinds of cooperativity a hierarchy of levels of interaction within neural masses has been suggested and in acknowledgment his name has been given to these levels.

species and small enough to represent the concentration across the element as uniform (Glansdorff & Prigogine, 1971).

(3) The time and distance scales of macroscopic neural events are much longer than the scales for individual neural events. We can say that the relaxation times for action potentials and synaptic potentials range from .5 to 5 msec, and that the periods over which ensemble averages exist range upward from 100 msec. Similarly, chemical reaction rates in general are slower than the relaxation times of reactive ionic collisions. Also the dimensions of a macroscopic event conform to those of a nucleus or area of cortex and not to the dendritic arbors of individual neurons.

(4) Differential equations can be constructed to describe macroscopic states of an interactive mass of neurons without explicit reference to action potentials, thresholds, refractory periods, etc., because the proportion of neurons generating pulses at any moment in the mass is small, and that proportion tends to be uniformly distributed through the mass. The typical cortical neuron receives pulses continually but gives pulses at rates less than 10/sec, and its pulses for the most part appear to occur randomly in time. Less than 1% of its lifetime is spent in the state of pulse transmission despite continual pulse input. This condition is analogous to the predominance in a chemical system of elastic over reactive collisions and the tendency toward a locally Maxwellian momentum distribution function of the reactants (Prigogine & Nicolis, 1973).

(5) The activity level of each neuron, to the extent that it is determined by the activity levels of the neurons in its surround, must on the average be consistent with the ensemble average of the activity level in the surround, because it is a part of the surround. This assumption of self-consistency (Prigogine & Nicolis, personal communication) enables us to describe neural interactions involving mutual excitation or mutual inhibition among large numbers of neurons with feedback equations (Section 1.3.4).

Cooperative activity is not unique to masses of neurons and can be inferred or observed to exist in neural networks. These assumptions, however, lead to expectations of neural activity quite different from the discrete characteristics of activity in networks. In other words, that which emerges from the study of neural mass action is not merely an extension of current understanding; it is revolutionary in the sense defined by Kuhn (1970). In each field science grows not by continuous evolution, but by discontinuous stages. Each stage can be characterized as having a paradigm, which consists of a set of elements and assumptions, a collection of techniques, some characteristic observable events, classical experiments, and agreed-upon methods of description and proof. Most scientific efforts are directed toward the extension and elaboration of established paradigms. It is only when substantial experimental data are accumulated that are incompatible with or are unexplained by an accepted paradigm that a need for a new paradigm becomes clear. Once established, a new paradigm either replaces an older one or incorporates it into a broader view. The change is often marked by confusion and misunderstanding, because the techniques, data, and methods of proof may be so different that logical confrontation is not feasible.

To illustrate this point, a short list of the attributes that characterize the neural network paradigm is given in Table 1.1. This paradigm was introduced

TABLE 1.1

PARADIGMS IN NEUROPHYSIOLOGY

Attributes	Sherringtonian	Neural network	Mass action
Elements	Center	Neuron	Neural set
Techniques	Inductorium, focal electrode, ablation	Oscilloscope, microelectrode	Electrode array, computer
Characteristic observable events	Muscle twitch	Action potential	EEG waves, pulse probabilities
Classical experiments	Antagonist inhibition of stretch reflex	Receptor field of retinal ganglion cell	(?) Changes in evoked potentials with learning
Preferred method of description	Algebraic summation	Pulse logic	Nonlinear partial differential equations

by McCulloch & Pitts (1943), was elaborated principally by Hebb (1949) and Eccles (1957), and has become the mainstay of contemporary studies of sensory and motor mechanisms. It has by no means completely replaced the Sherringtonian paradigm that preceded it, nor is it likely to be replaced by a paradigm for mass action. The list of attributes shows that paradigms need not be considered as true or false, but they are more or less appropriate in addressing certain questions, particularly those concerning the relation of brain to behavior. The way in which the questions arise or are cast depends on the techniques of observation, the part of the brain under study and the kind of behavior being pursued. In the best examples from the Sherringtonian paradigm the properties of the spinal cord, brainstem, and cerebellum in relation to postural and locomotor reflexes are studied with the techniques of stimulation and ablation. In the network paradigm the properties of single units are observed with microelectrodes in sensory and motor systems, in relation to sensory processing and the formation of stereotypic movements. There are, of course, as yet no classical experiments in the mass action paradigm, though a likely candidate is listed in Table 1.1 as the study of averaged evoked potentials (AEPs) and poststimulus time histograms (PSTHs) in relation to the formation of conditioned reflexes (John, 1967).

In the following chapters some evidence that macroscopic neural activity exists in the brain is presented and the methods by which the evidence is obtained is shown and evaluated. Descriptions are given for topological, time-, amplitude-, and space-dependent properties, starting with single neurons and parts of neurons and progressing to macrostates by use of the concept of neural sets. Formal descriptions of dynamics are restricted to lumped sets, because the data concerning spatial distributions of neural activity are still largely inadequate to guide the construction and conditions of solution of explanatory partial differential equations. In this and other respects, the more pressing needs and promising opportunities for further development are noted along the way.

1.2. Single Neurons

1.2.1. THE STRUCTURES OF NEURONS

The foundation of neurophysiology is the neuron doctrine. According to this concept the tissues of the central and peripheral nervous systems are composed of great numbers of tiny compartments or cells. Each cell consists of a collection of chemically active structures embedded in a watery medium called the *cytoplasm*, and it is bounded over its entire surface by a thin layer of fatty material called the *membrane*. Though it is very thin, the membrane is a relatively strong diffusion barrier and separates the intracellular compartment of each cell from the extracellular compartment common to all the cells.

There are two kinds of cells. First, the neuroglia in the brain and spinal cord and the Schwann cells of the peripheral nerves, which predominate numerically, are subsidiary cells serving to separate the neurons from widespread contact, to maintain the constancy of the chemical composition of the extracellular compartment, and possibly to effect slow or long-term changes in the functional properties of the neurons in the brain. Second, the neurons are the transactional cells, which receive input from peripheral and central receptors or other neurons, and which transmit over short and long distances within the brain or to peripheral effectors.

Each neuron has a spheroidal nucleus embedded in the cytoplasm, which serves to specify the location of its home base. The nucleus is essential for long-term survival and functioning, but it does not enter into the transactions discussed here. The expanded region of cytoplasm including the nucleus is the *cell body* or *soma*. From the soma extend one or more filaments or "processes" for varying distances, which usually branch repeatedly and taper as they do so. The entire set of branching trees is covered with the continuous membrane including the tips of the branches. Two types of cell filaments are distinguished on morphological grounds. The *axon* has more watery cytoplasm, a smoother surface, fewer branches, greater length, and commonly a laminar coat of fatty material called *myelin*. The *dendrite* or dendritic tree has denser cytoplasm, an irregular surface, and more branches, which are often studded with small protrusions called *spines* and *gemmules*. There is only one axon for each neuron (though a few types have none), but a neuron may have one or several dendritic trees (though some have none).

The filaments of a neuron are not randomly distributed in the brain. Though there is considerable variation in the size and shape of neurons, there is sufficient regularity to classify neurons into types. For each type there is a characteristic location, orientation (with respect to the brain), and length of axon, and a pattern of distribution of its branches. The branches may be distributed along a line, in a surface, or in a volume, and there is a measure for the width of distribution in each dimension. The dendrites also have reproducible characteristics in terms of the number of dendritic trees, orientation, length, degree of branching, etc. For each type of neuron, however, there is variation in the locations of terminal branches. The detailed geometry is known for only a very few neurons among the billions that comprise the brain. For most neurons we must work with averages of measured distributions. We assume as the null hypothesis that the local distributions around the means are random, in the sense that the precise locations of endings are neither predictable nor knowable and do not affect the performance of neurons. This is a working hypothesis (Section 1.1.3) that is continually subjected to challenge and restriction (Sholl, 1956).

1.2.2. THE OPERATIONS OF NEURONS

The typical neuron has a dendritic tree as its receptor pole and an axon conjoined to the dendrite at or near the soma as its effector pole. The dendritic membrane forms specialized membranous contacts with the axon tips of other neurons, which are the *synapses*. The membranes are closely apposed, but with few exceptions there is no cytoplasmic bridge between them. The dendrites receive input from as many as 10^5 axon tips from other neurons, combine the input, and deliver the resultant to the initial segment of the axon. The axon transmits the resultant to other parts of the nervous system, near or far, and distributes it in accordance with its pattern of branching.

The modes of operation of axons and dendrites are diametrically opposed. Dendrites receive pulse input and convert it to a continuously varying *graded* wave of ionic (synaptic) current (Bullock, 1959), which is manifested in the form of extracellular dendritic potentials or intracellular synaptic potentials. The *pulse to wave conversion* takes place at each synapse, whenever a pulse arrives on the axon terminal. The wave takes the form of a field of ionic current, which is distributed along the dendritic shaft. The output of the dendrites is the sum of waves resulting from all pulse inputs, which is delivered to the initial segment of the axon. Due to the electrical character- istics of the dendritic membrane and cytoplasm the sum is smoothed and attenuated (filtered), so that the irregularities resulting from trains of single pulses are minimized. The sum is *transmitted* (in the sense of translation in space and delay in time) to the initial segment of the axon. The amount of smoothing and attenuation of the part of the wave attributable to each pulse depends on the distance from the synapse to the initial segment. Due to the fact that synapses are distributed over the branches, the sum- mation is carried out over space as well as over time. The convergence of the dendritic branches to the soma provides for the *convergence* of the wave activity in each neuron.

The axon responds to this wave input by generating a pulse train. Each pulse has a relatively fixed amplitude and duration. It is actively transmitted or propagated. It is said to be all-or-none because, except at the axon branching points, it tends to have constant velocity and amplitude. However, the peak amplitude of transmembrane potential for each pulse does vary depending on the resting amplitude of transmembrane potential just before the pulse and on other factors. The effectiveness of the pulse in synaptically generating a wave also depends on this and other factors, so the output of the axon is not really all-or-none, in terms of either the effect of single pulses or the frequency of pulses. Moreover, the output is distributed through the volume of the brain in accordance with the location of the axon branches and terminals. This constitutes *divergence*. Due to variation in lengths of axon branches or collaterals and to variation in conduction velocities in proportion to axon diameters, there is variation in the times of arrival of pulses at the terminals of branches of the same axon. This constitutes *temporal dispersion.*

Whereas dendrites provide for convergence, summing, and smoothing of their input, axons chop the resultant into pulses of relatively fixed size and varying interval, multiply it by means of branching and the state of its terminal membranes, and disperse it both temporally and spatially. The prime function of the dendrites is integration (the weighted summation of small quantities) in the wave mode, and that of the axon is transmission in the pulse mode. The model neuron representing the "typical" neuron is a localized unidirectional integrator and transmitter having several operations. It receives pulses and converts them to waves, sums and filters the waves over space and time, focuses the resultant, reconverts it to pulses, and transmits the pulses with delays, multiplication, and divergence (spatial dispersion).

1.2.3. THE STATE VARIABLES OF NEURONS

Each of these operations is dependent on the existence in the membrane of electromotive forces (emfs) that can move ions across the membrane in either or both directions. When an input activates a neuron, it causes the neuron from its metabolic energy sources to build emfs in some part of the membrane. That part of the membrane is said to be *active*, whereas the rest of the membrane is *passive*. When the emfs move a net electrical charge across an active part of the membrane, the same quantity of charge must move in the opposite direction across the passive membrane of another part of the same neuron (Section 4.1.2). This gives rise to a loop current in which current flows from the active region to the passive region inside the neuron and in the reverse direction in the extracellular space, or vice versa. The loop current is the only means by which one part of a neuron affects other parts of the same neuron in the operations of integration and transmission. (Metabolic and trophic phenomena are not at issue here.) For this reason the existence of a neural loop current is a necessary and sufficient condition for a neuron to be active. If there is no loop current, either the neuron is at rest, or it has uniform emf over the membrane and is neither transmitting nor integrating.

It is not possible to measure the strength of a loop current of a neuron unless the neuron is isolated in a closed chamber. However, the loop current is accompanied by changes in potential at points both in and around the neuron, with respect to a reference potential at a point some far distance from the neuron. Measurements of these potential differences are the main source of information about the properties of intact neurons. It is important to realize that all such measurements are indirect with respect to the state of a neuron. If it is active, there must be one or more loop currents, but these may or may not be detectable as potential differences with electrodes placed in and outside the neuron. The degree of activity of a neuron is dependent on the distribution and intensity of all its loop currents. However, the degree of activity is in no way the simple sum of the current loops, which are the basis for the activity.

In order to describe, measure, and predict the activity of a neuron, we need to define precisely what is meant by its active state and not merely say that it is or is not generating synaptic currents and pulses. In the most general terms we must choose a set of measurements of potential differences (in the wave and pulse modes) and their rates of change, which are believed to manifest the activity of the neuron as a matter of inference and judgement based on extensive knowledge of the geometry and dynamic properties of the neuron. The loop currents vary with time, location, etc., and so do the numerical values derived from measurement.

By definition each ordered *sequence of values* constructed from the measurements of potential differences over time, distance, etc. constitutes a *state variable*. The set of all possible values of a state variable is called the *state space* of that variable. Any subset of values serves to define a *domain* in the state space of that variable. Then the state of the neuron is given by the minimal number of state variables necessary to describe the state uniquely. It should satisfy the following two conditions. First, the state at any time t_1 determines uniquely the state of the neuron at any time t other than t_1. Second, given the state at time t_1 and the inputs at t_1, which comprise the complete past history of the neuron, all of the state variables are uniquely determined. The set of all possible values of the minimal state variables constitutes the state space of the neuron.

The state of a neuron is more general than its active state. Other state variables may consist in the intracellular concentrations of various inorganic ions, ATP, protein, RNA, etc., their rates of turnover, size, length, location and rates of growth of fiber systems, and many others. We are not concerned with these, except indirectly to the extent that we can use them to explain in chemical and anatomical terms the loop currents already specified as essential to activity and the active state. Even with respect to loop currents, there are indefinitely many ways of constructing the minimal state variables in order to represent the same neuron uniquely with respect to its active state. We consider this in the next section. The important point here is that the active state of the neuron is given by an organized set of measurements, that describe its past input and its present levels of activity and their rates of change in such a way that the future activity of the neuron is uniquely predicted. The principle is exemplified in the measurement of action potentials by means of the Hodgkin–Huxley equations.

The problem of specifying the active state denoted $o(t)$ can be greatly simplified when we adopt the postulate that if a neuron has only one output channel, then in so far as a neuron in a network is concerned, specification of only one state variable in terms of history comprising the initial conditions, present level, and rates of change suffices to determine its active state. If each input axon to the neuron is the output channel of another neuron, there is only one minimal variable for the active state of each input neuron. If the nonlinear transformations of pulse to wave and wave to pulse conversion are known, a set of measurements of either a pulse rate in the pulse mode $p'(t)$ or a potential difference in the wave mode $v'(t)$ provides the basis for evaluating the active state of each neuron.

If the neuron performs wave to pulse and pulse to wave conversions within its dendritic tree, or if it has more than one output channel, or if the nonlinear conversion functions are not known, then more than one state variable is minimally required to specify the active state of the neuron.

The reason for advancing the concept of the active state goes to the crux of the relation between a model and the thing it represents. In the real neuron, there is a dynamic on-going event of a certain magnitude, which is manifested by certain measurable physical quantities. The event and its manifestations are not identical. The event is represented in the model by a symbol, say $o(t)$, and an observable state variable such as a pulse rate is represented by another symbol, say $p(t)$. The experimental observations are measured and expressed as the state variable $p'(t)$. The test of the model is the comparison of the prediction $p(t)$ with the observation $p'(t)$, but inference as to what is actually happening in the real neuron is from $o(t)$ to $o'(t)$, where $o'(t)$ is the active state and $o(t)$ is its representation:

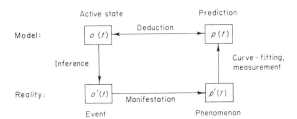

The active state has often been considered to be a form of energy, because it is a scalar having relative magnitude, is subject to operations such as transmission and transformation, and is dependent on metabolic energy. It is not a form of energy, however, because it is not conserved (Freeman, 1972f). The simplest proof is that two action potentials propagating toward each other on the same axon undergo annihilation. Moreover, both excitation and inhibition, which result in raised and lowered active states, make positive demands on metabolic energy sources. The active state is therefore uniquely defined in the relation of the neuron to the neuron model, which specifies the active state as a form of neural output $o(t)$, and it is not derived from or equivalent to analogous entities in any other physical system.

1.2.4. SPECIFICATION OF THE ACTIVE STATES AND OPERATIONS

Let us recall that the neuron can be viewed either as a collection of parts or as a part in a collection of neurons (Section 1.1.2). When we talk about the "function" of the neuron as determined by its parts, we must assign an active state variable to each of its parts, but when we are concerned with the "function" of the neuron in a system of neurons, we assign one active state variable to each neuron and identify that variable with an observable in either the pulse mode or the wave mode. The observable in the wave mode is usually taken to be the level of transmembrane potential difference at the soma, because it is most accessible to measurement with an intra-cellular electrode at that site, and because that is the site of maximal dendritic convergence. It is also the usual site of anatomical origin of the axon and therefore the site of wave to pulse conversion. The observable in the pulse mode is usually taken to be the recording from the soma indicating a pulse or pulse train. The level or amplitude of activity in the pulse mode can be expressed as an instantaneous value (whether or not a pulse is present), an average over a time period of observation (pulse rate), or as the instantaneous pulse rate (the reciprocal of the time interval between two pulses).[†]

However, when we treat the neuron as part of a system of neurons, the most significant aspect of its active state is the level of its output, meaning the amplitude of its effect on other neurons. This presents a major difficulty, because the amplitude of effect is determinable only by measurement on the observables of target neurons, except of course for the effector neurons in the motor and endocrine systems. A substantial part of our efforts in neurophysiology is explicitly or implicitly devoted to determining the relations between observables and active states (see Chapter 4). For example, the pulse rate or pulse probability of a neuron is generally valid as an index of its state, because once a pulse is formed, it usually sweeps the entire axon tree (the divergence property). Instances occur, however, in which transmission over some or all branches is completely blocked or is either more or less effective than normal. In other instances pulses are not detectable or do not occur, and yet transmission from the neuron takes place. Extracellular dendritic potential or the level of intracellular potential may then replace measurement of pulses as the basis for estimating the active state of a neuron. The cytoplasm of neurons is negatively polarized

---

[†] Alternatively, in an ensemble of observations made with respect to some repeated external event, such as the onset of a stimulus or the firing of some other neuron, the active state can be estimated from the probability of pulse occurrence in each of an ordered sequence of short time intervals during a designated postevent time period. The pulse probability is the number of times a pulse occurs during a short time interval (equal to pulse duration) divided by the number of events (see Chapter 3).

with respect to the extracellular space. An increase of active state is associated with decreasing intracellular negativity or depolarization, and a decrease in active state is manifested by hyperpolarization. Once again, these relations do not always hold, so that the observation must be tied to the state of the neuron by inference. The observable state variables must not be confused with the active state variables.

The dendrites perform the serial operations of pulse to wave conversion, convergence, summing over space and time, and filtering the resultant. The axons have the serial operations of wave to pulse conversion, transmission, multiplication, and divergence. It is logically possible to define a state variable specifying an active state of a neuron before and after each of these operations. However, the realizable state variables are those conforming to measurable quantities, which are usually the pulse rate at the initial segment and the level of dendritic polarization at the soma. When the operations listed above cannot be distinguished by experimental observation, they are combined together into a single operation.

An *operation* is specified by a certain kind of relation between any two state variables. Suppose that we measure state variables v and p in successive pairs and find that over a range of values of v, for each occurrence of the same value of v, there is the same value for p. We then say that p is a *function* of v, and that the function $p = G(v)$ represents uniquely the transformation of v to p by the operation G. This specification holds whether the state variables are from the same neuron or from two different neurons. Suppose that we make a surgical cut across a neuron or between two neurons and find that we cannot thereafter construct a function for v and p. Also suppose in the intact system that we can fix v experimentally at any value in a range and find that we can control p. Then we infer that p is caused by v. What is the entity that is transformed or transmitted? For each part of a neuron there may be a different entity, such as loop current for dendrites, pulses for axons, transmitter substance for synapses, etc. If the operation includes a sequence of differing entities, then it is convenient to represent only the magnitude of the entity by a generic abstraction, which we call *neural activity* denoted o. (An alternative abstract term, *signal*, is reserved for other use in Chapter 7.)

We can now say that neural activity is transmitted from one part of a neuron to another or from one neuron to another, and that it is transformed by a neuron or a part of a neuron. The level of each activity is a component of the active state, and the function of any two active states specifies a transmission or a transformation, which are *operations*. Operations are represented by equations that contain the state variables and certain fixed terms called the *parameters* of the neural system. The parameters are either time, space, or gain coefficients, which depend on the relation between the observed rates of change in the system and the choice of units for measurement of time, distance, and amplitude. When the units of measurement are taken from a particular set of operations of a neural system, the analysis is dimensionless. For example, if we construct a function to describe the operation of transforming dendritic current to a pulse train, we need a gain coefficient to relate microamperes to pulses per second. But if we measure dendritic current as a function of input pulse rate to the dendrites and arbitrarily express its amplitude in units of pulses per second, the gain coefficient is dimensionless.

To summarize, we postulate that the active state of a neuron is given minimally by a single state variable, provided the functions are known for pulse to wave and wave to pulse conversions. Measurements are made optimally at the soma on pulse and wave activities, partly because of experimental feasibility and partly because of the convergence–divergence properties of the neuron. Operations within and between neurons are described by constructing functions from sets of measurements of pulses and waves. The main sequence consists in pulse to wave conversion between neurons from the pulse variable of one neuron to the wave variable of another neuron, which is described by a time-varying nonlinear function $G_d(p, t)$, and in wave to pulse conversion within the neuron from the pulse and wave variables of the same neuron, which is described by a time-varying nonlinear function $G_s(v, t)$.

In applications this general form may require elaboration. The classic example of a neuron performing these serial operations is the spinal motorneuron (Eccles, 1957), and many neurons in other parts of the central nervous system conform to this type. However, there are also numerous variants, such as a variety of central neurons with electrical coupling or electrotonic synapses (Pappas & Purpura, 1972), neurons in the retina that do not generate detectable action potentials (Byzov et al., 1970; Werblin & Dowling, 1969), somatosensory neurons without dendrites but with peripheral axon terminals that operate like dendrites (Loewenstein, 1971), etc. The description of appropriate state variables and operations for these variants requires only minor modifications of the general form.

On the other hand, it is not always desirable to reduce the minimal data variables to the membrane potential or pulse rate at the soma. In some neurons, e.g., the hippocampal pyramidal cell (Kandel & Spencer, 1961) and the cerebellar Purkinje cell (Llinás & Nicholson, 1971), there are trigger zones located in the dendrites, which imply that intermediate stages of wave to pulse and pulse to wave conversion occur in localized parts of dendritic trees. The possible existence of pulses in apical dendrites (Gusel'nikova, Gusel'nikov, Tsytolovskii, Engovatov & Voronkov, 1970) of mitral-tufted cells in the olfactory bulb suggests that the active states of these neurons may not be minimally represented by two state variables in the pulse and wave modes. Moreover, both the mitral-tufted cells and the periglomerular cells have output by axons in conventional axodendritic synapses, and they also have output directly from their dendrites to the dendrites of other cells by dendrodendritic synapses (Rall, Shepherd, Reese & Brightman, 1966). There are, in effect, at least two synaptic output channels for each type of neuron. Consideration of these interesting arrangements is limited in order to simplify the development. The analytic approach being described here is competent to handle these problems, but detailed applications in these directions have not yet been undertaken.

1.2.5. INPUT–OUTPUT RELATIONS OF SINGLE NEURONS

There are two fundamental classes of neurons in terms of the nature or "sign" of their effects on other neurons. Synaptic inputs that depolarize a neuron and increase its pulse rate or pulse probability are called *excitatory* denoted e or +, and the input neurons and synapses are also called excitatory. Synaptic inputs that hyperpolarize a neuron and decrease its pulse rate or pulse probability are called *inhibitory* denoted i or −, as are the input neurons and their synapses. Most neurons receive input from both excitatory and inhibitory neurons, but with at least one exception (Kandel, Frazier & Coggeshall, 1967) their output is either excitatory or inhibitory, but not both. Obviously the active state of a neuron is independent of the polarity of its output, and the output can be given a positive sign if it is excitatory and a negative sign if it is inhibitory.

The sign of action is a higher-order property of a neuron, because it refers to other neurons rather than itself, in terms of how it influences or is influenced by those neurons. Attempts thus far have been unsuccessful in determining the structural or chemical properties unequivocally specific to excitatory and inhibitory neurons, and it is still unclear whether the specialization of excitatory and inhibitory synapses lies in the presynaptic (input) or postsynaptic (receiving) membranes of synapses, or (most probably) both. The designation of the output of a neuron as excitatory or inhibitory should always include specification of the target neurons or effectors to which the action refers. The designation of its state as excited or inhibited refers only to the neuron, but from that state and a preceding input we can infer the sign of input.

The operations of the synapse and of the initial segment are now considered in more detail. If a pulse is delivered to a neuron at rest by way of the axons ending on its dendrites and soma, a brief wave of dendritic potential occurs, which is a postsynaptic potential (PSP). If the input is excitatory, the PSP is a depolarizing or excitatory PSP (EPSP), and if it is inhibitory, the PSP is a hyperpolarizing or inhibitory PSP (IPSP). If the size of an afferent volley (the number of axons having input pulses) is increased over a relatively narrow range, the amplitude of the EPSP or IPSP increases in proportion to the number. If two or more small inputs are given simultaneously, the responses are simply added, and the system is said to be *linear*. If two otherwise identical inputs are separated in time, and if the responses are identical except for time of onset, the system is time invariant. If the size of the afferent volley is increased over a relatively broad range, the amplitude of the EPSP or IPSP fails to increase in proportion to the input. The pulse to wave conversion process saturates and is nonlinear and may be time varying. It functions in a linear, time-invariant range only for small active states with bilateral saturation outside that range on either excessive excitation or excessive inhibition.

Irrespective of the range of amplitude of activity, time variance is an important property of pulse to wave conversion and is commonly found in many synapses. Two easily observed forms are called *posttetanic potentiation* and *posttetanic depression*. Following a brief period of high-frequency electrical stimulation of an axonal tract, which is called the *conditioning* stimulus, the PSP in response to single test shocks is found to undergo a brief decrease in amplitude (depression) relative to the pretetanic control PSP and then a multifold increase (potentiation) lasting several minutes. The period of high-frequency pulse activity of the presynaptic axon terminals causes prolonged electrochemical changes in the membranes, which at first decrease and then increase the effectiveness of each test impulse.

The same or similar mechanisms are involved in the phenomena called *presynaptic inhibition* and *facilitation*. Axon terminals are subject to modification of their electrochemical properties, either by changes in the extracellular ionic concentrations or by other axon terminals, which form axoaxonic synapses on them. If an axon terminal is partly depolarized in a sustained manner (not below its threshold), then, when a pulse does occur, the amplitude of the PSP is decreased. If the axon terminal is hyperpolarized, the amplitude of the PSP is increased above the control amplitude. The event causing the presynaptic modification has no direct effect on the postsynaptic neuron. Although this event is called "inhibition," the use of the term is inappropriate. Whereas the combination of synaptic excitation and synaptic inhibition is additive, the combination of presynaptic inhibition with either is multiplicative. A better term is *presynaptic attenuation*, corresponding to *presynaptic facilitation*.

The levels of presynaptic attenuation or facilitation may depend on the history of the synapse or on a combination of inputs on different tracts. For example, an afferent volley evoked on one spinal nerve may diminish or block the PSP induced in a motorneuron by stimulation of an adjacent spinal nerve. In either case the amplification of the axon as a transmission channel is time varying.

The wave to pulse conversion process at the initial segment or trigger zone depends on the steady state level of dendritic polarization. If a neuron is at rest, an IPSP whether small or large does not induce a pulse. If the magnitude of a brief EPSP is increased on successive trials from a small to a large amplitude, then at some amplitude known as the *threshold* a pulse occurs. If the EPSP is suprathreshold, the resulting pulse has the same amplitude, irrespective of the amplitude of the EPSP (all-or-none). Once the pulse is begun, there is a brief period corresponding approximately to the duration of the pulse (about 1 msec), during which no amount of additional depolarization can induce another pulse. This is the absolute refractory period. Subsequently, there is a period lasting several milliseconds in which an additional EPSP can induce a second pulse, only if the second EPSP is larger than the first. This is the relative refractory period. For some neurons, the required amplitude of the second EPSP may be smaller. This reflects a period of potentiation or supernormality.

Because of the refractory periods and the threshold property of the axon, wave to pulse conversion by the resting neuron is nonlinear. If, however, the neuron is given a steady excitatory input, which provides a depolarizing bias, the neuron generates a pulse train at some mean rate. If the depolarizing bias is increased, the mean pulse rate increases, and if it is decreased, the mean pulse rate decreases. Over a relatively narrow range, the bias level and mean pulse rate are proportional. For two or more inputs (excitatory or inhibitory or both) the bias levels sum, and the mean pulse rate is proportional to the sum. In this mode, wave to pulse conversion is linear. Over a relatively wide range of bias level, the proportionality fails. At the lower end, the pulse rate is limited by threshold, and at the upper end it is determined by the relative refractory period, or by supernormality. Over many operating ranges of neurons, saturation is bilateral.

Wave to pulse conversion also can display time variance. For example, suppose that a steady depolarizing current is passed across an axon membrane at rest at a subthreshold level. Shortly after it is initiated, the apparent threshold for triggering a pulse on the axon is decreased, but after many seconds, the threshold returns to the resting value, even though the current continues. This phenomenon is called *accommodation*. If a steady suprathreshold current is passed across the membrane, the resulting pulse train initially has a high frequency and subsequently may diminish to a lower frequency. This is called *adaptation*.

1.2.6. MULTIPLE STABLE STATES OF NEURONS

The concepts of resting state and threshold lead to the concept of stability. If a neuron has no input, and if it settles to a low and unchanging active state (without pulses), it is at rest. Suppose that we stimulate the neuron repeatedly with electrical pulses, and that on each trial the amplitude of its transmembrane potential jumps to a new value and decays exponentially to the resting amplitude. Then we infer that the resting state of the neuron is stable, and that there exists a domain of stability in its state space. If, when it is stimulated, the neuron generates a pulse, then it has left this domain. By repeatedly observing the output of the neuron we define a new domain in its state space. Because events in this domain are both bounded and predictable we infer that there is a second stable domain. Further exploration may reveal three or more stable domains. The level of the active state or set of states at which a neuron changes domains is a *threshold*. If for any conditions the neuron does not sustain reproducible or controllable output, so that we cannot construct a function, we say that it is *unstable*. For example, a damaged neuron that emits a stream of impulses and is then silent is unstable until proven otherwise.

The multiple stable domains exist in a hierarchy, and the transition of the active state of the neuron from one domain to the next occurs only when there is external input to the neuron, which raises its level of excitation. The input may be a sustained, unvarying excitatory synaptic input, or it may be a nonsynaptic chemical or metabolic condition, which is sustained and unvarying, as in a stretch receptor or a pacemaker neuron. Because of specialized leakage channels across its membrane, this neuron undergoes steady depolarization until it reaches threshold, fires, repolarizes, and repeats the process at regular intervals. It generates a pulse train in the absence of external input, characteristically with constant interpulse intervals. In either case, for analytic purposes we do not treat the sustained input or condition as an input. We treat it as a parameter of the equation that describes the neuron.

For example, suppose that we apply sustained, unvarying excitation to a neuron, either by high-frequency electrical stimulation of an excitatory afferent tract or by passing outward direct current across its membrane with an appropriate set of stimulating electrodes. Suppose that we additionally apply transient or pulse inputs by either or both means. If there is zero steady stimulus and no transient input, and if the membrane potential is at a fixed, unchanging level, we assume that the neuron is at rest. In the classical theory of membrane function, the membrane and the neuron are at equilibrium. If small transient inputs are given to the neuron and its membrane potential is changed and then returns to the rest level, the equilibrium is stable. The domain of input values over which the membrane potential returns monotonically to rest is the domain of resting or *true equilibrium*.

If a small steady stimulus is given, the membrane potential is displaced from equilibrium to a new value, but its rate of change is zero. If a transient input is given, and if the membrane potential returns monotonically to the preinput level and remains there without further change, the neuron is stable but not at rest. The domain of inputs for which this holds we will call the domain of *stable zero equilibrium*. It includes the rest point and a certain range of membrane potential.

If there is a sustained, unvarying stimulus of sufficient amplitude, the neuron enters a domain of instability in which pulses occur at unpredictable times. With further increase in the stimulus, the neuron generates pulses at either fixed or randomly varying intervals but at a sustained, unchanging mean rate. Now the invariant is the mean pulse rate and not the membrane potential. This steady state constitutes another form of equilibrium for the neuron. If the mean pulse rate is transiently increased or decreased by excitatory or inhibitory pulse or current inputs, and if it then returns to the preinput mean rate and stays there, then it is a *stable nonzero equilibrium*.

If the steady stimulus is increased still further, the neuron no longer fires at a steady mean rate, but in short bursts at high frequency with intervening periods of low-frequency firing or silence. If the duration and interval of bursts is constant, there is a new invariant, which is the burst rate. If the burst rate changes following transient inputs and then returns to the preinput burst rate and stays there, the active state is stable. If there is a range of burst rates, such that the burst rate monotonically increases or decreases with the level of stimulation, and if each burst rate is stable, then there is a domain which we will call the *stable limit cycle domain*.

For each domain, zero equilibrium, non-zero equilibrium and limit cycle, there is a stable invariant, respectively, membrane potential, pulse rate, and burst rate. Each domain has an upper and lower boundary or threshold. For analytic purposes the level of the stable active state in each domain, determined by the level of stimulation (treated as a parameter), is at an equilibrium point. The three domains exist in a hierarchy, yet higher-order domains may be defined and demonstrated experimentally.

Most experiments are done when the neuron is found or placed in one of its stable states. The definitions can be extended to include time variance within a stable state. For example, the phenomena of adaptation and accommodation (Section 1.2.5) are examples of time variance of the neuron, respectively, in the zero and nonzero equilibrium domains, not of instability. Furthermore, the input–output operation of the neuron may be in the linear

range or in the nonlinear range in either of the three stable domains, depending on how the state variables are defined.

1.2.7. BASIC TOPOLOGIES OF NETWORKS OF NEURONS

There is no limit to the complexity of networks that can be constructed
by connecting the outputs and inputs of model neurons. When properly
interconnected and equipped with sensory and motor devices, as few as three
to seven model neurons can generate remarkably versatile adaptive behavior
simulating that of living animals, as shown by Walter (1953). The varieties
of logical, behavioral, and electrophysiological operations that can be
simulated with such networks have been described, respectively, by
McCulloch & Pitts (1943), Hebb (1949), Caianiello (1967), Liebovic (1969),
Brazier, Walter & Schneider (1973), and others.

The topological organization of a network is reduced to the set of lines
representing discrete channels by which the activity of each neuron effects
changes in the active states of other neurons. The lines connect nodes that
represent the individual neurons. Although there is evidence that real neurons
influence each other to some extent through diffuse chemical–electrical
changes in the extracellular compartment or through the neuroglia, most
such influences are considered here to be negligible. With few exceptions
(see Section 5.2.1) the only admissible transmission channels are those
corresponding to synaptic contacts between the filaments of neurons.

There are six basic patterns as shown in Fig. 1.1. *Convergence* (Fig. 1.1a)

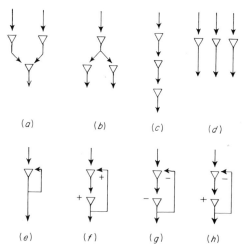

FIG. 1.1. Topological conventions representing patterns of connection among neurons.
(a) Convergence. (b) Divergence. (c) Serial transmission. (d) Parallel transmission. (e) Auto-
feedback. (f) Excitatory positive feedback. (g) Inhibitory positive feedback. (h) Negative feedback.

takes place when the axons of two or more neurons end on the dendrites and soma of one neuron. *Divergence* (Fig. 1.1b) occurs when the axon of one neuron ends on two or more neurons. If the output of each of several neurons is transmitted to the next in succession, they are in *series* (Fig. 1.1c). If two or more neurons all receive input from another group of neurons, and transmit in common to yet another neuron, they are in *parallel* (Fig. 1.1d). If no neuron by any series or parallel channel transmits output to itself, the channels are all *forward* (Fig. 1.1a–d). If the output of a neuron is returned by any channel or set of channels to its input, then one or more *feedback* channels exist (Fig. 1.1e–h).

A channel may be excitatory ($+$) or inhibitory ($-$). A neuron with feedback onto itself is said to be *autoexcitatory* or *autoinhibitory* (Fig. 1.1e). Two neurons each with input to the other form a feedback loop. If both are either excitatory (Fig. 1.1f) or inhibitory (Fig. 1.1g), there is positive feedback. If either is excitatory and the other is inhibitory (Fig. 1.1h), there is negative feedback.

These simple topological conventions are essential for the study of both networks of neural sets and networks of neurons. The description of the properties of neurons is also essential for both. The dynamic properties of networks of neurons, however, are quite different from those of networks of neural sets and need not be studied in preparation for the study of neural masses.

1.3. Neural Masses

1.3.1. A TOPOLOGICAL HIERARCHY OF INTERACTIVE SETS

The brain as a tissue consists of a vast number of neurons. Their processes are complexly interwoven with each other and form innumerable synaptic connections between neurons. The observed behavior of each neuron depends as much on the properties of its connections as on the properties of its parts. It is not possible to describe all connections of each neuron in the brain, but it is possible on the basis of connections to represent the brain as consisting of sets of neurons, and to describe the principal connections within and between sets. The formal description of the main connections within a neural mass takes the form of a network of sets.

A distinction must be made between anatomical and functional connections. An *anatomical connection* is a structural linkage, such as synapses or diffusion channels, between two sets of neurons. It implies the possibility of actions or interactions between the sets, but it cannot be used to infer that actions or interactions do occur, and it says little about the possible strength, spatial extent, or temporal course of actions or interactions.

A *functional connection* is predicated on the existence of a function describing the relations between active states of two sets of neurons. It implies the necessity of anatomical connections, with two possibilities. Either the two sets receive anatomical *forward connections* from some third set, or they have anatomical *interconnections* between them. Correspondingly there are functional forward connections leading to *coactive states* and functional interconnections leading to *interactive states*.

Networks of multiple neural sets are based on functional connections and not anatomical connections. A set of neurons having fixed anatomical connections may admit to several network representations, depending on the functional state of each of its anatomical connections.

The dynamics of networks of sets can rapidly become so complex that care must be taken to restrict consideration to those networks that represent experimentally realizable neural masses. The restriction is enacted by designating a topological hierarchy for neural sets. Each set has as parts the sets at the lower levels and is a part at the higher levels of the hierarchy. The levels are designated KO, KI, KII, ... (for Katchalsky), so that for example, a neural mass having a topology at the KII level of complexity is designated a KII mass, and its representation is a KII set.

We begin with the lowest levels of the hierarchy. A KO set is defined as any set of neurons numbering from 10^3 to 10^8 having a common source of input and a common sign of output ($+$ or e, excitatory; $-$ or i, inhibitory), and having no functional interconnections (Fig. 1.2a). The source of input may be a form of stimulus in relation to receptors, such as odor, white light, light of a particular wavelength, all cutaneous stimuli, a type of cutaneous stimulus such as heat or pressure, etc., or the source may be a set of primary sensory neurons previously defined, or it may be a bundle of axons, tract, or peripheral nerve at the convenience of the investigator. The set is not defined by a particular input but by a range of possible inputs from the common source. Once so defined, the set may be divided into subsets on the basis of location, grouping, or contiguity of its neurons, their cytoarchitecture or chemistry, their output paths and the locations of their target neurons, or their degree of accessibility to input at any moment in time or location in space. Such attributes define subsets but do not serve to define the set.

A common sign of output means that with respect to its effect on specified target neurons every neuron in the set is either excitatory (positive sign) or inhibitory (negative sign).

The first part of the definition is flexible in respect to particulars, so that the specifications for the input in any series of observations serves to define the set of neurons under observation. For example, if only a part of a central tract is accessible to stimulation, the number of neurons receiving

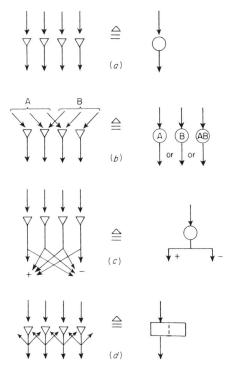

FIG. 1.2. Topological conventions representing KO and KI sets. (a) KO set with one input channel and one output channel. (b) KO sets with partially overlapping input channels and one output channel. (c) KO set with one input channel and two output channels. (d) KI set with one input channel and one output channel.

input from that part of the tract constitutes the set. If in later experiments a larger or different part of the tract is accessible, the set is redefined. Similarly a pair of sets may be redefined into three sets on the basis that a fraction of the neurons in each set receives input from a double source. Neurons receiving input from tract A form set A, and those with input from tract B form set B, whereas those with input from both tracts form set $A \cap B$ (where $\cap$ means intersection of the sets) as in Fig. 1.2b. Under this definition, however, $A \cup B$, the union of sets A and B, does not form a set.

The second part of the definition is rigid. If excitatory and inhibitory neurons both exist in a noninteractive mass, they must be treated as two sets, even if they have a common source of input. If they are not distinguished, the dynamics of the two types of neurons in higher-order networks are reduced to those of the type having the larger number, and the mixed nature of the mass is not recognizable. Special treatment is required for the case in which the neurons of a set A are all excitatory to set B, but all inhibitory to another set C, because the information concerning the dual sign of output of set A is preserved in the specifications of the signs of input to B (positive) and C (negative). In this case two output channels are assigned to the KO set (Fig. 1.2c).

A number of KO sets connected by forward channels in series or in parallel form a KO network. It is distinguished from networks of higher levels of complexity by the absence of functioning feedback channels between the KO sets.

Example A.   The proprioceptive afferent axons from each muscle run through the dorsal root into the spinal cord, where they form synapses on the dendrites of spinal motorneurons. The axons from muscle spindles are excitatory to motorneurons innervating the same muscle and are called Group 1A fibres. They form a KO_e set, which is designated KO_{1A} (Fig. 1.3a), which excites the KO_{M1} set of motorneurons. The axons from the tendon organs are inhibitory to the same motorneurons and are called Group 1B fibres. They form a KO_i set, or KO_{1B}. This is an example of parallel forward excitation and inhibition of the KO_M set (Sherrington, 1929).   ☐

Example B.   Group 1A axons are inhibitory to the set of motorneurons innervating antagonist muscles, KO_{M2}. According to Lloyd (1955) the actions are direct, in which case Group 1A axons constitute the KO_{1A} set

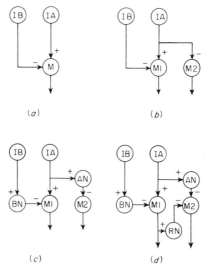

Fig. 1.3. Representations of the topology of the neural mass in the spinal cord by KO sets. (a) KO_M set with two input channels. (b) Model according to Lloyd (1955). (c) Model according to Eccles (1957). (d) Introduction of inhibition by Renshaw cells (RN).

with two output channels in parallel (Fig. 1.3b). The accepted view (Eccles, 1957) is that the inhibitory actions are mediated by sets of inhibitory inter-neurons KO_{AN} and KO_{BN} that form KO_i sets in parallel channels (Fig. 1.3c). □

Example C. When a motorneuron is excited by an *orthodromic* volley (in the normal direction of pulse conduction), its action potential is followed by a prolonged inhibitory event. That is lacking when the neuron is excited *antidromically* (in the direction opposite to normal pulse conduction) by electrical stimulation of its axon or by direct electrical stimulation of its soma. There is a set of neurons, called Renshaw cells, in the spinal cord located ventromedial to the motorneuron pool, which is excited by action potentials from motorneurons. The interneurons form a set designated KO_{RN}, which is inferred to deliver inhibitory activity to motorneurons (Fig. 1.3d). The output of each motorneuron delivers by this channel in-hibitory activity mainly to motorneurons other than itself. This is an example of parallel forward inhibition. It is called recurrent inhibition and is often cited as example of feedback. Doubtless under some experimental conditions the network of sets manifests feedback properties, but in the conditions in which it has been described, feedback is not manifested. □

A KI set is any set of neurons having a common source of input, a common sign of output, and dense interactions between neurons within the set (Fig. 1.2d). There are two types: The KI_e set consists of neurons which are mutually excitatory, and the KI_i set comprises mutually inhibitory neurons. Again, the restriction on sign of output is rigid, but the require-ments on specification of input are flexible. A number of KO and KI sets connected only by forward channels comprises a KI network.

Example D. The compound eye of the horseshoe crab *Limulus* consists of an array of photoreceptor neurons comprising a KO_e set designated KO_R and an array of neurons that are densely interconnected by axons forming inhibitory synapses. These neurons form a KI_i set designated KI_N (Fig. 1.4a). The set of efferent axons carrying pulse trains from all parts of the KI_N is shown as a pair of channels, on the basis that the positive feedback loop has two negative signs, and the output of the forward limb is opposite in sign to that of the feedback limb (Hartline & Ratliff, 1958; Knight, Toyoda & Dodge, 1970). □

Example E. Single-shock electrical stimulation of a dorsal root initiates a volley of action potentials on the primary sensory axons in the root forming a KO_R set. The collaterals of many of the axons initiate prolonged

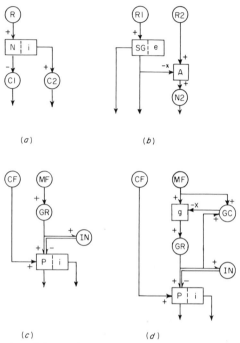

(a)   (b)

(c)   (d)

FIG. 1.4. Representation of the topology of (a) *Limulus* eye, (b) spinal cord, and (c) and (d) cerebellum by KO and KI sets.

activity of small neurons in the substantia gelatinosa in the dorsal sensory nucleus of the spinal cord, which is manifested by prolonged depolarization of the axons in the same KO_{R1} and adjacent KO_{R2} dorsal roots (Wall, 1962). The activity of the small neurons is presumably maintained by mutual excitation. If so, the neurons form a KI_e set designated KI_{SG} in Fig. 1.4b. Volleys from single-shock dorsal root stimulation of KO_{R2} normally excite a set of second-order neurons KO_{N2} and elicit output from them, which is measured in the wave or pulse mode. During the maintained activity of the KI_{SG} set, there is reduction in the amplitude of output from the KO_{N2} set, which is caused by presynaptic inhibition (attenuation) of the KO_{R2} axonal input by the KI_{SG} neurons. The attenuating effect by the KI_{SG} excitatory set is designated by $-x$. The locus of the action is shown by the square A, which is a topological element in the network and not a neural set. □

Example F. The efferent neurons in the cortex of the cerebellum are the Purkinje cells, which are inhibitory and are interconnected by inhibitory axon collaterals. They form a KI_i set (Fig. 1.4c). The KI_P set receives excitatory axons called climbing fibers from neurons in the inferior olivary nucleus. Although there is evidence for interaction of the neurons in the nucleus, in respect to electrical stimulation, the climbing fibers can be treated as the KO_{CF} set. Another cerebellar input channel consists of mossy fibers, the KO_{MF} set, which are excitatory to the cerebellar granule cells forming the KO_{GR} set. The granule cells emit axons called parallel fibers, which are excitatory both to Purkinje cells and to two types of inter-neurons. For simplicity these are represented as a single set KO_{1N}, which sends inhibitory axons to the Purkinje cells. This is an example of a network of sets having two converging inputs and output from a KI_i set (Eccles, Ito & Szentagothai, 1967; Bantli, 1974a, b).   □

Example G.   Another important set of neurons in the cerebellum consists of the Golgi cells, which can be represented as the KO_{GC} set (Fig. 1.4d). Axons from these neurons end in synaptic complexes called glomeruli (g in Fig. 1.4d), which consist of the axon terminals of mossy fibers, the dendrites of granule cells, and the axon terminals of the Golgi cells. The effect of Golgi cell input is to attenuate transmission through the mossy fiber–granule cell synapse, which is designated as $-x$. Because the input to Golgi cells is delivered through these synapses, the topology contains a feedback loop, which involves both excitatory and inhibitory neurons. However, the synaptic action is multiplicative rather than additive, so that special techniques are required to describe its dynamics. These are discussed in Section 5.2.2.   □

These examples are merely sketches that convey some of the main features of operation of the several mechanisms as they are described in the literature. They are not definitive models. For example, there is evidence that Renshaw cells interact with each other (Example C) and form a KI_i set, that cerebellar inhibitory neurons (Examples F and G) likewise form a KI_i set, and that motorneurons may form a KI_e set. These channels deserve careful experimental evaluation by the methods to be described.

The KII set is formed by the existence of dense functional interconnections between two KI sets. If both are excitatory, it is a KII_{ee} set, and if both are inhibitory it is designated KII_{ii}. If one component is KI_e and the other is KI_i, it is designated KI_{ei}, or KI_{ie}, or simply the KII set, irrespective of which set receives a specified input (Fig. 1.5a). In the KII set, each excitatory neuron interacts with inhibitory neurons as well as with other excitatory neurons, and each inhibitory neuron interacts with both excitatory and inhibitory neurons. Only for a special case, which will be discussed, can the functional topology be reduced to actions of excitatory neurons onto inhibitory neurons, and vice versa. This is the *reduced* KII set (Fig. 1.5b).

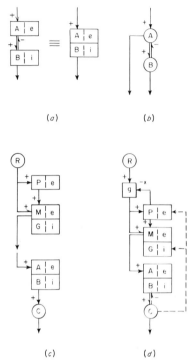

FIG. 1.5. Topological conventions representing (a) the KII set, (b) the reduced KII set, (c) the neural masses of the olfactory bulb and cortex at the KII level, and (d) the neural masses of the olfactory bulb and cortex at the KIII level.

Example H. The olfactory receptors in the nasal mucosa form a non-interactive set KO_R, and their axons are sent to the olfactory bulb in the primary olfactory nerve (PON). The terminals form excitatory synapses on the apical dendrites of mitral and tufted cells, which are excitatory to each other and form a KI_e set KI_M. The basal dendrites of the mitral–tufted cells form reciprocal dendrodendritic synapses with granule cells in the bulb, which have no axons, but which interact with each other, possibly through stellate cells, by mutual inhibition and form a KI_i set KI_G. The mitral–tufted cells excite granule cells and are inhibited by them. The interaction gives rise to the KII set KII_{MG}. The KII_{MG} set responds to electrical stimulation of the PON by generating a damped sine wave output, which arises from repeated cycles of excitation and inhibition (Fig. 1.5c) (Freeman, 1972c). ☐

The oscillation occurs only in waking or lightly anesthetized animals. Under deep anesthesia the evoked response may be reduced to a single cycle, which consists of initial excitation of each KI set followed by inhibition of each KI set. This so-called *biphasic evoked potential* is commonly observed on stimulation of many parts of the paleocortex and the neocortex. It is strong evidence that in most if not all types of cortices the excitatory neurons excite inhibitory neurons and are in turn inhibited by them. With few exceptions there is little or no experimental evidence for or against the occurrence of mutual excitation and mutual inhibition. In the absence of such evidence the excitatory neurons are treated as if they formed a KO_e set, and the inhibitory neurons are treated as if they formed a KO_i set. The interaction then forms a reduced KII set (Fig. 1.5b). This is useful as a first approximation for analyzing the KII set and in some conditions is a very good approximation, but no example has yet been demonstrated experimentally.

The biphasic evoked potential is the manifestation of recurrent inhibition, because the excitatory input is delivered to the KO_e set and, by its axon collaterals, to the KO_i set, which inhibits the KO_e set. This is not an example of negative feedback, because the recurrent inhibition initiated by each neuron in the KO_e set is returned mainly to neurons other than itself (see also Example C and Fig. 1.3d). Only if there is more than one cycle of the oscillation can feedback be said to occur (Section 5.1.1).

Example I. The PON input in Example H is also delivered to a set of mutually excitatory[†] neurons, the periglomerular KI $_P$ set, which delivers their output to the KII_{MG} set (Fig. 1.5c). The response of the KI_P set to a PON electrical stimulus is prolonged excitation, which causes prolonged secondary excitation of the KI_M and KI_G sets. The output of the KII_{MG} set consists of an oscillatory component resulting from its internal interaction and a nonoscillatory component resulting from the KI_P input. ☐

Example J. The prepyriform or primary olfactory cortex also contains a KII set that receives input from the bulbar KII set (Fig. 1.5d). The properties are analyzed in Chapters 5 and 6. This example is given in order to show how the graphic notation is used to describe complex topologies, including another example of multiplicative attenuation in the olfactory bulb. (See Figs. 1.4b and 1.4d.) ☐

The designation of KII_{ee} and KII_{ii} sets has been included for the sake of logical completeness, but as yet there are no physiologically verified examples. Networks of KII sets and lower-level sets occur at the KII level of complexity provided all of the sets have only forward connections as,

[†]For an alternate view of periglomerular neurons as inhibitory, see Pinching & Powell (1971d), Reese & Shepherd (1972), Shepherd (1972), and Freeman (1974e).

for example, in Fig. 1.5d (without the dashed lines). If there are one or more feedback channels (dashed lines), the network and the mass exist at the KIII level. KIII sets and higher- order sets have not been adequately studied and are not yet defined.

Three aspects of this hierarchical design deserve emphasis. The definitive attribute of the neural mass is its set of functional connections, which are the channels through which neural activity is transmitted. The assignment of a level of complexity depends on the number and the scope of feedback connections. The minimal elements for the analysis of neural masses are the KO or noninteractive set and the KI or interactive set.

1.3.2. The State Variables of KO and KI Sets

The neurons of a set are distributed in three dimensions, with afferent and efferent tracts approaching and leaving the same or different sides. For topological modeling a set is conceived as a surface distribution of model neurons. Afferent axons approach one face and efferent axons leave the other face, and both tracts are orthogonal to the surface. Divergence and convergence of afferent and efferent axons and the internal interconnections of axons and dendrites take place in distributions parallel to the surface.

The active state for a neural set must be assigned a value for each point of the whole surface. This cannot be done by measuring or assigning a value to each of the 10^3–10^8 neurons comprising a set, so an alternative approach must be used. We begin by assuming that the input activity to a KO set is *continuously distributed* in both time and space (Section 1.1.3).

The basis for this assumption is that most realizable inputs to a set consist of pulse trains on more than one afferent axon in the input tract. Characteristically the axons branch and the terminal branches diverge over the surface of the set, intersperse with branches of other axons, and end on multiple neurons in the set. Each neuron in the set shares with its neighbors some common input from afferent axons. To the extent that its active state is dependent on its input, its state will resemble that of its neighbors. The closer the spatial proximity of two neurons, the more similar is their state of activity. This implies that the active state of the set in the vicinity of a point is the average of the active states of the neurons of the same set in that vicinity. The value of the average may change as the location of the point is changed, but if the change in location is made vanishingly small, then it may be assumed that the change in the average will also be vanishingly small. The level of activity may then be said to change in a continuous manner across the surface.

At each time t_1 and point in the surface (x_1, y_1) there is an *activity density* denoted $o(t, x_1, y_1)$, which is the local active state of the set. It is manifested by the time sequence in mean local level of dendritic polarization or pulse rate divided by the surface area over which the mean is taken. Any set of measurements on the manifestation of activity density at a set of points in the KO set serves to describe a neural *activity distribution* in either the pulse mode $p(t, x, y, z)$ or the wave mode $v(t, x, y, z)$, which is a discrete sample from a continuously varying distribution. If the sample is adequate, then a continuous function may be derived by appropriate transformations to describe the active state of the whole surface. This time and space function is called an *activity density function* $o(t, x, y)$. It is the best attainable description of the active state of the set and may be expressed either in the pulse mode $o_p(t, x, y)$ or the wave mode $o_v(t, x, y)$.

If the active state is assumed to be uniform across the KO set, it has a single value for the set. It is then identical to the Sherringtonian (1929) central excitatory state (ces) or central inhibitory state (cis). Its value is the same as the mean of the states of all the neurons in the set. Any change in value may be due to a relatively large increase in depolarization or pulse rate of a few cells or to a relatively small change in many cells. In either case, the set can be modeled as if it were a single "average" neuron for the purposes of constructing a topological flow diagram. Examples are the "motorneuron pool" and the "respiratory centers," which are known to be sets, but which in networks can be represented by single model neurons.

The KI_e set, which is the interactive set of excitatory neurons, requires no restrictions on the continuity of its input activity. The existence of excitatory interconnections implies that if any neuron receives input and becomes active, its output is delivered to many neurons in its vicinity. Those neurons in turn deliver input to the initiating neuron in varying degree and with varying delay. This interaction implies that the active states of neurons in the vicinity of a point tend to the same value, and that the active state of an interactive set can be described in terms of a continuum. Therefore we describe the active state of a KI_e mass by means of a continuous activity density function $o(t, x, y)$, which is evaluated by inference from measurements of the manifestations of neural activity density at selected points.

Continuity need not hold for the KI_i set if it receives input from a KO set. If, however, it receives input from a KI_e set, or if the activity distribution from a KO set is continuously distributed, then its activity density function is also continuous.

In the event that continuity holds, the state variables of a KI set, which are functions of time and distance, are evaluated from multiple sequential measurements on averages across neurons of dendritic potentials and axonal pulse rates in the vicinity of each of a number of recording sites in the set.

Interaction implies that variation in the active states of neurons in the set with time occur in a coordinated manner, though not necessarily in synchrony. The sequences of values for the active states of any two neurons in a KI set, which constitute their state variables, are correlated or covariant to a degree depending on the level of interaction in their vicinity of the KI set and not on their private interaction. While interaction implies covariance, the converse is not valid, because the activity of two neurons may be correlated, if they have some degree of common input and are not members of a KI set.

Because interaction exists in a KI set, the active state of neither the set nor any of its subsets can be represented as that of an "average" neuron, as in the instance of the KO set. By virtue of the interaction a new entity arises that has properties peculiar to itself. These properties are to some extent manifested in the behavior of single neurons in the set, but they cannot properly be considered as properties of the single neurons. In the first place the state variables are predictable and measurable only for averages across numerous measurements on the activity of many single neurons. The averages are taken either across ensembles of neurons at any time, or across ensembles of observations on one neuron at a set of times, or both. In the second place the cooperative states are incommensurable with single neural events. They last longer, are more widespread, and have slower rates of change than events from single neurons and cannot exist in the time and space dimensions of activity in single neurons. In the third place the KI set has stable domains of operation in its state space, which are qualitatively different from those of single neurons.

The state variables of KII and higher-order sets and networks are given only by the state variables of the KO and KI component sets. For this reason, the KO and KI sets are essential parts in KII and higher-order sets. The definition of the state space for a single neuron requires that a minimal number of state variables be known, such that every state variable can be uniquely predicted from knowledge of the history contained in the initial conditions and the values at any time. For a neuron the active state can be given by a single state variable. The same definition holds for the neural set with the following difference. The activity of a set is an activity density function, and the state of the set is given by a state variable, which is a time function for the entire surface of the set. One activity density function is sufficient for each KO and KI set, irrespective of the organization of the KO and KI sets into KII and higher-order sets. The KO_μ and KI_μ activity density functions $o_\mu(t, x, y)$ are the minimal state variables that define the states of KII and higher-order sets. The $o_\mu(t, x, y)$ for the KO and KI sets comprising a neural mass such as the olfactory bulb constitute together the *macrostate* of the mass.

1.3.3. THE OPERATIONS OF NEURAL SETS

Neural activity in masses occurs in the wave mode o_v referring to synaptic current or potential v and in the pulse mode referring to action potentials p. Either or both forms are denoted by u. As in the case of single neurons the operations of masses include conversions of activity between the two modes. Integration occurs predominantly in the wave mode, and transmission takes place mainly in the pulse mode. Integration comprises weighted summation over both space and time, including filtering in both dimensions; transmission in either mode comprises translation, delay, dispersion, convergence, and divergence. Each operation in a mass is specified by measurement of a pair of input and output state variables and by construction of a function describing their relation to each other.

The most easily controlled form of input to a neural mass is the volley of action potentials induced in a tract or nerve by an electrical stimulus or impulse, which is given once on each of a sequence of trials. The measured output in the wave mode is an average of the extracellular potential recorded at an appropriate point in the mass on a sequence of trials, each serial trial beginning with the time of onset of the stimulus. This output is known as an *averaged evoked potential* (AEP). It reflects an average of the dendritic currents from many neurons in accordance with their cellular geometry and an average across the ensemble of trials. The measured output in the pulse mode is a histogram in which time after the stimulus is divided into intervals minimally equal to the duration of the action potential. On sequential trials the occurrence of a pulse in a given interval on any trial is noted by adding a unit to that interval. Over a stated number of trials, a poststimulus time histogram (PSTH) emerges. If the recording electrode in the set is optimally positioned with respect to one neuron, so that its pulse can be clearly distinguished, the output is a unit PST histogram, which is an average over an ensemble of trials. If the pulses are counted from more than one neuron, the result is a multiple unit cluster PSTH, which is an average over ensembles of trials and the neurons in the vicinity of the recording site.

The AEPs and PSTHs from an appropriate set of points spaced in a mass describe the neural activity distribution, from which activity density functions for the KI sets in the mass can be determined. The functions are generated by equations, which are the solutions to differential equations proposed to describe the dynamics of the interactive sets. They are tested and evaluated by fitting curves to the AEPs and PSTHs. The variables in the equations fitted to the AEPs and PSTHs, which represent potential or pulse density as functions of time and distance, $v(T, X)$ or $p(T, X)$, respectively, represent state variables of the neural sets. In accordance with the definition of state variables in Section 1.2.3, the value of $v(T, X)$ or $p(T, X)$ at any time T uniquely determines the value of $v(T_1, X)$ or $p(T_1, X)$ at another time T_1 at that place.

In general there are two minimal state variables required to specify the active state of each KI set, one in the wave mode $v(T, X)$ and one in the pulse mode $p(T, X)$. The function G, which is given by the relation between any two state variables, defines an operation between two KI sets or within a KI set. For example, suppose we have two sets KI_1 and KI_2, which generate the state variables $v_1(T, X)$, $p_1(T, X)$, $v_2(T, X)$, and $p_2(T, X)$. We can construct four functions. Two of these are functions representing operations between the sets $v_1 = G_{12}(p_2)$ and $v_2 = G_{21}(p_1)$. The other two functions represent operations within sets, $p_1 = G_{11}(v_1)$ and $p_2 = G_{22}(v_2)$. If the function G_{11} or G_{22} has been determined, then the minimal number of state variables required to specify the active state of set KI_1 or set KI_2 is one, in either the wave or pulse mode. Typically the input $p_1(T, X)$ on the axons of set KI_1 is known, because it is the response to an electrical stimulus. The observed output of the target set KI_2 is $v_2(T, X)$ or $p_2(T, X)$ or both, which gives the means for determining G_{21} and G_{22}. That is, each fixed electrical stimulus and AEP or PSTH constitutes an input–output pair, from sets of which the operations $G_d(p)$, $G_s(v)$ or more generally $G(u)$ within and between KI sets can be determined.

When a large number of input–output pairs have been collected over a sufficient range of variation of input, a state space is defined for the state variables. The extent and complexity of the state spaces of even the simplest neural masses are staggering. We cannot hope to describe all the operations the masses are capable of, nor do we wish to. We restrict consideration to certain limited domains in several ways. The choice of inputs is limited to those that give reasonable opportunities for measurement and control of input. The permissible domain of input amplitude is limited, so that the range of output is similar in terms of amplitude, spatial extent, rates of change, etc. to the output observed from the same masses when the same or a similar animal is engaged in normal behavioral activity, presumably involving activity of the mass. The state of the animal under observation is kept as close to that of appropriately defined behavior as the recording conditions allow. Unstable or nonreproducible responses are not considered as an explicit basis for modeling.

Following these limitations, the resulting domain of the state space is subdivided by separating the main independent variables. If responses are observed in spatially uniform activity distributions, the relations between state variables are reduced to operations only in the time domain. If they are measured at many sites and are constant over some time period Δt, the state variables yield operations in the space domain. Most of our discussion will be concerned with time-dependent operations.

1.3.4. FEEDBACK GAIN AS A PARAMETER FOR INTERACTION

Even the foregoing restrictions are insufficient to limit the field of study of a set, because there are too many unspecified degrees of freedom in the choices of the nature and location of the input, the precise definition of the set, the location of recording sites, the procedures for averaging, and many aspects of the condition of the animal. We must have precise predictions on what to look for, so that these circumstances of indirect observation can be properly controlled. Our best recourse is to the theory of neural masses. As it is thus far developed, the theory can be used to generate elementary curves or functions. These elementary forms we call *basis functions*, and they tell us what AEPs and PSTHs ought to look like if our theory of neural masses is valid. We adjust our experimental conditions until the expected response forms are observed and then fit the predicted curves to the response forms.

In order to apply the theory, we must convert our topological model to a computational model, in the following way. We note in Section 1.2.5 that when operations of the neuron are described in the form of equations, certain fixed terms emerge as the parameters. The time and space coefficients have values reflecting the relation between the natural rates of change of the neuron and the units of measurement of time and distance. The gain coefficients reflect the relative amplitudes of output and input state variables and are given by the ratio of output to input amplitude. If both active states are measured with the same units, the gain is dimensionless. The gain for the single neuron is forward gain. For any desired interval of time if the neuron transmits as many pulses as it receives, its gain is 1. If it transmits more than it receives, its gain exceeds 1, and if less its gain is less than 1.

The KO set and the KI set have time, space, and forward gain coefficients g as parameters in equations describing their operations. The KI set has one additional parameter, which is called its *feedback gain K* and which describes the level of interaction within the set. The feedback gain at each point in the set is defined by the ratio of the activity density at the point for any two successive time intervals of appropriate separation and duration, provided there is no external input. If the activity density is constant but not zero, feedback gain is 1. If the activity is decreasing, gain must be less than 1, and if the activity is increasing, gain must be greater than 1. Moreover, the feedback gain is always dimensionless, because it is a measure of increment or decrement in a closed loop.

Feedback gain is a pure collective property that cannot be reduced to or measured as the level of transmission between any two neurons. It is locally specified as a dimensionless quantity for every subset having sufficient density of functional interconnections to sustain an average over the subset. It is a continuous variable over the surface of a set with a value at each point on the surface equal to the mean over the vicinity of the point. Specification of the level of interaction for a set is by a surface function $K(X)$. If the level of interaction is sufficiently uniform over the set, then it has a single value for the set.

For the purpose of evaluating feedback gain, a KI set can be divided into two KO subsets on the following basis. In the presence of ongoing activity of unspecified origin, in which each neuron generates pulses at random at some mean rate, at any moment some neurons are giving pulses and most are not. Those neurons transmitting pulses are unable to receive pulses at that time because they are refractory. The other neurons are receiving pulses but are not transmitting pulses. The transmitting and receiving subsets are mutually exclusive and together include all members of the set. The neurons in the two subsets are homogeneously distributed over the surface. Each neuron in the set switches at random between the two subsets, and across the set the switching is continuous in time and uniform in space. By this definition an external input must go to the receiving subset. If the input is effective, a transmitting subset emerges from within the receiving subset and transmits to the continuously reconstituted receiving subset.

By this partitioning (see also Section 1.1.3) the KI set can be reduced to a single feedback loop between two KO sets (Fig. 1.6b) in a topological flow diagram. The level of interaction is the feedback gain of the loop. Because the neurons all have the same sign of output, the feedback gain of a KI set is always positive $K \geq 0$, whether the set is excitatory with $K_e \geq 0$

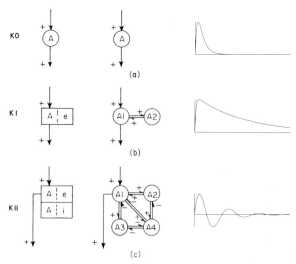

FIG. 1.6. Representation of (b)KI and (c)KII sets by networks of (a) KO sets.

or inhibitory with $K_i \geqq 0$. For uniformly distributed activity in the steady state its value must be unity. Otherwise, for the set having a spatially non-uniform active state, which is continuously varying with time and distance, the feedback gain is a space–time-dependent variable. For present purposes, the representation of the spatially uniform interactive set as a single feedback loop without spatial dimensions with fixed feedback gain (not necessarily unity) suffices as a topological model. It is called the *lumped circuit model*.

The topological representation of the KI set does not include channels for autoexcitation or autoinhibition. These are excluded on the premise that the proportion of its total input that each neuron receives directly from its own output in the interactive set is vanishingly small. In this respect the KI model differs from other proposed interactive neural models (e.g., (Wilson & Cowan, 1972; Grossberg, 1973a; also see Section 6.2.5). Further, the exclusion of autoexcitatory and autoinhibitory channels makes it possible to include the refractory periods with other determinants of interaction strength and to avoid having to specify channels in which they play special roles. Then, both kinds of nonlinear conversions $G(u)$ can be conceived to occur instantaneously at points and are independent of time and distance. The activity density function of the μth set $o_\mu(t, x, y, u)$ is dependent on time, distance, and amplitude in either or both modes. Operations on the activity density function, which take place in the Cartesian dimensions of the neural set $X = x, y, z$, are denoted by capital letters as in $O_\mu(s, X, U)$, where s is a complex frequency (see Section 2.2.3) replacing time t or T. Because the amplitude-dependent nonlinearity is independent of time and distance, we can separate $O_\mu(s, X, U)$ into an equivalent sequence of a linear space–time operation $FH(s, X)$ and a nonlinear operation $G(U)$ as in $O_\mu(s, X, U) \propto G_\mu(U)FH_\mu(s, X)$, where $G(U)$ incorporates the feedback gains.

From this analysis we can predict that the observed output of a KI set (in the form of AEPs or PSTHs) should conform to the output of two identical KO sets with positive feedback between them. This can be tested by measuring the response of a KO set to impulse input to evaluate its time constants and calculating the expected impulse response (a set of basis functions) for a KI set by means of a feedback equation. The set of basis functions then consists of a sum of exponential terms. The impulse response of a KO set closely resembles the impulse response of a single neuron in its fast rise and less rapid decay (Fig. 1.6a). The impulse response of a KI set has a still faster rise and very slow monotonic decay (Fig. 1.6b). This conforms to the prediction from the set of basis functions. The predicted curve is fitted to the AEP or PSTH. The value for feedback gain can be calculated from the required decay rate of the fitted curve.

The impulse responses of both forward and feedback elements of the KI_e set are both upward for excitatory input or downward for inhibitory input. On focal excitation of the distributed KI_e set the activity density must either be increased in or around the region of input, or be at background level at sufficient distances. For the KI_i set the output of the feedback element is inverted in sign from the output of the forward channel. On focal excitation the KI_i set can display surround (locally distributed) inhibition and possibly secondary surround excitation with increasing distance from the center of the focus. That is, for brief focal excitation the impulse response of the KI_e set decays monotonically from the input with both time and distance, whereas the impulse response of the KI_i set decays monotonically with time but may oscillate with distance. Therefore, complex spatial frequencies can be expected from KI_i sets but not from KI_e sets.

There is a wide range of experimental conditions in which the KII set may also be represented by interacting KO_e and KO_i sets (Fig. 1.6c). In addition to positive feedback there is negative feedback denoted by K_n. The sign of action by convention is incorporated into the topological representation of the feedback loop so that K_n is a real number ≥ 0. The predicted impulse response or set of basis functions contains a sum of damped sine waves, which conforms to observations on KII sets. In this case, three gain coefficients can be evaluated: positive excitatory feedback K_e, positive inhibitory feedback K_i, and negative feedback K_n, representing the three interactions of excitatory and inhibitory neurons.

A beginning analysis should give two very general results. First, we should have a realizable point in the state space of a KI or KII set. Around this point, we can expect to develop domains of increasing scope, in which the activities of these sets can be predicted and understood. Second, we should obtain values for the essential parameters of interactive sets. As we find other means for evaluating the same parameters, we can hope to establish both their ranges and their significance in relation to larger aspects of brain function.

1.3.5. MULTIPLE STABLE STATES AND THE LEVELS OF INTERACTION

We have seen that in theory a KI set or a KII set can be described by means of a network of KO sets with feedback between them. The solutions to the appropriate equations describing the dynamics of feedback for impulse input specify a set of basis functions, respectively, a sum of real exponentials for a KI set, and a sum of damped sine waves for a KII set. We shape the experimental conditions so that an AEP or PSTH conforms to the set of basis functions. We fit the observed wave form with a set of basis functions and evaluate the coefficients in the basis functions. The coefficients then serve to evaluate the feedback gains, which are the numerical estimates of the interaction levels.

Next we systematically vary one of the experimental conditions, such as input amplitude or depth of anesthesia. We observe changes in the AEP or PSTH. We fit the changed wave forms with the same basis functions to obtain sets of rate coefficients, and from the sets we calculate sets of feedback gain coefficients. With each experimental variable we deduce that a systematic change occurs in the value of one or more feedback gain coefficients.

We infer that the levels of interaction in KI and KII sets are dependent on input amplitude, on depth of anesthesia, and on many other experimental variables. The changes in levels of interaction are continuous in the sense that each change can be made as small as desired by reducing the change in experimental variable to a small step. Three facts emerge. First, there is virtually no range of output of KI and KII sets over which superposition holds and which can be said to be linear. Second, over small domains of change in input about many amplitudes of input, the range of output can be treated as if it were linear with a fixed value for the feedback gain coefficients. Third, we can combine a set of linear domains in the form of a continuous successive linear approximation by describing the feedback gain coefficients as functions of the relevant experimental variable, such as input amplitude, etc.

These facts imply that we can predict the shapes of sets of AEPs and PSTHs by using three equations to describe the dynamics of KI and KII sets: a linear equation in time, a linear equation in space, and a nonlinear equation in amplitude. We can separate the linear time- and space-dependent properties from the nonlinear amplitude-dependent properties. We use linear analysis to treat the dynamics in the time and space domains by means of linear operators $F(s)$ and $H(X)$, where $FH(s, X) \propto H(X)F(s)$. This frees us to examine the nonlinear properties $G(p)$ and $G(v)$ in greatly simplified form. When the feedback gains are written as functions of some controlled experimental variable, we can make direct inference from an experimental manipulation to its effect on the levels of interaction in KI and KII sets. For example, we can measure the set of AEPs from a KI or KII set for a set of pulse stimuli over a domain of input amplitudes, and from the measurements we can calculate how the change in input amplitude affects the levels of interaction in the KII sets. Then $O_\mu(s, X, U) \propto G_\mu(U)H_\mu(X)F_\mu(S)$ in the serial order of operation $F_\mu(s)$, $H_\mu(X)$, and $G_\mu(U)$ for each set and mode.

The value of this approach stems from the definition of the KI and KII sets as interactive. If interaction is so basic as to be definitive, we must have direct access to the defining characteristic in the form of a measure as our first major step toward understanding.

There is good reason to expect the levels of interaction in KI and KII sets to vary. As noted in Section 1.3.1 the existence of anatomical inter-connections does not imply interactions but only their possibility. If the neurons in an anatomically interconnected set are in a resting state, which is so far below their thresholds that no available input can cause them to transmit pulses to each other, they form a KO set. A set of neurons that normally functions at the KI or KII level can be reduced to the KO level by a strong general anesthetic. In this state the set has no interaction and therefore its feedback gain is zero. It is said to be in the *open loop state*. This is a useful state because the rate constants of the neurons in the set can be measured in the open loop state.

The open loop state provides the starting point for description of the multiple stable states of KI and KII sets, which are analogous to the stable states of the neuron (Section 1.2.6). For each KI or KII set there is at least one sustained, unvarying input, or a combination of such inputs, which can be treated as a parameter of the system. The parameter may be a sustained synaptic excitatory input, or an electrochemical property of the membranes of the constituent neurons, or some combination of these. It is a principal determinant in KI or KII sets of the steady state magnitude of interaction. When that magnitude serves as a reference magnitude with respect to gain changes induced by transient input, it is designated K_o.

If there is no sustaining input, the value of K_o is zero. If K_o is zero and there is no transient input, the KI or KII set is at the resting equilibrium, and the active states are all zero. If for small transient inputs the active states of sets are displaced and then return to their zero state and stay there, the resting equilibirium is stable. If there is a nonzero value for K_o that is not too great, one or more of the active states in the wave mode (but not the pulse mode) may be nonzero, but the rates of changes of all the active states are zero. That is, some or all neurons in the sets in the steady state may have steady membrane potentials other than resting, but none has pulse trains. The range of values for the parameter and the transient input conforming to this condition defines the stable zero equilibrium domain of the KI and KII sets. It includes the open loop state but is not identical with the open loop state, in which feedback gain is zero at all times and neither transient nor steady transmission can occur in any loop channel in the sets. The zero equilibrium range of outputs includes responses to transient inputs, which may consist of short trains of pulses and waves, but which terminate in zero pulse rates and unvarying wave amplitudes.

If, when K_o is increased sufficiently, the KI and KII active states are increased and are manifested by pulse trains and wave amplitudes at steady, nonzero mean rates, the sets are at a new equilibrium. If the active states are changed by transient inputs and then return to the preinput levels and stay there, the equilibrium is stable. This is the stable nonzero equilibrium state of KI and KII sets. Within this domain, the constant values of the mean pulse rates and the wave amplitudes depend on K_o and increase with increasing K_o.

For the KII set and the KI sets within KII sets, there is another state, which is induced by yet further increase in K_o. This state is characterized by limit cycle oscillation of the active states of subsets in the domains of the component KI sets in both the wave and pulse modes. The value for the frequency of the oscillation may or may not depend on the value of K_o over a limit cycle domain. It is in the limit cycle state that certain types of electroencephalographic potentials (EEG waves) arise. It the oscillatory active state has a certain frequency and amplitude in the absence of input, and if activity manifested in the EEG is changed by transient input and then returns to the same frequency and amplitude, the limit cycle is stable. For example, in certain unusual conditions, such as following a period of hyperthermia with brain temperature of about 42°C, the KII set in the prepyriform cortex generates sustained high-amplitude sinusoidal EEG waves at a frequency of about 28 Hz. This EEG activity manifests a limit cycle. The activity is only briefly altered by strong electrical stimulation of the afferent path to the cortex. It is totally suppressed by a brief period of asphyxia, but it recurs at the same frequency and amplitude on recovery from asphyxia. Therefore, the limit cycle is stable.

The existence of nonzero equilibrium and limit cycle stable states depends on the presence of sufficient sustaining excitation represented by the parameter K_o. If K_o is decreased sufficiently following the induction of a limit cycle state, the KII set returns to the nonzero equilibrium state or further to the zero or resting equilibrium states. Whether the thresholds for K_o and the active states are the same for entering and leaving each of these states is not known from experimental data. The possibility that the entering and leaving thresholds may differ significantly and give rise to hysteresis effects has been shown by theorists (Section 6.2.5). Such effects may occur in both KI and KII sets.

To summarize, multiple stable states can exist in the activity of neural sets, which are characterized by the stable invariance of one or more state variables. In the zero equilibrium state the pulse density function and the rate of change with time of wave amplitude are everywhere zero. In the nonzero equilibrium state the rates of change with time of pulse densities and wave amplitudes are zero. In the stable limit cycle state the pulse densities and wave amplitudes vary at a fixed frequency. These stable states are the set of conditions in which the KI and KII sets are placed or are assumed to be prior to measurement of their observable state variables. The experimental evidence and the neural mechanisms for these stables state are described in Chapter 6.

1.3.6. THE RELATION OF MULTIPLE STABILITIES TO NEURAL SIGNALS

The importance of sustained excitatory input as a determinant of the properties of neural sets is well known. For example, the interesting linear interactive properties of the *Limulus* eye depend on the presence of diffuse illumination of the photoreceptors that provides background excitation to the KI_i set and places it in a stable nonzero equilibrium state.

It is not generally appreciated that these stable states are ubiquitous in the mammalian central nervous system, lasting for time periods ranging from 0.1 sec to many seconds, as shown by the near-universal presence of background activity in the form of seemingly random pulse trains. If we use the concept of multiple stable states to interpret our electrophysiological and behavioral data, we open a new approach to understanding the neural dynamics reflected in these data.

For example, suppose that the neurons in a KI_e set at rest in a zero equilibrium stable state are brought sufficiently close to threshold by a brief excitatory input so that each neuron giving a pulse to its neighbors excites them and receives more than one pulse in return. The feedback gain is greater than unity, and the active state of the mass must increase. The increase continues until the pulse rate of each neuron is high enough to be limited by the relative refractory period of each neuron. Under certain conditions corresponding to a normal physiological state of the animal, the input can be terminated, and a new steady state develops. In this state each neuron in the set fires at nearly random intervals of time and independently of its neighbors but at a steady mean rate. If the set is further perturbed by input, the active state of the set changes momentarily but returns to the prestimulus steady state. It is therefore a self-sustained, nonzero equilibrium stable state. It may be terminated by a brief inhibitory pulse.

This mechanism involving one KI_e set with output to a motorneuron pool can account for an action in which a limb or an eye is moved to a certain position, held there for a certain time, and then returned to its starting point. The actual position may depend on the value for K_o in the KI_e set, which may be determined by the membrane properties of the neurons in the KI_e set or by sustained input from a KO set or another KI set.

In the absence of sustained excitatory input the KII set stabilizes in the stable zero equilibrium domain. The introduction of an excitatory bias from a KO, KI_e, or another KII set can induce stable nonzero equilibrium and limit cycle states in the KII set. Examples are given in Chapters 5 and 6.

In order to explore these possibilities to maximal advantage, however, we must pause to recognize the complexity of the undertaking and to adopt some guidelines for experimental analysis. The most important restrictions are: (1) We must have clearly in hand the topological and electrophysiological data on a neural mass before proposing a K-set analysis, in order to specify the number of sets involved, the constraints on the operations of each set, and the K-level of analysis; and (2) we must know the behavioral correlates of the activities of the neural mass so as to determine the domains of normal function.

As stated in Section 1.3.1 the combination of KII and lower-order sets having feedback between them gives a system at the KIII level. This approaches in complexity the level of the classical sensory, motor, or corticonuclear systems. An example is shown in Fig. 1.5d of the primary olfactory system, consisting of the receptors (the KO_R set), the olfactory bulb (the KI_P and KII_{MG} sets), the olfactory cortex (the KII_{AB} and KO_C sets), and the anterior olfactory cortex (N, an unidentified set). These sets together with their forward connections and feedback interconnections (as well as others not shown) comprise the mass of the primary olfactory system.

Whereas KO, KI, and KII are the levels of electrophysiological analysis, KIII is the lowest level of behavioral analysis. At this level a space–time pattern of neural activity, which is represented by an activity density function, can be said to be a *neural signal*, in the sense that it constitutes a unique effect and correlate of an external stimulus. For example, an odor (which, as distinct from an odorous substance, is an effective stimulus) must be represented by a space–time pattern of activity in each KO and KI set in the olfactory system, including the receptors, the bulb, and the cortex. Each pattern is a signal at a particular stage in a transmission sequence through the olfactory system. When these patterns have been described and measured in order to specify activity density functions, the operations within and between the sets can be determined, including transmission or translation and delay, transformation, storage, comparison, classification, and elective readout from stage to stage.

A concluding hypothesis of this monograph is that some neural signals may exist by virtue of the interactions of neurons in masses, and they may then be identified with specific active states (macrostates) of neural sets at the KO and KI levels. The complex space–time dynamic patterns of the active states, which are the neural equivalents to dissipative structures, are the result of stable limit cycle states in KII sets. Such states arise primarily because of continuing input from a KI_e set into a KII set, which drives the KII set from a nonzero equilibrium range into a limit cycle state, in which the signal is held for as long as transforming operations require.

1.3.7. THE CONDITIONS FOR REALIZABILITY

In order for the function of a KO, KI, or KII set to be observable, four conditions must hold. First, it must be possible to isolate the set, so that the pattern of transmission within it conforms to the proposed topology.

This can be done by control of input or by use of a variety of surgical or pharmacological techniques. When it is not possible to do this, it may be possible to dissect a complex pattern of responses into components, one of which represents the operation of the set in the designated mode. If neither approach is feasible, there is no alternative except to construct a higher-order model.

This condition may be very difficult to satisfy by surgical isolation of a part of the brain such as cortical undercutting, because the sets in such a part may depend on an external bias for maintenance of certain internal connections in a functional state. A KII set that is normally capable of oscillation may be reduced by deafferentation to the functional level of its KO components, and the analysis may reveal little more than the properties of its component neurons. In general it is necessary to work mainly with intact preparations, to propose a set of alternative models based on local or more distant topologies, and to weed out alternatives as opportunities arise.

The second condition is that the component neurons must generate detectable forms of activity, either in the form of dendritic potentials or pulse trains or preferably both. Many and perhaps most neurons in the brain are too small to permit intracellular recording. Many do not generate extracellularly detectable pulses and may not generate pulses at all. Others generate no extracellularly detectable dendritic potentials. In some instances there may be no measurable extracellular potential for a set, and its existence and actions must be inferred from the behavior of other sets with which it is connected anatomically. Analysis of an unknown mass into sets requires formulation of several simple alternative topologies and dynamics on the basis of anatomical examination, which can predict the existence of classes of responses of the mass and its neurons for specified input. The failure of predicted classes of response to exist and the existence of supernumerary classes give clues as to how the simple models are to be modified or elaborated. This is the dialectical process between theory and experiment.

Third, the experimental techniques must permit multiple simultaneous measurements at different points in the mass. (Uncommonly, the function of the mass may be shown to be sufficiently constant in time that sequential sampling at different points is permissible.) This condition follows from the definition of a set as a number of neurons, which must have a certain distribution in space. The existence of cooperative activity cannot be inferred without demonstration of correlated activity at many points in the set.

Fourth, the measurements of active states of single neurons must be averaged over time and space to give estimates of the active states of sets of neurons. The duration of observation or time window ΔT for averaging and the size of the domain of spatial averaging cannot exceed the temporal size and spatial limits (lower as well as upper) of the extent of a cooperative event. This condition severely limits the usefulness of the pulse train or intracellular dendritic potential of a single neuron. It places the greater value on the extracellularly recorded dendritic potentials and groups of action potentials p called *unit clusters*, which result from the weighted sum of extracellular currents near a recording site. Such events represent spatial averages that in the appropriate experimental situation can be interpreted as or used to infer the time-varying means for the active states o_v and o_p of a set or a subset near the site.

For example, one of the manifestations of a limit cycle in a KII mass is the occurrence of extracellular fields of potential that vary in amplitude in a rhythmic manner—the EEG waves. They can occur as background activity without reference to a specific external stimulus. The background pulses of single neurons in such a mass may appear to occur at random, but if their times of occurrence are averaged in an appropriate way with respect to the ensemble mean taken from the EEG, it is seen that the probability of pulse discharge may oscillate in time at the frequency of the EEG. This oscillation is called the *pulse probability wave* of the neuron. Although the pulses are generated by a single neuron, the pulse probability wave is a collective property of the KII set within which the neuron is embedded.

1.3.8. THE USE OF DIFFERENTIAL EQUATIONS

An overview has now been given in general language for analysis of neural masses along with a proposed set of models to describe them. Each of these models is described in detail in subsequent chapters. As noted above each has four aspects.

First, the anatomical structure is reviewed and expressed in the form of a geometry and a topological flow diagram. The geometry is important with respect to observation and measurement, and the topology is essential for the dynamics.

Second, the input–output relations are summarized and expressed by means of generic wave forms in pairs. These input–output pairs serve to classify the system under study in relation to certain general properties, such as linearity, time invariance, and level of complexity. They serve to specify the kind of descriptive equation needed for each set and its degree of complexity.

Third, a set of differential equations is constructed to represent the dynamics of the mass. The class of each equation is determined by the input–output relations, and its internal structure and parameters are chosen in accordance with the topology. The solution of the equations for the initial conditions prescribed by the input is compared with the output of each input–output pair. The differential equations are modified until the solution conforms to the output, and they are then said to represent the dynamics of the set.

Fourth, the parameters of the equation are interpreted in terms of the parts at the lower levels in the hierarchy. The differential equations are then simplified, so that they can serve as a part in relation to models of sets at higher levels in the hierarchy.

The mathematical approach is required for two reasons. It is the only means by which quantitative comparisons can be made between the observed and predicted responses of selected sets, so that proposed dynamics can be accepted or rejected. Also it is the easiest way to combine the models constructed at one level of the hierarchy to formulate a model for testing at the next level. Because the mathematics is a means and not an end, the forms of the equations and the means of solution have been kept as simple as the experimental observations would allow. The peculiar properties of neural masses even in multiple stable states have lent them to an unanticipated degree to the use of linear differential equations with amplitude-dependent co-efficients. Therefore, the analysis of the dynamics of masses is not limited by the intractibility of nonlinear equations but by the need for better definitions and measurements of observable events. Much of the material in this monograph is devoted to the problems of how to observe and how to measure events in neural masses, so that proposed models can be adequately tested.

CHAPTER 2

Time-Dependent Properties

The activity of neurons is manifested by time-varying neural fields of potential. The procedure for analysis of a temporal sequence of magnitudes for a source for an electrical field consists of (1) repeated measurement of the field potential, (2) postulation of a model expressed in the form of a differential equation, (3) solution of the equation for specified initial conditions and input to obtain the time response of the system, and (4) comparison of the observed and computed field potentials. For the simplest class of neural events the models can be based on ordinary and partial differential equations with constant coefficients. In this chapter the experimental conditions are described for which such equations are applicable, and an operational method for solution is demonstrated with neural phenomena.

2.1. Measurement of Neural Events

2.1.1. REPRESENTATION OF EVENTS BY FUNCTIONS

Electrophysiology is based on observations of continuously varying currents and potential differences in and around neurons. Such observations are usually made in simultaneous pairs over specified durations of time ranging from milliseconds to hours or more. Because neural systems under study have causal dynamic processes, each pair is inferred to have an antecedent or input member and a subsequent or output member. If the observer has adequate or complete control of the input member, it is called a *stimulus,* and the output member is a *response.* This may be called a *stimulus–response pair.* If control is inadequate or not imposed, the pair should be called an *input–output pair.*

Each member varies with time. It is measured by assigning to it a real number at each moment in time and a real number to that moment. The set of real numbers assigned to time forms a domain, and the set assigned to the variable forms a range. The relation between the pairs of real numbers constitutes a function. A function is defined as the relation between a set of ordered pairs of real numbers in which no two numbers in the range correspond to the same number in the domain. In the case of neural events no variable has two values at the same time, but the same value of the variable can occur at two or more times. The input functions and output functions constituting input–output pairs are represented by symbols, such as v for potential, i for current, p for pulse, and f for any of these and are called *functions of time,* such as $v(t)$, $i(t)$, $p(t)$, and $f(t)$.

The process of measurement by which the sets of real numbers are derived has two requirements. The first is a set of *basis functions.* A basis function is an elementary function of time that is defined over all time. Some examples of common basis functions that we will use are the exponential

$$v(t) = \begin{cases} v_0 e^{-\alpha t}, & t \geqq 0, \\ 0, & t < 0, \end{cases} \tag{1}$$

the sine wave

$$v(t) = v_0 \sin \omega t \quad \text{for all } t, \tag{2}$$

and the rectangular pulse

$$p(t)\Delta t = \begin{cases} v_0, & t_1 \leqq t < t_2, \\ 0, & \text{elsewhere}, \end{cases} \tag{3}$$

with $\Delta t = t_2 - t_1$. The typical output functions of K-sets are complicated functions, which we like to express in a simpler way. One possibility is by using sums of simple functions such as exponentials and sine waves. A *family* of basis functions that lets us do this is a *basis.* A *set of basis functions* is a specified number of basis functions that is added together to fit or reproduce a function being measured.

The second requirement is for units of measurement, such as seconds, volts, amperes, pulses per second, etc., and their submultiples. When a unit of time has been selected, such as a millisecond, an appropriate real number for α, ω, and Δt in Eqs. (1)–(3) is then assigned to each basis function in the set. When the unit of the variable has been selected, such as millivolts, a real number is assigned to v_0 in each of the basis functions. The real numbers must be chosen so that the sum of basis functions optimally represents the observed function.

Example A. An event is observed in the nervous system that consists of a stimulus current $i(t)$ and response potential difference $v(t)$. The period of observation from $t = 0$ to $t = T\,msec$ is divided into N time intervals (commonly $N = 100$), so that $\Delta t = T/N\,msec$. Each basis function is a rectangular unit pulse $p_n(t)\Delta t$, having duration Δt, location in time t_n, and amplitude of $1\,\mu A$ or $1\,\mu V$.

$$p_n(t)\,\Delta t = \begin{cases} 1, & \leqq t_n \quad t < t_n + \Delta t, \\ 0, & \text{elsewhere.} \end{cases} \tag{4}$$

Each basis function is multiplied by a real number $i(t_n)$ or $v(t_n)$, so that the amplitude of the rectangular pulse optimally approximates the amplitude of the input or output member at t_n. The set of basis functions is added over time

$$i'(t) = \sum_{n=1}^{N} i(t_n)\,p_n(t)\,\Delta t, \qquad v'(t) = \sum_{n=1}^{N} v(t_n)\,p_n(t)\,\Delta t, \tag{5}$$

where $p_n(t)\Delta t$ is a unit vector and $i(t_n)$ and $v(t_n)$ are real numbers. □

This procedure is called *digitizing*. We use primes to designate events measured in this way. The process is complete when the set of real numbers suffices to reconstruct an event to any specified degree of precision.

Example B. Suppose that an input–output pair is observed to undergo periodic oscillation in time. We can measure each function by digitizing to obtain $i'(t)$ and $v'(t)$. We can then fit these functions with another basis function.

$$i(t) = i_0 \sin(\omega_i t + \varphi_i), \qquad v(t) = v_0 \sin(\omega_v t + \varphi_v). \tag{6}$$

The process of measurement of the two functions consists of finding values for i_0, v_0, ω, and φ, such that

$$i(t) = i'(t) + \varepsilon_i(t), \qquad v(t) = v'(t) + \varepsilon_v(t), \tag{7}$$

where $\varepsilon_i(t)$ and $\varepsilon_v(t)$ are minimized deviations (errors) between $i(t)$ and $i'(t)$ or $v(t)$ and $v'(t)$. The usual criterion is least mean squares deviation. This aspect of measurement is a problem in curve-fitting, and is treated in many statistical texts. For some basis functions, such as straight lines and single exponentials, we can use linear regression. For most sets of basis functions, such as sums of exponentials and sine waves, we use nonlinear regression (Section 2.5.1). □

Each basis function has one or more parameters other than its amplitude. These may be fixed as is, for example, the duration of the rectangular digitizing pulse. When we vary the parameters, as in the case of ω and φ in Eqs. (6), we have an *adaptive* basis function. A basis function can be considered to establish a coordinate space for measurement, similar to a unit of length, volume, pressure, etc. Some set of basis functions is necessary and sufficient to represent any observable neural event.

The nature of the representing function depends on the choice of basis functions. The outstanding virtue of the rectangular basis function or digitizing interval is that it permits measurement to any desired degree of precision without the restriction as to the nature of the wave form being measured, and without inference regarding the underlying dynamics. All of the measurements from electrophysiological observations described in this study, which are the data, have been made by digitizing. They are represented graphically by points.

Other basis functions are derived from two sources. Theoretical basis functions result from solving differential equations representing the dynamics of neural systems. Experimental basis functions are derived by inspection of observed events in time. All of these basis functions are displayed graphically as smoothed curves.

Example C. Two microelectrodes are inserted into a neuron, and two electrodes are placed in the tissue outside it. A brief current pulse is passed between one inside and one outside electrode, and the potential difference is recorded between the other inside and outside electrodes. If the duration of the current pulse is shorter than the digitizing interval, the stimulus member of the input–output pair can be represented as

$$i_f(t) = \begin{cases} 0, & t \neq 0, \\ i'(0), & t = 0, \end{cases} \tag{8}$$

where $i'(0)$ is the amplitude of the applied transmembrane current pulse in microamperes. The response member is represented by

$$v_m(t) = \begin{cases} 0, & t < 0, \\ v'_m(t), & t \geq 0, \end{cases} \tag{9}$$

where $v_m(t)$ is a continuously varying transmembrane potential difference, and $v'_m(t)$ is the sequence of digitized values of amplitude of transmembrane potential difference in millivolts.

By inspection the sequence $v'_m(t)$ often takes the form of an exponential decay. A new basis function is chosen, such that

$$v_m(t) = \begin{cases} 0, & t < 0, \\ v_0\, e^{-t/\tau}, & t \geq 0, \end{cases} \tag{10}$$

where v_0 is amplitude in millivolts at $t = 0$ and τ is a time constant in units of milliseconds. By proper choice of v_0 and τ, $v_m(t)$ may be fitted to $v'_m(t)$ to an acceptable degree of approximation. □

Unless otherwise stated, the values of stimulus–response pairs are always zero for times less than zero. In order to simplify the notation, the functions of input and output are represented as

$$i_f(0) = i', \qquad t = 0, \tag{11}$$

and

$$v_m(t) = v_0\, e^{-t/\tau}. \tag{12}$$

Zero values for $t < 0$ are implied if not stated. Equation (12) may not represent $v_m(t)$ as precisely as Eq. (9), but it reduces the parameters of the output to two, as opposed to the number of digital values, and it suggests something about the nature of membrane dynamics, which Eq. (9) does not.

2.1.2. INPUT–OUTPUT FUNCTIONS

Multiple observations of input–output pairs are made in an experiment or a set of experiments. A set of ordered input–output pairs constitutes a function. Again, no two different output members can have the same input member. That is, the same input repeated two or more times cannot result in two or more different outputs. If it does, then either there is some other uncontrolled input, such that the input members are not completely described, or the neural system is changing with time, so that the set of input–output pairs does not constitute a function.

If the variation of the input or the system is not of interest, then we average across repeated trials. We can do this by digitizing the input or output functions on each trial w so that, for example,

$$\mathscr{E}\,[i'_w(t)] = \hat{i}_w(T) = \sum_{n=1}^{N} i'_w(T_n)\, p_n(T)\, \Delta T,$$

$$\mathscr{E}\,[v'_w(t)] = \hat{v}_w(T) = \sum_{n=1}^{N} v'_w(T_n)\, p_n(T)\, \Delta T, \tag{13}$$

where $\Delta T = T/N$ and $\mathscr{E}$ denotes the ensemble average. We average the values of $i'_w(T)$ or $v'_w(T)$ over W trials for each n to estimate the ensemble average (Fig. 2.1):

$$\hat{i}_w(T) = (1/W) \sum_{w=1}^{M} \sum_{n=1}^{N} i'_w(T_n) p_n(T) \Delta T,$$

$$\hat{v}_w(T) = (1/W) \sum_{w=1}^{M} \sum_{n=1}^{N} v'_w(T_n) p_n(T) \Delta T. \tag{14}$$

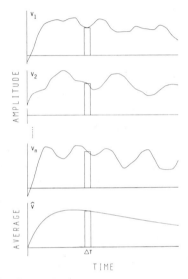

FIG. 2.1. Derivation of an ensemble average.

If on repeated trials the measurements either of input or output are randomly distributed, then the mean $\hat{v}_w(T)$ is the most reasonable estimate for $v'_w(T)$ and $\hat{i}_w(T)$ is likewise for $i'_w(T)$. The ordered pairs then constitute a function F such that

$$\hat{i}_w(T) = \mathscr{E}[i'_w(t)], \qquad \hat{v}_w(T) = \mathscr{E}[v'_w(t)], \qquad \hat{v}_w = F(\hat{i}_w). \tag{15}$$

If the variation is of interest, or if the measurements cannot be averaged, then the input–output pairs must be ordered into more than one set, so that other functions are defined.

Example A. Suppose that in Example C (Section 2.1.1) the measured output v_0 is found to very randomly on successive trials but without variation in or observable variation in $i'_f(t)$. We may ignore the variation by taking ensemble averages $[\cdot]$ as in Eq. (14) or we may infer that there is unexplained variation in our input and look for it by describing another set of functions

$$i'(t) = \hat{i}(t) + i_\varepsilon(t), \qquad v'(t) = \hat{v}(t) + v_\varepsilon(t), \qquad (16)$$

where $i_\varepsilon(t)$ and $v_\varepsilon(t)$ are random variables. We may infer that

$$\hat{v} = F(\hat{i}), \qquad v_\varepsilon = F(i_\varepsilon), \qquad (17)$$

or more generally

$$v = F(i). \qquad (18)$$

We may also infer time variation in the system, which is formulated in a way depending on the results, one of which might be

$$i_f(T) = i'(T), \qquad \hat{v}(T) - \mathscr{E}[v'(t)] k_\varepsilon(T), \qquad \hat{v} = F(i_f), \qquad (19)$$

where $k_\varepsilon(T)$ may be a randomly varying parameter. $\square$

If a system gives the same responses on successive trials of the same input, or the same mean responses on successive sets of trials with the same input, then it is time invariant. If it is rapidly time varying, then an explicit time-dependent function of a variable or parameter is required, as above. If the time variance is slow with respect to the duration of each trial, the input–output pairs are ordered into a sequence of sets or functions, each function being valid only for a limited time, and only by approximation. This condition holds for most physiological research.

2.1.3. LINEAR INPUT–OUTPUT FUNCTIONS

The order in a set of input–output pairs is imposed by ranking them with regard to one or more of the variables describing the input members, such as stimulus or amplitude. The entire sample of input–output pairs is never complete, because new pairs can always be added. The set can be divided into subsets by imposing other constraints. The input members of a subset constitute a domain of input, and the corresponding output members define a range of output.

The most important subset for our purposes is established by imposing the constraints of proportionality and additivity. Proportionality or homogeneity means that the input and output increase by the same factor:

$$v(\alpha i) = \alpha v(i). \qquad (20)$$

Additivity means that when two inputs are given at the same time, the output is equal to the sum of the outputs of the two inputs given separately:

$$v(i_1 + i_2) = v(i_1) + v(i_2). \qquad (21)$$

These two conditions are equivalent to the single condition of super-imposibility:

$$v(\alpha_1 i_1 + \alpha_2 i_2) = \alpha_1 v(i_1) + \alpha_2 v(i_2). \tag{22}$$

This condition establishes a domain of input and a range of output that are said to be linear. This subset of input–output pairs defines a linear function, and the neural dynamics are said to be linear in this range. The linear domain of input for membranes and for neurons is a small part of the total input domain, comprising inputs with low amplitudes and relatively short durations. However, a large part of neural activity takes place within the linear range, and, in fact, the range is broader than it at first appears.

Example A. A pair of electrodes 3 mm apart is placed on one end of an axon suspended in mineral oil, and a second pair 3 mm apart is placed 20 mm down the same axon. A single shock consisting of a brief current pulse with a fixed amplitude is delivered to the axon at one end, and the external potential difference is measured further down the nerve. The input amplitude is varied on successive trials. Below a certain input level, there is no output; above that threshold there is an action potential, the amplitude of which is independent of the input. This so-called all-or-none property is an example of nonproportionality of output to input. Such a system cannot be linear.   □

Example B. Paired shocks are given, the first or conditioning shock being supra threshold, the second or test shock being adjusted to threshold. With decreasing interval between the two shocks, the amplitude of the second must be increased in order to obtain a second response (relative refractory period), and for an interval corresponding approximately to the duration of the first response (the action potential) there is no second response for any intensity of input (absolute refractory period). This is an example of nonadditivity of output for the sum of two inputs displaced in time and is evidence for nonlinearity in the system. It is also evidence for time variance.   □

Example C. Let the conditioning stimulus current be considerably below the amplitude for threshold (thr) i_{thr} and have amplitude i_1. At times long after the first shock, the required threshold amplitude for the second shock i_2 to elicit a response is that threshold value i_{thr} needed in the absence of the conditioning shock. For shorter intervals, the experimental evidence (Katz, 1939) is illustrated in the relation

$$i_{thr} - i_2 = i_1 e^{-t/\tau} \tag{23}$$

where τ is a constant that depends on the nature of the axon and the external medium. Now let i_1 be either negative (cathodal) or positive (anodal) but not be given values near i_{thr}. In a certain small domain, the required amplitude of the test shock i_2 is linearly dependent on the amplitude of the conditioning shock i_1 by Eq. (23). This is an example of proportionality. □

Example D. Let two subthreshold conditioning shocks, i_1 and i_2, not necessarily equal in sign or magnitude, be given at an interval T. The threshold voltage i_{thr} and test input i_3 required to trigger the impulse are experimentally determined as before. They conform to the relation

$$i_3 = i_{thr} - i_1 e^{-\alpha t/\tau} - i_2 e^{-\alpha(t-T)/\tau}. \tag{24}$$

The effect on the nerve produced by the second conditioning shock adds to that produced by the first. Both effects decay independently of each other, and the time course depends only on the initial amplitude and time of onset of each. This is an example of additivity. □

In these examples the nerve axon responds linearly to subthreshold inputs, and its main nonlinear characteristic (the threshold) can be used as a tool for measuring its function in this range.

Example E. Let a number n of suprathreshold stimuli in a train be given the same intensity $i(t_n)$ at times t_n, separated by an interval greater than the relative refractory period. A set of n action potentials $p(t_n)$ results which is identical to the sum of the responses of n single stimuli given at times t_n. This is an example of additivity. Now let us redefine the input variable, calling it the *average number of stimuli per second* in each second $\hat{i}(T_n)$, and the output variable, calling it $p(T)$ the *average number of action potentials* or *pulses per second*. Output is then proportional to input, and it is additive for two or more inputs, provided that no interval between two or more stimuli is less than the refractory period or greater than the averaging period, and provided that the amplitude of each stimulus train is fixed above threshold. This defines a set of linear domains and linear functions for the axon, there being one domain for each suprathreshold amplitude of input. □

These examples show that the terms "linear" and "nonlinear" are applied to the domain of input, the range of output, and to the function in that range, but not to the neuron. A membrane or an axon is a system having both linear and nonlinear functions, and each function is nothing more than the description of the operation for transforming or mapping a subset of inputs into a subset of outputs with correspondence between pairs.

2.1.4.   THE IMPULSE AND THE IMPULSE RESPONSE

The single shock has long been recognized in physiology as a powerful driving energy applied for a time interval that is very brief in comparison to the duration of the response. The shock is measured by the product of its magnitude and duration if it is a rectangular function. More generally, it is the integrated area under the input curve.

The mathematical impulse or Dirac delta function may be defined as a rectangular pulse of unit area. Let $A_n(t) = n$ for $0 \leqq t \leqq 1/n$ (Fig. 2.2), and $A_n(t) = 0$ elsewhere. As the duration $1/n$ approaches zero, the unit impulse is

$$\delta(t) = \lim_{1/n \to 0} A_n(t). \tag{25}$$

Under certain conditions it is permissible to represent the single-shock input to a neural system by the delta function and call the output the *impulse response*. Experimentally, these conditions may be established by applying a rectangular pulse of appropriate magnitude and duration to an axon, nerve, or afferent tract. The duration is then decreased and the amplitude is increased in such fashion that their product is kept constant. For relatively long durations the system may show varying, mixed, or long latency components in the response, such that the form of the response changes as the pulse duration is decreased. Below some value for the duration, the output function is independent of the pulse duration. Below that value, the shock can be treated as an impulse and can be represented by the delta function $\delta(t)$ multiplied by a constant representing intensity.[†]

These concepts are particularly useful in neurophysiology for two reasons. First, the axon responds to a variety of input wave forms by generating one or more action potentials. If each action potential causes an event in other neurons that does not depend on the duration of the action potential, it can be treated as an impulse, so that irrespective of the nature of the input to the axon, the input to some further stage may be treated in terms

[†]This procedure should not be confused with that for determining the strength–duration curve. A rectangular current pulse I is applied to a nerve for a time interval T just long enough to elicit an action potential, i.e., threshold is determined. For low pulses, long durations are required. There is some level of current I_{thr} below which excitation will not take place for any duration (rheobase or threshold current). The values for I and T when plotted in rectangular coordinates conform to a hyperbola having the equation

$$(I - I_{thr})T = Q_{thr} \tag{26}$$

where Q_{thr} is the total charge displaced across the nerve membrane by the exciting current at threshold. The *chronaxie* is the duration required for a threshold current having twice the amplitude of the rheobase. It is an empirical measurement, and a pulse at chronaxie may or may not be regarded as equivalent to the impulse, depending on whether the response being observed is independent of changes in duration about the chronaxie.

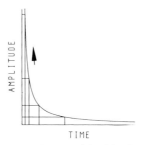

FIG. 2.2. Derivation of the delta function.

of impulse functions. Second, the impulse response $f(t)$ of a linear system consists typically of the sum of exponential terms (including the step and impulse) and damped sinusoids

$$f(t) = \sum_n A_n e^{\alpha_n t} + \sum_n B_n \cos(\omega_n t + \varphi_n) e^{\beta_n t}, \qquad (27)$$

where A_n and B_n are the initial amplitudes in volts, the α_n are rate constants in reciprocal seconds, ω_n are the frequencies of sinusoidal oscillation radians per second (equal to 2π times the frequency in cycles per second) φ_n are phase of onset expressed in radians or degrees of the sinusoid, and β_n are the rate constants in reciprocal seconds of the envelopes of the sinusoids. Both α_n and β_n are real numbers.

The term $\cos(\omega t)$ may be written

$$\cos(\omega t) = \tfrac{1}{2}\cos(\omega t) + \tfrac{1}{2}j\sin(\omega t) + \tfrac{1}{2}\cos(\omega t) - \tfrac{1}{2}j\sin(\omega t), \qquad (28)$$

where $j = (-1)^{1/2}$. Using Euler's theorem $e^{jy} = \cos y + j \sin y$ this may be written as

$$\cos(\omega t) = \tfrac{1}{2}e^{j\omega t} + \tfrac{1}{2}e^{-j\omega t}. \qquad (29)$$

Therefore the general form of the impulse response of a linear system may be written as

$$f(t) = \sum_n A_n e^{\alpha_n t}, \qquad (30)$$

where α_n may be either real or complex, and the complex terms occur always in conjugate pairs.

2.2.   Linear Models for Neural Membrane

2.2.1.   THE TOPOLOGY OF THE MEMBRANE

The anatomical structure of each neuron generating or affecting a field of potential consists of a closed surface (the membrane) across which ionic currents flow in closed loops. The internal and external compartments and the currents have three dimensions, and there is great variability in their geometries. In two dimensions the structure and the flow can be represented by an arbitrary closed boundary and by closed lines of current (Fig. 2.3). For topological purposes, the structure and lines are reduced to linear configurations. Two patterns of current are distinguished. Transmembrane current i_m flows across the membrane and longitudinal current flows parallel to the membrane. By convention, inward flow and flow to the right are positive (Fig. 2.4).

From Kirchhoff's current law, the sum of currents entering and leaving every node at all times is zero:

$$\sum_n i_n(t) = 0. \tag{31}$$

From Kirchhoff's voltage law around any closed path in a topological representation the sum of potential differences at all times is zero:

$$\sum_n v_n(t) = 0. \tag{32}$$

The properties of the system are derived by describing the relation between current and voltage for each node and path in the topological diagram.

How do we know what properties to assign to the current paths across the membrane and in the two compartments? Our best information comes

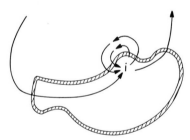

FIG. 2.3. Topological representation of loop current for a neuron of arbitrary shape.

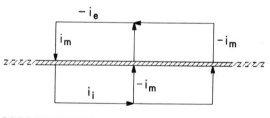

FIG. 2.4. Reduction of loop current to transmembrane, extracellular, and intracellular geometrical channels.

from input–output pairs. We know that when the input member is a sub-threshold step or a pulse, the output member can be measured with a set of basis functions containing at least one exponential term with a real rate coefficient α. Further, we know that the exponential function is the solution to a first-order differential equation. We infer that the dynamics of passive membrane can be described by such an equation.

From elementary circuit theory we know that current paths exist in which the current $i(t)$ is proportional to the rate of change of potential difference $dv(t)/dt$ by a fixed parameter called *capacitance* C:

$$i(t) = C\, dv(t)/dt. \tag{33}$$

We know that other current paths exist in which current is proportional to potential difference by a fixed parameter called *resistance* R:

$$v(t) = Ri(t). \tag{34}$$

Here C and R are defined by Eqs. (33) and (34) where R is measured in units of ohms (volts per ampere) and capacitance is measured in farads (volts per second per ampere) or in microfarads ($10^{-6}\,F$).

Salt solutions have pure resistance over all rates of change of potential that concern us here. Because the inner and outer compartments usually behave like salt solutions, and because the membrane has an appropriate molecular structure, we infer that an element behaving like a capacitance is in the membrane. Electrodes can be represented by an equivalent circuit composed of resistors and capacitors, but attempts to approximate this circuit by a single resistor R and a single capacitor, C in parallel yield a circuit element for which R and C increase with decreasing frequency or rate of change of potential (Cole & Curtis, 1939). Thus, a parallel combination of fixed R and C is merely an approximation for the elements of an electrode. Similarly, the equivalent resistance and capacitance of the membrane depend on the rate of change. At relatively low or high rates of change, they are treated as fixed parameters. They are functions describing the relations between current and voltage in limited domains, and should not be identified literally with physical circuit elements.

The topology of the membrane is elaborated to introduce the specific functions that are assigned to each current path. As shown in Fig. 2.5, R_m designates transmembrane resistance and C_m the transmembrane capacitance of each part of the membrane, R_e is extracellular resistance, and R_i is intracellular resistance.

An element across which the voltage is proportional to the rate of change of current is an *inductance* measured in henries:

$$v(t) = L\, di(t)/dt. \tag{35}$$

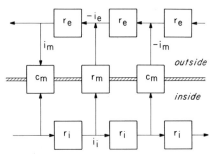

FIG. 2.5. Representation of channels for loop current by dynamic elements defined by functions.

Although this has been introduced several times into physiology in the past half century, its use has been discarded in favor of nonlinear circuit elements that is, variable voltage-dependent membrane conductances (Hodgkin & Rushton, 1946). The present discussion is restricted to the linear range of neuron function and does not require use of an equivalent inductance.

2.2.2.   DIFFERENTIAL EQUATIONS

A set of examples is given to illustrate several aspects of analysis of the model for neural membrane.

Example A.   Electrodes are placed in an axon as in Example C, Section 2.1.1, and are used to pass a unit current impulse $\delta(t)$ across the membrane to a distant external electrode. The output function to be predicted is transmembrane potential $v_m(t)$ and its dependence on the input current. A simplified representation is shown in Fig. 2.6. From the definition of the impulse, we assert that the input pulse lasts for a negligibly small time interval during which the capacitance is charged to a certain potential v_0. After the pulse ends, current flows only as indicated by the arrows in Fig. 2.6. By Kirchhoff's laws, in Section 2.2.1,

$$i_r(t) = \begin{cases} 0, & t < 0, \\ -C_m \, dv_m(t)/dt, & t > 0, \\ v_m(t)/R_m, & t > 0. \end{cases} \qquad (36)$$

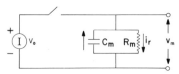

FIG. 2.6. Reduction of representation of loop current to lumped circuit model for membrane.

Therefore

$$dv_m(t)/dt = -av_m(t) + \delta(t), \tag{37}$$

where the rate constant is given by $a = 1/R_m C_m$ in units of reciprocal seconds. The solution is

$$v_m(t) = v_0 e^{-at}, \qquad t > 0, \tag{38}$$

where v_0 is the voltage across the capacitor at time $t = 0$ by the impulse $\delta(t)$. The charge q delivered by a unit current impulse is one couloumb:

$$v_0 = q/C_m = 1/C_m. \tag{39}$$

Thus the response for a unit current impulse is

$$v_m(t) = (1/C_m) e^{-at}. \quad \square \tag{40}$$

The same model holds to a first approximation for the response of a synaptic membrane to an afferent volley in which the current source is a region of activated membrane and the RC network is the passive membrane. This is discussed in Section 2.3.4.

Example B. The same electrode is used to pass a current step $\mu(t)$ across the membrane. The external resistance R_e is included in the model (Fig. 2.7). Again by Kirchhoff's laws

$$v_c(t) = v_r(t), \qquad\qquad i_c(t) + i_r(t) = i_e(t),$$
$$i_c(t) = C_m dv_c(t)/dt, \qquad i_r(t) = v_r(t)/R_m. \tag{41}$$

The input is

$$i_e(t) = \begin{cases} 0, & t < 0, \\ I, & t \geqq 0. \end{cases} \tag{42}$$

Therefore

$$dv_c(t)/dt = -av_c(t) + (I/C_m), \tag{43}$$

where a is a rate constant in seconds and $a = 1/R_m C_m$. The solution is

$$v_c(t) = IR_m(1 - e^{-at}). \tag{44}$$

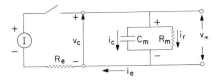

FIG. 2.7. Elaboration of Fig. 2.6 by introduction of longitudinal resistance.

The ratio of output to input is

$$v_c(t)/I\mu(t) = R_m(1 - e^{-at}),$$ (45)

in volts per unit current step. □

This model is used to measure the parameters of membrane with intracellular stimulation and recording. As $t \to \infty$, $v_c(t) \to V_\infty$, and $R_m = V_\infty/I$ in ohms. When $t = 1/a$ in milliseconds, $v_c(t) = V_\infty(1 - 1/e)$. Then $C_m = 1/aR_m$ in microfarads.

Example C. The same circuit is used as in Example B, but the input is a step voltage $v_i(t) = V_0 \mu(t)$. From Kirchhoff's laws,

$$i_c(t) + i_r(t) - i_e(t) = 0, \qquad\qquad v_r(t) + v_e(t) - v_i(t) = 0,$$

$$i_c(t) = C_m dv_c(t)/dt, \qquad\qquad v_c(t) = v_r(t),$$ (46)

$$i_r(t) = v_r(t)/R_m, \qquad\qquad i_e(t) = v_e(t)/R_e.$$

Therefore

$$\frac{dv_c(t)}{dt} + \frac{v_r(t)}{C_m}\left(\frac{1}{R_m} + \frac{1}{R_e}\right) - \frac{v_i(t)}{C_m R_e} = 0.$$ (47)

Let

$$b_1 = \frac{1}{C_m}\left(\frac{1}{R_m} + \frac{1}{R_e}\right), \qquad b_2 = \frac{1}{C_m}\cdot\frac{1}{R_e}.$$ (48)

Equation (47) then becomes

$$dv_c(t)/dt = b_1 v_c(t) + b_2 V_0 \delta(t).$$ (49)

The solution has the same form as for Eq. (42),

$$v_c(t) = V_0(b_1/b_2)(1 - e^{-b_1 t}),$$ (50)

or as the ratio of output to input,

$$v_c(t)/V_0 \mu(t) = [R_m/(R_m + R_e)](1 - e^{-b_1 t}).$$ (51)

The impulse response for a voltage pulse can be found by differentiating Eq. (50) with respect to time and is

$$v_c(t)/V_0 \delta(t) = b_2 e^{-b_1 t}.$$ (52)

The rate constant b_1 is not that for passive membrane a, because when the output in response to a voltage input V_0 depends on both the transmembrane and external resistances, the external path short-circuits the membrane and causes the potential to change at a more rapid rate. This model conforms to the conditions obtaining with stimulating electrodes commonly used in which the output voltage and not the output current is regulated (characteristic of transformers, batteries, and other sources with low internal impedance), or to extracellular stimulation in vivo when the extraneuronal fluid short-circuits the stimulating current. ☐

Example D. Let two widely spaced electrodes be placed on a nerve in air and be connected through a switch to a battery (Fig. 2.8). It is proposed that the transmembrane voltage v_2 at the cathode can be predicted as a function of $v_1(t)$, i.e., the ratio $v_2(t)/v_1(t)$. From Kirchhoff's laws,

$$v_1(t) = v_{in}(t) - v_2(t),$$

$$i(t) = \begin{cases} C_1 \dfrac{dv_1(t)}{dt} + \dfrac{v_1(t)}{R_1}, \\[2mm] C_2 \dfrac{dv_2(t)}{dt} + \dfrac{v_2(t)}{R_2}. \end{cases} \tag{53}$$

Because of the rectification characteristic of nerve membrane, $R_1 \neq R_2$ and the classical methods exemplified here are very cumbersome. The solution is deferred to Section 2.2.4. ☐

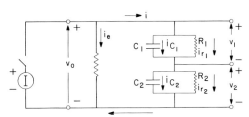

FIG. 2.8. Elaboration of Fig. 2.7 by introducing a difference in the membrane at site of current inflow i_1 and outflow i_2.

These examples illustrate the general property that in the linear range of function, neuron systems are described by linear differential equations in the input and output. The solutions represent predictions of what the output will be for a specified input. For realistic problems representing more complex topologies, the solutions are too difficult to obtain by the conventional methods described. An operational method will now be introduced to provide solutions to such problems more easily.

2.2.3. THE LAPLACE TRANSFORM

The study of a neuronal system consists of analysis of its output for specified input conditions and synthesis of a model expressed by differential equations. In diagrammatic form there is an input $u(t)$ and an output $v(t)$, both functions of time, which are related to yield a statement about the intervening transforming process F.

$$
u(t) \longrightarrow \boxed{\quad F \quad} \longrightarrow v(t)
$$

In Section 2.1.4 it is stated that for an impulse input, the output of a linear system has the form

$$
v(t) = \sum_{j=1}^{m} B_j e^{-\beta_j t}, \tag{54}
$$

which is the sum of the exponential and sinusoidal components. This holds for a variety of inputs including impulses, steps, exponentials, etc., so that for all commonly used inputs

$$
u(t) = \sum_{j=1}^{n} A_j e^{-\alpha_j t}. \tag{55}
$$

In Section 2.2.2 it was stated that the characteristics of a linear system can be described using ordinary differential equations in the input and output functions. The generic form is

$$
a_n \frac{d^n}{dt^n} u(t) + \cdots + a_1 \frac{d}{dt} u(t) + a_0 u(t) = b_m \frac{d^m}{dt^m} v(t) + \cdots + b_1 \frac{d}{dt} v(t) + b_0 v(t) \tag{56}
$$

where the a_j and b_j, $0 \leq j \leq n$, $0 \leq j \leq m$, are constants. The problem for analysis is to evaluate A_j, B_j, α_j, and β_j from observation of the neural system. The problem for synthesis is to set up Eq. (56) in the effort to bring together all sources of information about the system in a form suitable for comparison of predicted output with measured output.

In the event that all initial conditions are zero as with impulse input, we can think intuitively (for our present purposes) of a variable s as an operator,

$$
s \propto d/dt, \tag{57}
$$

expressing the operation of taking the derivative with respect to time. This operator s has the dimensions of reciprocal seconds. Substitution of s for d/dt in Eq. (56) yields a polynomial in s:

$$
a_n s^n U(s) + \cdots + a_1 sU(s) + a_0 U(s) = b_m s^m V(s) + \cdots + b_1 sV(s) + b_0 V(s), \tag{58}
$$

where the input and output are expressed as functions of s rather than of time. This can be rewritten by collecting terms:

$$(a_n s^n + \cdots + a_1 s + a_0) U(s) = (b_m s^m + \cdots + b_1 s + b_0) V(s). \qquad (59)$$

The ratio for output to input is then

$$\frac{V(s)}{U(s)} = \frac{a_n s^n + \cdots + a_1 s + a_0}{b_m s^m + \cdots + b_1 s + b_0}. \qquad (60)$$

The substitution of s for d/dt when the initial conditions are all zero constitutes the Laplace transformation of Eq. (56) to Eq. (58), which is expressed in generic form as

$$\mathscr{L}[u(t)] = U(s), \qquad \mathscr{L}[v(t)] = v(s). \qquad (61)$$

The inverse transform is by reverse substitution:

$$\mathscr{L}^{-1}[U(s)] = u(t), \qquad \mathscr{L}^{-1}[V(s)] = v(t). \qquad (62)$$

The *transfer function* of a linear system can now be expressed as a function of s and is defined as the ratio of the input function to the output function,

$$F(s) = V(s)/U(s), \qquad (63)$$

so that

$$F(s) = \frac{a_n s^n + \cdots + a_1 s + a_0}{b_m s^m + \cdots + b_1 s + b_0}.$$

The differential equation is now in the form of the ratio of two polynomials. The next step toward solution is to factor these polynomials into the form

$$F(s) = k\frac{(s + c_1)(s + c_2) \cdots (s + c_n)}{(s + d_1)(s + d_2) \cdots (s + d_m)}, \qquad (64)$$

where c_j and d_j are real or complex, and where complex numbers always occur in conjugate pairs (see Section 2.1.4). When m or n is equal to 2, the quadratic formula is used. For higher-order polynomials, other methods are required (e.g., DiStefano et al., 1967, pp. 64–80).

Because the roots in Eq. (64) take the form of complex numbers, the operator s may be given values in the form of complex numbers. When s approaches $-c_j$ for $0 \leqq j \leqq n$, then $F(s)$ approaches zero. Characteristically, the output of a system does not contain frequencies for inputs whose frequencies are such that s approaches $-c_j$ for some j where $0 < j \leqq n$. On the other hand, when s approaches some $-d_j$, $0 \leqq j \leqq m$, then $F(s)$ approaches infinity. This represents a characteristic or natural frequency or rate of change for the system. The values for $s = -c_j$ are known as the *zeros* and the values for $s = -d_j$ are known as the *poles* of the system.

The poles and zeros together completely describe the characteristics of a linear system. The values for the poles and zeros are readily susceptible to graphic display in the coordinates of α and ω, which is known as the s plane, where α is the real part and ω is the imaginary part of $s = -\alpha \pm j\omega$.

The ratio of factored polynomials provides the solution to the differential equation. The inverse transform, Eqs. (62), yields the output function for the impulse input. This consists of the sum of exponential terms having rate constants specified by the poles

$$v(t) = B_1 e^{-d_1 t} + B_2 e^{-d_2 t} + \cdots + B_m e^{-d_m t}. \tag{65}$$

The amplitude coefficients B_m are found by the method of residues (DiStefano et al., 1967). Let the value of s approach the value of one of the coefficients in the denominator

$$B_1 = k \cdot \lim_{s \to -d_1} [(s + d_1) \cdot F(s)]. \tag{66}$$

Therefore

$$B_1 = k \frac{(-d_1 + c_1)(-d_1 + c_2) \cdots (-d_1 + c_n)}{(-d_1 + d_2)(-d_1 + d_3) \cdots (-d_1 + d_m)}. \tag{67}$$

The procedure is repeated m times to find the m values for B_m. Conjugate pairs of complex exponentials are transformed to sinusoids by use of Euler's theorem (see Section 2.1.4).

2.2.4. APPLICATION OF THE LAPLACE TRANSFORM TO THE MEMBRANE

The operational method is now demonstrated using the examples in Section 2.2.2.

Example A. This is the same as Example A in Section 2.2.2, Fig. 2.6. The equation relating input to output is

$$dv_m(t)/dt = -av_m(t) + (1/C_m)\delta(t). \tag{68}$$

The Laplace transform of the impulse function $\delta(t)$ is equal to unity (see Section 2.3.2). Therefore the Laplace transformation of Eq. (68) is

$$sV_m(s) + aV_m(s) = 1/C_m. \tag{69}$$

Algebraic reformulation to solve for the ratio of output $V_m(s)$ to input, which is $F(s) = 1$, gives

$$V_m(s)/1 = (1/C_m)/(s + a). \tag{70}$$

The inverse transform is

$$\mathscr{L}^{-1}[V_m(s)] = (1/C_m)e^{-at}. \quad \square \tag{71}$$

Example B.   The system (Fig. 2.7) in Example B, Section 2.2.2, has the input function

$$i_e(t) = I \cdot \mu(t),$$

a constant times the unit step function. The Laplace transform for $\mu(t)$ is $1/s$ (see Section 2.3.2). Therefore, from (43)

$$sV_e(s) + aV_e(s) = \frac{I}{C_m} \frac{1}{s}. \tag{72}$$

By rearrangement

$$\frac{V_e(s)}{I} = \frac{1/C_m}{s(s+a)}. \tag{73}$$

The solution is

$$\frac{v_e(t)}{I\mu(t)} = \frac{1}{C_m}(B_1 + B_2 e^{-at}), \qquad B_1 = \frac{1}{a}, \qquad B_2 = -\frac{1}{a}, \tag{74}$$

or

$$v_e(t) = I \cdot \mu(t) \cdot R_m(1 - e^{-at}). \qquad \square \tag{75}$$

Example C.   Equation (47) in Section 2.2.2 can be rewritten as

$$dv_e(t)/dt + b_1 v_e(t) = b_2 V_0 \cdot \mu(t). \tag{76}$$

This transforms to

$$V_e(s)/V_0 = b_2/s(s+b_1). \tag{77}$$

The solution is found as for Eq. (73), and it is identical to Eq. (51) in Section 2.2.2. $\square$

Example D.   Equations (53) in Section 2.2.2 are written as time functions and combined (see Fig. 2.8):

$$v_1(t) = v_0(t) - v_2(t), \tag{78}$$

$$C_1 \frac{dv_1(t)}{dt} + \frac{v_1(t)}{R_1} = C_2 \frac{dv_2(t)}{dt} + \frac{v_2(t)}{R_2}. \tag{79}$$

The Laplace transform gives

$$V_1(s) = V_0(s) - V_2(s), \tag{80}$$

$$\left(C_1 s + \frac{1}{R_1}\right) V_1(s) = \left(C_2 s + \frac{1}{R_2}\right) V_2(s). \tag{81}$$

By substituting Eq. (80) into Eq. (81) and regrouping,

$$\frac{V_2(s)}{V_0(s)} = \frac{C_1}{(C_1 + C_2)} \cdot \frac{(s + b_1)}{s(s + b_2)},$$

(82)

where

$$b_1 = 1/R_1 C_1, \qquad b_2 = (R_1 + R_2)/R_1 R_2(C_1 + C_2).$$

(83)

The solution by inverse transform is

$$\frac{v_2(t)}{v_0(t)} = \frac{C_1}{C_1 + C_2}(B_1 e^{-b_1 t} + B_2 e^{-b_2 t}), \qquad B_1 = \frac{b_1}{b_2}, \qquad B_2 = \frac{-b_2 + b_1}{-b_2}.$$

(84)

This reduces to

$$\frac{v_2(t)}{v_0(t)} = \frac{R_2}{R_1 + R_2}\left[1 - \left(\frac{1 + (R_1/R_2)}{1 + (C_2/C_1)}\right)e^{-b_2 t}\right].$$

(85)

For the case where $R_1 = R_2$ and $C_1 = C_2$,

$$v_2(t)/v_0(t) = \tfrac{1}{2}. \quad \square$$

(86)

Further examples of lumped circuit analysis using conventional and operational methods can be found in any of several texts on linear analysis. The examples selected here represent common problems in the analysis of neural membrane dynamics, particularly in regard to whether the input is a current or voltage, when the output is measured as a potential difference across the membrane or across the external resistance of the medium.

2.3.   Linear Models for Parts of Neurons

An operational method has now been demonstrated for solving simple differential equations from the network model of passive membrane. Before the method is applied to more complex systems, of which the membrane is a part, the operation must be defined, and some of its basic properties must be clarified.

2.3.1.   CONVOLUTION

A property of a system in a linear, time-invariant range is that when the impulse response is known, the output can be predicted for any other input. This is done by treating the input as if it were an ordered sequence of impulses and adding the sequence of impulse responses.

In Section 2.1.1 we note that a neural event $i(t)$ can be measured by using a set of N digitizing basis functions (Fig. 2.9) $p_n(t), n = 1, ..., N$. Each rectangular pulse has unit amplitude, time of occurrence t_n, and

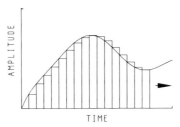

FIG. 2.9. Representation of continuous activity in the wave mode $i(t)$ by a sequence of pulses $i'(t)$ as the basis for constructing a wave function.

duration Δt. The value of an input function $i'(t)$ representing an input event, is equal to the sum of the set of basis functions.

$$i(t) = \sum_{n=1}^{N} i(t_n) p_n(t) \Delta t, \qquad (87)$$

where $p_n(t) = 1$ for $t = t_n$ and $p_n(t) = 0$ elsewhere.

Here we can treat the input as if it consisted of an ordered sequence of delta functions or impulses with amplitude $u(t_n) \Delta t$. If each input impulse occurs at time T measured with respect to a reference time t the amplitude of the input function at time T_n is $u'(T_n) \Delta T$. The function $u'(t)$ is given by

$$u'(t) = \sum_{n=1}^{N} u(T_n) \Delta T \, \delta(t - T_n), \qquad (88)$$

where $\delta(t - T_n)$ replaces $p_n(t)$. Each impulse initiates an impulse response at $t - T_n$, which has the value $f(t - T_n)$, because the system is time invariant. For any time t the predicted output $v(t)$ is the sum of all the impulse responses weighted by $u(T_n) \Delta T$, because the system is linear.

$$v(t) = \sum_{n=1}^{N} u'(T_n) f(t - T_n) \Delta T, \qquad t \geqq T > 0. \qquad (89)$$

This is illustrated in Fig. 2.10.

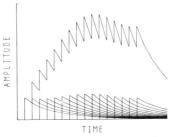

FIG. 2.10. Representation of a wave function by the sum of a set of impulse responses in convolution.

If the input function and impulse response are both measured by digitizing at n intervals, $u'(T_n)$ and $f'(t_m - T_n)$, then the output $v'(t_m)$ is predicted by a set of discrete sums

$$v'(t_m) = \sum_{n=1}^{N} u'(T_n) f'(t_m - T_n) \Delta T. \qquad (90)$$

If the input function and impulse response are represented by sets of continuous basis functions, we allow the duration of the unit impulse to approach an infinitesimal value $\Delta T \to dT$. The summation becomes the convolution integral

$$v(t) = \int_0^t u(T) f(t - T) dT. \qquad (91)$$

It is easily seen, also, that Eq. (91) is equivalent to

$$v(t) = \int_0^t f(T) u(t - T) dT. \qquad (92)$$

Example A.　A well-known use of convolution is the synthesis of the compound action potential that results from stimulation of a nerve (a bundle of axons) with an extracellular current pulse, while recording the potential difference from an extracellular electrode on the nerve with respect to a reference electrode on the cut end (Gasser & Grundfest, 1939). Both the conduction velocity and the extracellularly recorded amplitude of the action potential of each component axon vary in proportion to the fiber diameter of the axon. The duration of the action potential of single fibers is independent of diameter. The wave form of the action potential is the impulse response for a single fiber recorded in air $f(t)$, and is approximated by a triangle. The input function $u(t)$ is obtained from the histological enumeration, measurement, and classification of fibers in accordance with diameters in the form of a histogram. The contribution to the potential for each group of fibers (e.g., 9–11 μm) in arbitrary units is the number times the diameter, e.g., $100 \times 10\,\mu$m = 1000, or $20 \times 20\,\mu$m = 400, etc.

The value for T for each group that appears in Eq. (90) is obtained by measuring the latency for the first or largest group at a recording site 40 mm from the stimulus site. This is 4 msec, giving a velocity of 100 m/sec for a diameter of 14 μm. The factor for converting diameter to velocity is 7.14 m/sec/μm.[†] The velocity for each group divided into the distance gives the latency T for each group, this defines $f(t - T)$.

[†] Conduction velocity is proportional to diameter in myelinated and small unmyelinated axons (Freeman, 1972a) and to the square root of diameter in large unmyelinated axons (Hodgkin & Huxley, 1952).

The solution in these terms for Eq. (90) has been obtained by graphic summation as shown in Fig. 2.11, where it is shown as a dashed line superimposed on a recorded potential from the same nerve (saphenous nerve of the cat.) The underlying mathematical assumption in the representation is that although the stimulus impulse is given at one point of the fiber, and the action potentials travel from that point, this is equivalent to giving a series of impulses to the appropriate fiber groups at the recording site, but with a delay for each specified by its conduction velocity. □

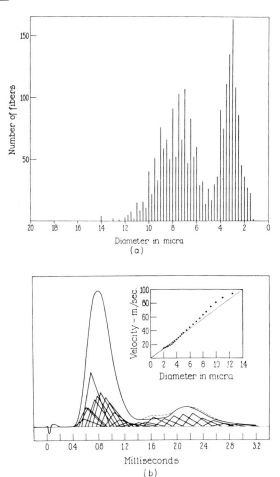

FIG. 2.11. (a) Distribution of fibers according to size in the saphenous nerve of the cat; total is 2119. (b) Use of convolution to predict the compound action potential (Gasser & Grundfest, 1939).

Example B.   Suppose that the subthreshold impulse response of an axon is represented by the function

$$f(t) = (1/C)\,e^{-t/RC}, \qquad t \geq 0. \tag{93}$$

We want to predict the output function for a current step applied across the membrane.

$$u(t) = \begin{cases} I\mu(t), & t \geq 0, \\ 0, & t < 0. \end{cases} \tag{94}$$

From Eq. (91)

$$v(t) = \int_0^t (I/C)\,e^{-(t-T)/RC}\,dT. \tag{95}$$

The solution is

$$v(t) = IR(1 - e^{-t/RC}), \qquad t \geq 0. \tag{96}$$

Observation is then made to determine whether $v'(t)$ in response to a current step conforms to Eq. (96).   □

The convolution integral lies at the heart of linear systems theory, for it describes in specific terms what a system will do in response to any input function, once the impulse response is known. The labor required for use in this form is too great, however, for routine application. An alternative approach is described.

2.3.2.   THE CONVOLUTION THEOREM

The Laplace transform has been introduced as a method for converting differential equations to algebraic equations in order to simplify the task of solution. Here we begin with the formal definition, particularly in order to introduce the convolution theorem on which we will depend heavily.

The Laplace transform is defined by

$$\mathscr{L}[f(t)] = \int_0^\infty f(t)\,e^{-st}\,dt, \tag{97}$$

in which the term e^{-st} has been selected from among numerous possibilities, because it leads to the useful properties already described as well as others still more useful. A given function of time $f(t)$ has the transform $F(s)$ if and only if the integral converges. In each case the inverse transform

$$\mathscr{L}^{-1}[F(s)] = (1/2\pi j)\int_{c-j\infty}^{c+j\infty} F(s)\,e^{st}\,dt \tag{98}$$

exists as well. Therefore, we have a set of functions in time $f(t)$ and a set of functions in the complex frequency $F(s)$ that form an ordered set of input–output pairs. The linear operator $\mathscr{L}$ is the symbol for the operation by which each member is transformed into the corresponding member.

Example A. Consider the Laplace transform of the exponential term

$$\mathscr{L}[e^{-\alpha t}] = F(s) = \int_0^\infty e^{-\alpha t} e^{-st} dt, \tag{99}$$

$$F(s) = -e^{-(s+\alpha)t}/(s+\alpha) \Big|_0^\infty = 1/(s+\alpha). \quad \square \tag{100}$$

Example B. The unit step function $\mu(t)$ transforms to

$$\mathscr{L}[\mu(t)] = \int_0^\infty 1 \cdot e^{-st} dt, \tag{101}$$

$$F(s) = -e^{-st}/s \Big|_0^\infty = 1/s. \quad \square \tag{102}$$

Example C. The delta function $\delta(t)$ can be transformed by breaking the integral into two parts:

$$\mathscr{L}[\delta(t)] = \int_0^\infty \delta(t) e^{-st} dt, \tag{103}$$

$$F(s) = \int_0^{\Delta t} \delta(t) e^{-st} dt + \int_{\Delta t}^\infty 0 \cdot e^{-st} dt. \tag{104}$$

From the definition of the impulse, the value for Δt can be made as small as desired, so that for all non zero values of $\delta(t)$, e^{-st} is 1. Therefore,

$$F(s) = \int_0^\varepsilon \delta(t) dt = 1. \quad \square \tag{105}$$

The direct and inverse transforms for large numbers of functions have been obtained by these and similar techniques and have been tabulated as transform pairs. If either the time response or the differential equation of a neuron system has been identified, these tables provide ready access to the desired transforms.

The next step is to show how two or more parts of a linear system independently described can be assembled into a total system. In Section 2.3.1 the procedure for obtaining an output $v(t)$ of a system from its input $u(t)$ is described as the convolution of the input function with the impulse response $f(t)$ of the system:

$$v(t) = \int_0^t u(T) f(t-T) dT. \tag{106}$$

In Section 2.2.3 the transfer function is defined as the ratio of output to input for each pair:

$$F(s) = V(s)/U(s). \tag{107}$$

If $u(t) = \delta(t)$, then $U(s) = 1$. Therefore the Laplace transform of the impulse response $F(s)$ is identical to the transfer function for the system $V(s)$:

$$F(s) = V(s). \tag{108}$$

Let us now take the Laplace transform of both sides of Eq. (106). The left side is

$$V(s) = \mathscr{L}[v(t)] = \int_0^\infty v(t) e^{-st} dt. \tag{109}$$

The right side is

$$V(s) = \int_0^\infty e^{-st} \left[\int_0^\infty u(T) f(t-T) dT \right] dt, \tag{110}$$

because $f(t-T) = 0$ for $T > t$. We can change the order of integration, so that

$$V(s) = \int_0^\infty u(T) \left[\int_0^\infty f(t-T) e^{-st} dt \right] dT, \tag{111}$$

by the same reason, i.e., $f(t-T) = 0$ for $T > t$. We hold T constant while integrating over time. Next, let $y = t - T$ and $dy = dt$, so that the quantity in brackets becomes

$$\left[\int_0^\infty f(y) e^{-s(y+T)} dy \right].$$

Because e^{-sT} is constant under the integration, it can be taken ouside the integral sign. From Eq. (97)

$$e^{-sT} F(s) = \left[e^{-sT} \int_0^\infty u(v) e^{-sy} dy \right]. \tag{112}$$

From Eqs. (111) and (112)

$$V(s) = \int_0^\infty u(T) [e^{-sT} F(s)] dT. \tag{113}$$

Taking the function of s outside the integral we have

$$V(s) = F(s) \int_0^\infty u(T) e^{-sT} dT. \tag{114}$$

The integral is again identical with Eq. (97) so that

$$V(s) = F(s) U(s). \tag{115}$$

This result is of fundamental importance in the study of linear properties of neuron systems for it offers a major simplification in the task of solving a convolution integral. Three steps are taken. The transforms are taken of the impulse response and of the input function. The two algebraic expressions in s are multiplied. The inverse transform of this product gives the desired result.

$$v(t) = \mathscr{L}^{-1}[V(s)] = \mathscr{L}^{-1}[F(s) U(s)]. \tag{116}$$

The theorem can be extended to a series of convolutions representing serial and parallel stages in a system, each described by linear equations. Moreover, multiplication of a time function by a constant is equivalent to multiplication of its transform by that constant:

$$\mathscr{L}[kv(t)] = kV(s). \tag{117}$$

Integration of an input function is equivalent to multiplication by $1/s$. Differentiation for zero initial condition corresponds to multiplication by s:

$$\mathscr{L}\left[\int_0^t v(t)\,dt\right] = (1/s) V(s), \tag{118}$$

$$\mathscr{L}[dv(t)/dt] = sV(s). \tag{119}$$

As a consequence of the linearity of $\mathscr{L}$, the output of parallel channels is represented by addition of their transforms

$$\mathscr{L}[v_1(t)+v_2(t)] = V_1(s) + V_2(s). \tag{120}$$

Example D. A unit current step is applied to two axons having differing rate constants. The axons cannot be separated, so that the common output is amplified by a known constant K and is electronically differentiated. The problem is to evaluate the two rate constants and the amplitudes of the two responses from measurement of the single output $v'(t)$.

From our understanding of the passive membrane, we postulate that the dynamics of the membranes of the two axons are given by

$$dv_a(t)/dt = A - av_a(t), \qquad dv_b(t)/dt = B - bv_b(t). \tag{121}$$

The Laplace transform gives

$$V_a(s) = A/(s+a), \qquad V_b(s) = B/(s+b), \tag{122}$$

where A and B are real constants. The Laplace transform of the input function, which is a unit step $\mu(t)$, is

$$U(s) = 1/s. \tag{123}$$

Multiplication and differentiation are represented, respectively, by multiplying by K and, recalling our assumption of zero initial conditions, by s. The multiplicative and additive operations determining the output are represented as

$$V(s) = Ks[V_a(s) + V_b(s)]. \tag{124}$$

Substituting Eqs. (121)–(123) into (124), we obtain

$$V(s) = \frac{Ks}{s}\left(\frac{A}{s+a} + \frac{B}{s+b}\right). \tag{125}$$

The inverse transform is

$$V(t) = K(Ae^{-at} + Be^{-bt}). \tag{126}$$

The predicted output is the sum of two exponential basis functions, which is fitted to $v'(t)$ to evaluate the four unknown parameters. □

The order of operations is unimportant and may be interchanged in solving the equations in principle, but this does not carry back to the original system. One serial arrangement may permit operation in the linear range of all components, while another may not.

2.3.3. Transfer Functions for Pulse Transmission

The characteristic mode of transmission for axons is by trains of pulses. Instances are known in which transmission occurs without pulses, but these are not treated here (see Section 6.2.4). Each pulse is commonly found to have unchanging shape and amplitude at successive points along the axon. Though exceptions occur, it is reasonable to treat the pulse as a time function $v(t)$ that is invariant under translation $v(t-T)$ by a conduction delay T. Because the pulse is the response to a fixed suprathreshold shock $I\delta(t)$, it is an impulse response. With respect to a postsynaptic event, which lasts much longer than the axon pulse and is not dependent on the duration of the pulse, the pulse of a single axon can itself be treated as a unit impulse. The axon impulse response in the time domain (though not in the spatial domain) is

$$f(t) = \delta(t - T) \tag{127}$$

for any assigned conduction delay T. This holds only for a linear domain as described in Section 2.1.4. The Laplace transform of Eq. (127) is

$$F(s) = \int_0^\infty \delta(t - T) e^{-st} dt. \tag{128}$$

Let $y = t - T$. Then $dy = dt$ and

$$F(s) = \int_0^\infty \delta(y) e^{-(y + T)s} dy. \tag{129}$$

Taking the term e^{-sT} before the integral sign we have

$$F(s) = e^{-sT} \int_0^\infty \delta(y) e^{-sy} dy. \tag{130}$$

The integral is equal to unity, so the axon transfer function is

$$F(s) = e^{-sT}, \tag{131}$$

which is delay without change in amplitude. Thus a function of a single unbranched axon can be described in terms of the operator s, although the expression does not take a rational form.

It is reasonable to believe that the magnitude of the synaptic effect of an axon varies with its diameter, though its intracellular pulse amplitude does not. Moreover, most axons branch repeatedly before sending multiple endings to their target neurons. Each branch causes an increase in the number of action potentials, though not in the amplitude of the total extracellularly recorded action potential. The branches are smaller in diameter than the parent axon, and the extracellular pulse amplitude of each branch is proportionally smaller. The cumulative output onto target neurons of a densely branched axon must be greater than that of a sparsely branched axon. Therefore, for any axon we can assign a dimensionless real number K_a, which represents the relative magnitude of output. If we assume that all branches have the same delay, the transfer function is

$$F(s) = K_a e^{-sT}. \tag{132}$$

The assumption does not hold in general. Because conduction velocity is proportional to axon diameter, the arrival times of action potentials on branches of varying diameter and length are dispersed.

Dispersion also occurs in a nerve consisting of a bundle of axons having a distribution of diameters. The effect on the compound action potential following single-shock stimulation has been shown by means of the convolution integral (Example A, Section 2.3.1). The same problem can be analyzed by using the Laplace transform.

The distribution of diameters of axons in a typical nerve is multimodal (Fig. 2.11a), but around each mode, and in the PON over the entire nerve, the axon diameters D are normally distributed (Fig. 2.12a). The mean diameter $\bar{D}$ is $0.276\,\mu m$, and the coefficient of variation σ_a is the standard deviation S_a divided by $\bar{D}$, $\sigma_a = S_a/\bar{D} = 0.20$. The axons are excited by single-shock stimulation with an extracellular cathode in the PON and an anode on the skull. There is a set of fixed conduction distances up to $\eta = 2.5\,mm$ to an extracellular electrode on the PON for monopolar recording with respect to a reference electrode on the skull. The arrival time t_a for the pulse on each axon depends on the distance η divided by the conduction velocity θ of each axon, $t_a = \eta/\theta$. From the linear relation between axon diameter and conduction velocity (Section 2.3.1) we infer that $\theta/D = \bar{\theta}/\bar{D}$, where $\bar{\theta} = .42\,m/sec$ is the mean PON conduction velocity. Then the pulse arrival time for each group of axons in the histogram in Fig. 2.12b is

$$t_a = (\bar{D}/\bar{\theta})\eta/D. \tag{133}$$

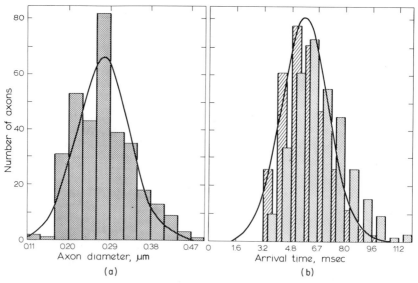

FIG. 2.12. (a) Distributions of axon diameters and (b) predicted arrival times for PON (Freeman, 1972a). (a) Mean diameter = $.276\,\mu m$, $S_a = .055\,\mu m$, and $\sigma_a = .20$. (b) Hatching: weighted by square of diameter; dotted areas: not weighted. Mean arrival time $T_a = 56\,msec$, $\bar{\theta} = .42\,m/sec$, and $\eta = 2.5\,mm$.

The distribution of arrival times is slightly skewed, but it is sufficiently close to a normal distribution to be treated as such (Fig. 2.12b), with a mean T_a, a standard deviation $\sigma(T_a)$, and a coefficient of variation $\sigma_t = \sigma(T_a)/T_a$. That is, the normal density curve is selected as the basis function.

Both T_a and $\sigma(T_a)$ increase with increasing conduction distance η, so that dispersion, like delay, is a distance-dependent parameter. The coefficient of variation σ_t is not, however, and in fact depends only on the variation of axon diameters. For this reason, $\sigma(T_a)$ is expressed as the product $\sigma_t T_a$. The function for the arrival times (Fig. 2.12b) can be written

$$p(t, T_a) = 1/[(2\pi)^{1/2} \sigma_t T_a] \exp[-(t - T_a)^2/2(\sigma_t T_a)^2]. \tag{134}$$

A table of Laplace transforms[†] gives

$$P(s, T_a) = \exp[(s\sigma_t T_a)^2/2] \exp(-sT_a). \tag{135}$$

If each axon pulse can be treated as an impulse with an amplitude weighted according to the square of its diameter (Fig. 2.12b), then

$$f(t) = K_a \delta(t), \tag{136}$$

and

$$F(s) = K_a. \tag{137}$$

By the convolution integral, the transfer function $A_k(s, T_a) = F(s)P(s, T_a)$ for a compound nerve is

$$A_k(s, T_a) = K_a \exp[(s\sigma_t T_a)^2/2] \exp(-sT_a). \tag{138}$$

The compound nerve and by inference the branches of a single axon do more than multiply and delay pulse input. Dispersion transforms the input in a way that is dependent on the mean and variation of axon diameter and the mean length of axon.

Example A. Qualitatively, the effect of dispersion can be seen in Fig. 2.13a. The compound action potential recorded in the brain has a triphasic configuration, as does that of single axons when the recording site is not too near either end of the axon. Whereas the action potential of the single axon shows negligible attenuation of amplitude with distance along the axon, the compound action potential undergoes rapid attenuation with

[†] The Laplace transform of the normal density function cannot be expressed in closed form and in fact is

$$P(s, T_a) = \exp[(s\sigma_t T_a)^2/2] \exp(-sT_a) \operatorname{erfc}(\sigma_t T_a/2^{1/2}).$$

The complementary error function term refers to the tail of the normal distribution of a set of action potentials extending beyond the time origin $t < 0$. This part of the tail physiologically does not exist, so the erfc term can be omitted without affecting the results.

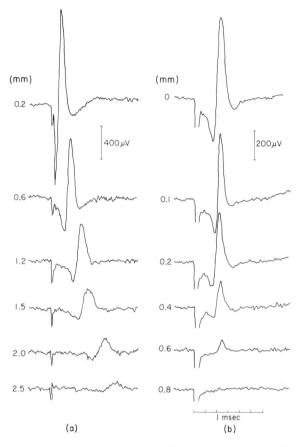

Fig. 2.13. Compound action potential of PON as (a) a function of distance from the stimulus site in the direction of propagation (horizontal), and (b) as a function of distance perpendicular to the axis of propagation (vertical) (Freeman, 1972a).

conduction distance. Both responses show attenuation with distance perpendicular to the axon or the axon bundle (Fig. 2.13b), yet the axon pulses in the compound nerve are still present, because a postsynaptic event is found in the vicinity of the axon terminals.

Quantitatively, the effect of dispersion can be predicted by treating the compound action potential recorded very near the stimulus site not as an impulse but as a brief sine wave $K_a \sin(\omega t)$. The frequency ω can be estimated from the duration of the main upward peak, which is 8 msec. Twice this value, i.e., 1.6 msec, gives the wavelength, and the reciprocal gives the frequency about 600 Hz. The angular frequency is $2\pi \cdot 600$ or about 3700 rad/sec. (Advanced students will recognize that a more accurate estimate can be obtained by using numerical integration to obtain the Fourier transform $V'(j\omega)$ of the digitized action potential $v'(t)$.)

The value for s in Eq. (134) is set equal to $j\omega = j4000\,\text{rad/sec}$, $\alpha = 0$.

Then

$$P(s, T_a) = \exp[(j\omega\sigma_t\,T_a)^2/2]\exp(-j\omega T_a). \tag{139}$$

The transfer function is split into the real and imaginary parts to give the gain $P(j\omega)$ and the phase $\Phi(j\omega)$:

$$P(j\omega, T_a) = \exp(-\omega^2\sigma_t^2\,T_a^2/2), \qquad \Phi(j\omega, T_a) = -\omega T_a. \tag{140}$$

There is a phase lag in proportion to the delay. The attenuation depends on the square of frequency, axon variation, and mean delay. For $\sigma_t = .19$ and $T_a = 1\,\text{msec}$, $P(j\omega, T_a) = e^{-.25}$ or .8. For $T_a = 4\,\text{msec}$, $P(j\omega, T_a) = .02$. Figure 2.14 shows sets of measured amplitudes $v'(t)$. The lower curve shows the predicted function $P(j\omega, T)$ from Eq. (140), where $\sigma_t = .19$. The upper curve is for a lower value of σ_t. $\square$

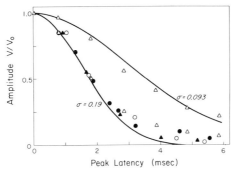

FIG. 2.14. Effect of temporal dispersion on the amplitude of the PON compound action potential. Curves are from Eq. (140). $\triangle$: amplitudes predicted by numerical technique of convolution; remaining symbols: three sets of observations (Freeman, 1972a).

The result holds for the extracellularly recorded compound action potential, but it is not applicable to the volley of impulses in the nerve.

Example B. The treatment in Example A is based on the use of the normal density function for measuring the distribution of arrival times. Even though there is reason to believe that the axon diameters vary at random, we are free to choose other basis functions to meet our computational needs. Provided the same precision of measurement is obtained, the conversion from one set of basis functions to another can be regarded in much the same way as a transformation from Cartesian to polar coordinates.

Moreover, if we are not interested in the details of a function, such as axon diameters or pulse arrival times, but only in the mean and variance, then approximating representations can be greatly simplified. For example, the arrival times in Fig. 2.12 can be approximated by an exponential basis function

$$\psi(t, T_a) = \frac{K_a}{2\sigma T_a} e^{-(t-T_a)/(2\sigma T_a)}. \tag{141}$$

This function represents the essential features of dispersion which are the broadening of the time distribution with mean conduction delay and the constant area under the curve representing the fact that none of the pulses is lost (see Section 4.5.1).

The Laplace transform yields a first-order approximation for the impulse response of a dispersive neural tract.

$$\Psi(s, T_a) = \frac{K_a e^{-sT_a}}{2\sigma T_a s + 1}. \tag{142}$$

The conditions in which this is used are discussed in Sections 2.4.2, 5.2.2, 5.3.2, and 5.4.3. □

As a rule, dispersion in branched axons and compound nerves attenuates rapidly varying events and smooths complex sequences of observed potentials. It is a powerful high-frequency cutoff filter, and its presence should be expected whenever the latency of an event exceeds its duration. It is an essential property of nerve tracts in the brain, and it is one of the main factors that reduces the rates of change of events in neural masses to such low frequencies, that the single action potential can be treated as an impulse in the mathematical sense.

2.3.4.   The Core Conductor Model

We consider the topology, the parameters, the state variables, and the differential equation and a set of solutions that represent problems of physiological interest.

The axons and dendrites of neurons consist of long threads of electrically conducting material that are sheathed with a poorly conducting material in the membrane and are embedded in a widespread medium with a high conductance—the extracellular space. Each filament resembles an insulated electrical cable and is called a *core conductor*. Whereas the topology of the lumped circuit model for membrane is described in terms of discrete channels, the topology of the core conductor requires treatment of continuously distributed parameters and state variables in the long dimension of the cable.

It is assumed that the core conductor is infinitely long and that the diameter is very small compared to unit length. Each unit length of cable is assigned the parameters of specific transmembrane resistance r_m, specific transmembrane capacitance c_m, and specific longitudinal resistance, r_1 the internal and external specific longitudinal resistances are designated r_i and r_e. The parameters are conventionally assumed to be independent of time and location.[†]

At any time t the external and internal longitudinal currents have a single value for each point x along the cable $i_i(x, t)$ and $i_e(x, t)$. The transmembrane current is a state variable which is a function of the spatial variable x and is designated current per unit length or current density $j_m(x, t)$ in units of amperes per centimeter. The sum or integral of $j_m(x, t)$ over all x is zero. The transmembrane potential v_m has a single value at each point along the cable $v_m(x, t)$. For present purposes we assume that the external and internal specific resistances are $r_e = 0$, $r_i = r_1$, and that the internal and external $v_i(x, t)$ and $v_e(x, t)$ are measured with respect to the far distant point at $x \rightarrow \infty$, respectively, inside and outside the cable. Therefore,

$$v_i(x, t) - v_e(x, t) = v_m(x, t).$$

These six state variables at each point in x are also functions of time t, but at present we are concerned with $v_i(x, t)$ for a fixed value of t.

From Kirchhoff's current law we know that for each point on the cable the rate of change of longitudinal current is equal to the transmembrane current density.

$$j_m(x, t) = - \partial i_i(x, t)/\partial x. \tag{143}$$

By our convention, positive longitudinal current is to the right and positive membrane current is outward, so with an increasing value of x, the value for i_i must decrease, and the derivative is negative.

The product of the longitudinal current i_i with the internal specific longitudinal resistance r_i equals the negative of the gradient of the potential

---

[†]The conventional unit for specific transmembrane capacitance c_m is microfarads per centimeter (μF/cm), and the total capacitance C_m in microfarads is given by the product of c_m and the length L of the axon membrane in centimeters. The unit for specific transmembrane resistance r_m is ohms · centimeters (ohm · cm). Alternatively, the unit for specific transmembrane conductance $g_m = 1/r_m$ is mhos per centimeter (mho/cm) and the total conductance G_m in mhos is given by the product of g_m and L. The total transmembrane resistance in ohms is $R_m = 1G_m = r_m/L$. The unit for specific longitudinal resistance r_1 is ohms per centimeter (ohm/cm), and the total longitudinal resistance is $R_1 = r_1 L$. Similar conventions are used to evaluate specific surface resistance and capacitance (e.g., μF/cm^2 and ohm · cm^2) and volume specific resistance (e.g., ohm · cm^2/cm) when the descriptive differential equations require this (see Section 3.1.4).

in volts per centimeter:

$$\partial v_i(x, t)/\partial x = -r_i i_i(x, t). \tag{144}$$

Combining Eqs. (143) and (144), we have

$$\frac{1}{r_i} \frac{d^2 v_i(x)}{dx^2} = j_m(x, t). \tag{145}$$

From Kirchhoff's laws, the transmembrane current is equal to the sum of a resistive fraction and a capacitative fraction:

$$j_m(x, t) = \frac{v_i(x, t)}{r_m} + c_m \frac{\partial v_i(x, t)}{\partial t}. \tag{146}$$

The membrane model is now incorporated into the core conductor model by combining Eqs. (145) and (146) and rearranging the parameters to obtain a partial differential equation:

$$\lambda^2 \frac{\partial^2 v_i(x, t)}{\partial x^2} = \tau \frac{\partial v_i(x, t)}{\partial t} + v_i(x, t). \tag{147}$$

This is the cable equation or core conductor equation, where λ is a length constant in centimeters and τ is a time constant commonly given in milliseconds:

$$\lambda = (r_m/r_i)^{.5}, \qquad \tau = r_m c_m. \tag{148}$$

It has many solutions that depend upon the boundary conditions imposed.

Example A.   Two electrodes are placed on an axon suspended in air several millimeters apart, anode on the left and cathode on the right, and a current step $I\mu(t)$, beginning at $t = 0$, is passed between them. The potential is measured on the membrane very near the cathode and at points to the right of the cathode (not between them) with respect to a far distant point on the axon. At $t = 0-$, the axon is at rest, so that $j_m(x) = 0$ and $v_e(x)$ and $v_i(x)$ are everywhere zero, as are their derivatives. At $t = 0+$, all the current flows through the membrane capacitance adjacent to the electrodes, inwardly at the anode and outwardly at the cathode. As the membrane capacitance becomes polarized with the passage of time, the transmembrane current is distributed along the axon. Longitudinal current is established, and both internal and external longitudinal gradients of potential $v(x, t)$ occur (Fig. 2.15a). The gradients are observed as potential differences $v'(x, t)$ between each point along the axon and a distant reference site. For each point x there is a time function $v(x, t)$ that predicts the observed potential difference. What is the predicted spatial function $v_e'(x, t_\infty)$ in the steady state?

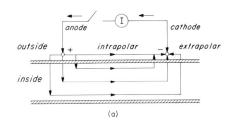

(a)

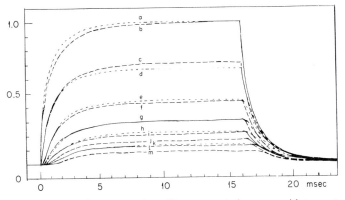

FIG. 2.15. (a) Geometrical representation of loop current of an axon with two extracellular stimulating electrodes. (b) Experimental and theoretical curves [Eq. (154)] showing rise and fall of extracellular potential at different distances from the cathode (Hodgkin & Rushton, 1946).

For this input the time derivative in the steady state is zero, so Eq. (147) becomes an ordinary differential equation

$$\lambda^2 \, d^2 v_e(x)/dx^2 = v_e(x). \tag{149}$$

The general solution is

$$v_e(x) = A e^{-x/\lambda} + B e^{x/\lambda}. \tag{150}$$

One of the boundary conditions is that $v_e(x)$ must go to zero as x goes to infinity, so that $B = 0$. At $x = 0$ at the cathode, $v_e(0) = A$. Therefore,

$$v_e(x)/v_e(0) = e^{-x/\lambda}. \tag{151}$$

If an exponential basis function is fitted to the data $v'(x, t_\infty)$, the value for λ serves to evaluate the length constant of the axon. This is the distance over which $v(x, t_\infty)$ falls to $1/e$ of its value at the cathode. The length constant is useful as a parameter for estimating how far an axon or dendrite can transmit in the passive mode. Typical values for large myelinated axons are 1–2 mm. For small unmyelinated axons and dendrites the values range upward from $30 \, \mu m$. $\quad \square$

Example B. In the more general case, we want to know the function of potential in time at any point on the axon. The Laplace transform provides a convenient method of solving the cable equation.[†] By replacing $\partial/\partial t$ with s in Eq. (147), we obtain an ordinary differential equation.

$$\lambda^2 d^2 V(x,s)/dx^2 = (s\tau + 1)V(x,s). \tag{152}$$

For the same boundary conditions as in Example A, the solution is

$$V(x,s) = V(0,s)\exp[-(x/\lambda)(s\tau + 1)^{1/2}], \tag{153}$$

where $V(0,s)$ is the value at $x = 0$. The inverse transform is obtained from a table of transform pairs. In terms of dimensionless units, $X = x/\lambda$ and $T_c = (t/\tau)^{1/2}$, and for $v(0,T) = 1$,

$$v(X,T_c) = \tfrac{1}{2}\{e^{-x}[1 - \mathrm{erf}(X/2T_c - T_c)] + e^x[1 - \mathrm{erf}(x/2T_c + T_c)]\}. \tag{154}$$

It is evaluated by use of tables of the error function erf. A set of curves generated by Eq. (154) fitted to measurements of the external potential of axon are shown in Fig. 2.15b (Hodgkin & Rushton, 1946). □

Example C. A double-barreled microelectrode is placed in the soma of a large neuron. A current step is passed through one electrode and the transmembrane potential is measured with the other. What are the total transmembrane resistance R_m and capacitance C_m?

The heuristic assumption is often made that the neuron soma can be treated as a lumped circuit, particularly if the current stimulus and recording sites are close together. The asymptotic change in potential is measured, and R_m is calculated from Ohm's law. The rising phase of the step response $v_m(t)$ is measured with an exponential basis function to give an estimate of $\tau = R_m C_m$ [see Eq. (43)]. □

Rall (1960) has shown that the dendrites provide a low-resistance shunt through which the capacitance of the soma is charged. The time function of the step response is not exponential but takes a form related to Eq. (154). If the time function is fitted with an exponential basis function, and this can easily be done, the resulting value for τ' is as little as half the time constant defined as $\tau = R_m C_m$.

Specific membrane resistance r_m and capacitance c_m are found by dividing R_m and C_m by the estimated anatomical surface area of neurons in the same population as those from which recordings have been made, and in many instances from the same cell. It is generally believed that c_m is invariant

---

[†] For the axon suspended in a nonconducting medium such as air or oil, the forms of the internal and external potential functions are mirror images (see Section 4.1.3).

during action potentials (though Cole & Curtis, 1939, reported changes on the order of 2%), and that the value for most neurons is about $1 \mu F/cm^2$. The estimates for r_m range from under 2000 ohm·cm² to over 10,000 ohm·cm². The variation is partly intrinsic, partly due to cell damage on penetration, and partly from the use of improper basis functions and a model inadequate for the purpose.

The good approximation of the predicted curves to the experimental results from many types of nerve fibers has led us to conclude that the core conductor model is a valid representation for axon and dendritic dynamics in the linear range. The model has been extended by Rall (1962) to treat fibers corresponding to cylinders with taper, cut ends, sealed ends, multiple successive branches of diminishing size, varying parameters of r_m and r_e, etc. For our purposes however, the homogenous, unbranched, unterminated cylinder will suffice.

2.3.5. SYNAPTIC DELAY

The cable equation is formally identical to the one-dimensional heat or diffusion equation. It can be used to describe the first-order dynamics of diffusion at chemical synapses. Each presynaptic terminal contains a specialized transmitter substance contained in small packets known as *synaptic vesicles*. When the terminal is depolarized during an action potential, some of these packets discharge their contents into the synaptic cleft between the pre- and postsynaptic membranes. The release can be shown to be quantal in special conditions at some synapses, but ordinarily the discharge can be treated as continuous. The substance diffuses across the cleft, acts on the postsynaptic membrane surface to alter its conductance, and is then converted to an inactive form.

Most central transmitter substances are either unverified or unknown, and their concentrations have not been measured in the synaptic clefts. Instead, the time course of their effects on postsynaptic membranes have been measured. From these indirect observations it is thought that, following a presynaptic action potential there is a brief delay. The concentration at the postsynaptic membrane rises rapidly to a peak within clefts and then more slowly decays. There is evidence that traces of the substance may linger for many milliseconds or tens of milliseconds after the onset.

Synaptic delay is usually treated as a simple dead time. The estimates very from .2 to over 1.0 msec, depending partly on intrinsic variability and partly on the end points used to specify the time interval, such as the crest of a presynaptic action potential and the start of a postsynaptic potential or a conductance change. This approach is inadequate, because it does not allow for the distributed nature of the event in time and particularly for the possibility of a long tail.

An alternative form of the cable equation (147) is

$$\frac{\partial^2 v(x,t)}{\partial x^2} = r_i c_m \frac{\partial v(x,t)}{\partial t} + \frac{r_i}{r_m} v(x,t).$$ (155)

For simplicity it is assumed that the parameter r_m is infinite. In the cable this means that there is negligible leakage across the membranes and in synaptic diffusion it means that there is no loss of substance from backward or lateral diffusion or inactivation in excess of that corresponding to diffusion beyond the fixed distance x.

The Laplace transform is taken as before,

$$d^2 V(x,s)/dx^2 = r_i c_m s V(x,s).$$ (156)

The solution for conditions corresponding to those previously given is

$$V(x,s) = \exp[-x(r_i c_m s)^{1/2}],$$ (157)

where $V(0,s) = 1$. The distance x is fixed, so that there is a lumped resistance $R_i = r_i x$, and a total capacitance $C_m = c_m x$. Their product defines a *lumped delay* parameter $T_b = R_i C_m$ in seconds. Thereby,

$$V(T_b, s) = \exp[-(sT_b)^{1/2}].$$ (158)

From a table of transform pairs, the impulse response is

$$v(T_b, t) = \begin{cases} \dfrac{1}{2\pi^{1/2} t}\left(\dfrac{T_b}{t}\right)^{1/2} e^{-T_b/4t}, & t > 0, \\ \delta(t), & t = 0. \end{cases}$$ (159)

A set of solutions for values of T_b in milliseconds is shown in Fig. 2.16. Each curve has brief apparent delay in onset, rapid rise to a peak at $t = T_b/6$, relatively slow decay, and a long tail.

The inverse transforms of the trancendental expressions in the operator s are much too cumbersome for routine use. Instead, a rational approximation is introduced that takes the form of a ratio of poles and zeros. The

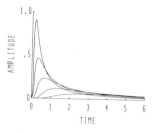

FIG. 2.16. Predicted impulse responses from Eq. (159) for $T_b = 1, 2, 4, 8,$ and 16 msec.

derivations for the approximations can be found in advanced texts on systems theory. The grounds for making these approximations can be seen in terms of the measuring process.

The transfer function for delay in onset is approximated in the simplest mode by one pole and one zero

$$V(s) = e^{-sT_c} \approx (c-s)/(s+c), \tag{160}$$

where $c = 2/T_c$ in reciprocal seconds. This gives delay without attenuation and holds for values of T_c that are much shorter than other time constants in the system. There are other rational approximations for larger values of T_c (e.g., Smith, 1958). In the time domain Eq. (160) gives the inverse transform

$$v(t) = \delta(t) + 2ce^{-ct}, \tag{161}$$

which is shown in graphic form in Fig. 2.17. It is compared with a unit pulse at $T_c = 2$.

A rational approximation of the transfer function for a normal distribution, Eq. (135), is

$$V(s) = \exp\left(\frac{s^2\sigma^2 T_a^2}{2} - sT_a\right) \approx \frac{1}{2\sigma T_a s + 1}\, e^{-s(T_a - \sigma)}. \tag{162}$$

The inverse transform is

$$v(t) = (1/2\sigma)\exp[-(t - T_a + \sigma)/2\sigma]. \tag{163}$$

The normal density curve and the rational approximation from Eq. (163) are shown in Fig. 2.17.

The transfer function for one-dimensional diffusion is approximated in the simplest mode by two poles and two zeros:

$$V(s) = \exp[-(sT_b)^{1/2}] \approx \frac{d_1 d_2}{z^2}\frac{(s-z)^2}{(s+d_1)(s+d_2)}, \tag{164}$$

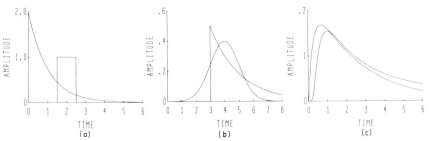

FIG. 2.17. Comparison of impulse responses specified by transcendental operators and by rational approximations for them: (a) dead time, (b) normal distribution, (c) cable lag.

where $d_1 = (\pi/2)^2/T$, $d_2 = (3\pi/2)^2/T$, and $z > d_2$ is given a large positive real value. Equation (164) has the inverse transform

$$v(t) = V_1 \, e^{-d_1 t} - V_2 \, e^{-d_2 t} + \frac{d_1 d_2}{z^2} \delta(t), \tag{165}$$

where V_1 and V_2 depend on the values of d_1, d_2, and z in partial fraction expansion. That is, the impulse response specified be Eq. (159) is approximated by the sum of two exponential terms, one for the rising phase and one for the falling phase (Fig. 2.17).

The use of rational approximations is required by the facts that the existence of synaptic and cable delays cannot be neglected in modelling neural masses, but in order to solve feedback equations their expressions must be reduced to simplified forms that retain the essence of their contributions.

Equations (164) and (165) approximate the one-dimensional diffusion process and can be used to describe and measure synaptic delay and cable delay with a single delay parameter for each or for both together. For these delay elements in series, the exponents in the cascaded transfer functions are additive, and the form of the delay is invariant. This expression for delay has also proven useful for modeling temporal dispersion and, in the early stages of developing a model for a complex neural mass, for modeling with a single delay parameter an unknown topological channel, in which serial undefined delays occur. That is, Eq. (164) is a highly versatile descriptive tool, and we will use it in several ways in Chapter 5.

2.4. Linear Models for Neurons

We follow our standard procedure. A topology of functional connections is described, and the sets of state variables and observables are specified. Samples of input–output pairs are given, a linear domain is established, and the basis functions for measurement are chosen and applied. From these elements, a differential equation is constructed to represent the dynamics. The parameters of the equation are interpreted in terms of the parts comprising the neuron.

2.4.1. FORMULATION OF THE TOPOLOGY

The anatomical concept of a neuron is a bounded protoplasmic unit with a soma, an axon, and a dendritic tree. To set up the dynamic concept of a neuron, we take a slightly different view. The input consists of activity on an axon or a set of branched axons that extends to the dendritic tree of a neuron and forms synapses at numerous sites on the dendritic membrane. The dendritic branches converge to the soma. The initial segment of the axon projects from the soma or a main dendritic trunk and continues into the efferent axon, which carries the output of the neuron. Hence we analyze the dynamic neuron from afferent axon to efferent axon rather than from postsynaptic membrane to presynaptic membrane.

The state variables are specified in terms of the activity occurring within each stage. The dendritic tree receives terminals from numerous axons, and the input $p_d(t, n_d)$ is specified by the presence or absence of an action potential on each afferent axon n_d at any time t. The axon terminals release transmitter substances at rates dependent on the rates of occurrence r of action potentials. The transmitter substances cause changes in dendritic membrane conductance $g_d(t, n_d)$ at each synapse n_d. These changes either depolarize the dendritic membrane and decrease transmembrane potential $v_d(t, n_d)$ and are called *excitatory*, or they hyperpolarize the membrane and are called *inhibitory*. In some conditions they appear to stabilize the transmembrane potential below threshold in which case they are also called *inhibitory*. The depolarization or hyperpolarization of the membrane results in dendritic current that is transmitted to other parts of the dendritic tree by its cable properties.

All parts contribute current by summation in greater or lesser degree to a convergence point at or near the soma. This summation determines the transmembrane potential of the soma $v_s(t)$. At or near the convergence point lies a region of the neuron membrane that has a lower threshold in relation to excitatory dendritic current than any other part of the neuron. This is called the *trigger zone*, and it is usually identified anatomically with the initial segment. There can be only one trigger zone at any time, by definition, but its location may vary. If $v_s(t)$ exceeds the threshold amplitude, an action potential $p_a(t)$ results that propagates forward or orthodromically into the efferent axon, and often propagates backwards or *antidromically* (in reverse of the direction of flow of activity) into the soma and proximal dendritic tree.

This topology consists of forward transmission through several serial stages or transformations. That which is transmitted is an active state, and is identified seriatim with $p_d(t, n_d), r(t, n_d), g_d(t, n_d), v_d(t, n_d), v_s(t)$, and $p_a(t)$, each being dependent on the preceding active state through an operation. This constitutes a causal flow for which the dynamics are to be specified. Unlike the models for dispersion and for membrane and the core conductor, which describe the flow of a single element, respectively, pulses or electric current, we must now deal with multiple elements. In order to specify the relation between measured antecedent and consequent state variables, we must use empirical conversion factors to reconcile the units of measurement. In other respects the procedure for analysis is the same.

The observable or controllable events in the sequence are the mean rates of action potential formation on one or more subsets n of afferent axons $p_d(t)$, the level of transmembrane potential in the soma $v_s(t)$, and the rate or probability of action potential formation on the efferent axon $p_a(t)$. In some instances, the total transmembrane conductance is estimated from measurements at the soma, but this will not be considered here. In the usual case there are only $n + 2$ observables, so the model can admit only that number of state variables representing real quantities. There is no restriction on the number of state variables defined for heuristic or computational purposes, but they cannot be used for validation of the model.

2.4.2. INPUT–OUTPUT PAIRS AND THE DIFFERENTIAL EQUATION

The choice of input is usually limited to extracellular single-shock electrical current stimulation of carefully defined afferent peripheral nerves and central tracts. This is because the transformations of sensory stimuli to afferent action potentials are too complex in themselves to provide reliably quantifiable input. Stimulation with improperly placed electrodes causes activation of multiple serial and parallel chains of neurons leading to a neuron under study, which gives a poorly defined or unknown input. In optimal cases, however, the input can be reduced to a volley of action potentials on a homogeneous afferent axon subset with minimal temporal dispersion. The input amplitude and delay in onset are measured from the compound action potential $p_z(t)$ with an extracellular monopolar recording microelectrode in the set of target neurons. The output is measured as the intracellular potential in the soma of a representative target neurons for both $v_s(t)$ and $p_a(t)$.

Before stimulation, the observables are allowed to come to resting levels at which the derivatives are zero. These levels are the baseline and may be assigned zero values. The input function is treated as an impulse $I\delta(t)$. The latency to the crest of $p_d(t)$ recorded presynaptically defines the afferent conduction delay T_a. In general the relation between the amplitude of the stimulus pulse I and the amplitude of the afferent volley $p_d(t)$ is nonlinear. We separate the linear and nonlinear parts of the input system by defining a nonlinear input–output function G_d such that p_a is some monotonic function of I and t:

$$p_d(t, I) = G_d(I)\delta(t - T_a). \qquad (166)$$

The function G is not treated analytically here.

For small values of I, the postsynaptic potential (PSP) $v_s(t)$ is unchanged for a short time T after T_a, and then it rapidly increases or decreases to a crest and decays monotonically to baseline (Fig. 2.18). For a limited range

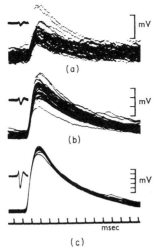

FIG. 2.18. EPSPs in a spinal motorneuron with afferent volleys of different size. Insets at left show the compound action potential in the dorsal root (Coombs, Eccles, & Fatt, 1955).

of I the crest amplitude of the PSP changes in proportion to I. When it is sought, a long-lasting shallow overshoot is commonly seen (Fig. 2.19). There is no action potential for this input domain. For small inputs on two afferent subsets, $p_{a1}(t)$ and $p_{a2}(t)$, it is found commonly that $v_{s1}(t)$ and $v_{s2}(t)$ are additive, though not invariably so. On repeated trials over minutes to hours, the PSP crest amplitude is often found to be constant for constant I. When these conditions hold, the input–output pairs define a linear domain of input and a linear range of output.

When output is a linear function of input, the optimal basis functions for measuring the impulse response are exponentials. Inspection of PSPs shows that two terms will usually suffice. The rising phase of the PSP corresponds to e^{-at}, and the falling phase corresponds to e^{-bt}, where a and b are rate constants with real values in reciprocal seconds. Alternatively,

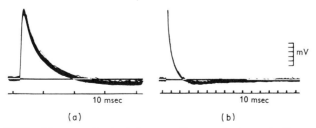

FIG. 2.19. EPSPs of large amplitude at slow recording speeds, demonstrating an overshoot (Coombs et al., 1955).

we can say that the PSP contains little consistent information besides its delay in onset, rate of rise, rate of fall, and amplitude (including polarity). That is, the shape of the start of the PSP, which is a concave upward curve, is treated as a sharp break at $t = T_c$, for which the derivative is infinite, and the overshoot is not considered. By these simplifications the impulse response of the linear part of the neuron can be fitted with the sum of two basis functions

$$v_s(t) = ab(e^{-a(t-T_c)} - e^{-b(t-T_c)}), \qquad t \geq T_c, \tag{167}$$

where the synaptic delay time T_c is measured from the presynaptic action potential (Fig. 2.18, insets) to the foot of the PSP. The afferent delay T_a is not included in the delay attributed to the neuron.

The Laplace transform of the sum of the exponential basis functions used to measure the impulse response is

$$V_s(s) = abe^{-sT_c}/(s+a)(s+b). \tag{168}$$

The transfer function can be broken into three operations, V_c, V_a, and V_b, in series:

$$V_c(s) \triangleq e^{-sT_c}, \qquad V_b(s) \triangleq \frac{b}{s+a}, \qquad V_a(s) \triangleq \frac{a}{s+b}, \tag{169}$$

where

$$V_c(s) = \frac{V_1(s)}{P_d(s, I)}, \qquad V_b(s) = \frac{V_2(s)}{V_1(s)}, \qquad V_a(s) = \frac{V_s(s)}{V_2(s)}, \tag{170}$$

and

$$V_s(s) = V_a(s) V_b(s) V_c(s). \tag{171}$$

Both $V_1(s)$ and $V_2(s)$ are inaccessible state variables.

In the form of a flow diagram, where input is $P_d(s, I)$,

The corresponding equations in time are

$$v_1(t) = p_d(t, I)\delta(t - T_c),$$

$$\frac{dv_2(t)}{dt} + bv_2(t) = bv_1(t), \qquad \frac{dv_s(t)}{dt} + av_s(t) = av_2(t). \tag{172}$$

Therefore the operation of the neuron in the linear range can be approximated by a delay in onset and two first-order rate processes in series.

2.4.3. INTERPRETATION OF THE PARAMETERS

The dynamics of the membrane model are expressed by a first-order differential equation that is based on sets of input–output pairs. The parameters of the equation are interpreted in terms of equivalent resistances and capacitance. These in turn are lumped circuit models that are described in terms of ionic channels and electrically polarizable molecular structures in membrane. Similarly the neuron model is expressed by a differential equation based on sets of input-output pairs, and its parameters are interpreted in terms of models of its parts: axon tract, synapse, core conductor, and membrane.

The rate constant a is interpreted as representing the reciprocal of the time constant of passive membrane τ. This is because the values for τ, commonly ranging from 4 to 10 msec, are similar to those found by passing current steps across the membrane (Section 2.2.2, Example C).

The rate constant b and the delay T_c are lumped representations of serial distributed delays, including temporal dispersion in the afferent tract, synaptic diffusion, and resistive–capacitative delay in the dendritic cable. They are lumped together because the rising phase is brief, seldom exceeding 1–4 msec, and the several processes are so similar that they cannot readily be distinguished. Moreover, there is usually no means for measuring them separately in order to evaluate the parameters of their operations. Finally, they depend mainly on structural and chemical properties of the neuron, which are relatively invariant for a given input subset.

These interpretations however are subject to error in any particular case. This uncertainty always holds when inferences are made from one level in a hierarchy to another. If, for example, the rate constant for a passive membrane is less than the lumped input delay, then the rate of rise b in Eq. (167) is determined by τ, and the rate of fall a is dependent on input delay. This may occur when any one or all of the sources of input delay is unusually large. (The reader should note that for describing events in neural sets, the above convention for a, b, and c is not adhered to.)

Example A. A set of excitatory of EPSPs $v'_s(t)$ obtained (Eccles, 1957) with an intracellular electrode in the soma of a motorneuron is fitted with an exponential basis function $v_s(t)$ yielding a crest latency of 1.0–1.5 msec and an exponential decay time constant τ_s of 4–7 msec with an average of 4.7 msec. The passive time constant is measured by passing current in steps across the membrane and measuring the rise time of transmembrane potential. The estimated value is $\tau_m = 2.5$ msec. The dynamics of membrane potential $v_m(t)$ are represented by a first-order differential equation

$$\frac{dv_m(t)}{dt} + \frac{1}{\tau} v_m(t) = 0. \tag{173}$$

For the initial condition $v_m(0)$, the solution is

$$v_m(t) = v_m(0)e^{-t/\tau}, \qquad t \geq 0, \tag{174}$$

where $t = 0$ at the foot of the PSP. An input function $i_d(t)$ is then found, which, on convolution with the impulse response, yields the observed response

$$v_s(t) = \int_0^t i_d(t - T)v_m(T)\,dT. \tag{175}$$

The time course of this hypothetical state variable is shown in Fig. 2.20 and represents the flow of synaptic current required to generate the output of the neuron when modeled by Eq. (173). □

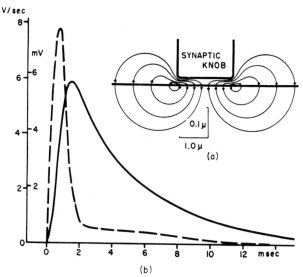

FIG. 2.20. (a) Solid curve: ensemble average of several EPSPs; dashed curve: synaptic current required to generate the potential change by convolution. (b) Schematic representation of loop current for a single synapse (Eccles, 1957).

The use of convolution in Example A is formally equivalent to measurement of the PSPs with Eq. (167) instead of Eq. (173) (see Sections 2.3.1 and 2.3.2), in which case the synaptic and dendritic delays are approximated by a single rate constant. The cause of the long-lasting synaptic current is suggested (Eccles, 1957) to be a "lingering" transmitter substance, though there is no means for distinguishing the effects of temporal dispersion in the terminal branches of the afferent axons, diffusional delays of substance across the synaptic cleft, and cable delays in terminal dendrites from the effects of residual transmitter substance on or in the postsynaptic membrane.

2.4.4. LINEAR FUNCTION FOR WAVE TO PULSE CONVERSION

If the output of the neuron is defined as a continuous function of axon transmembrane potential in time $v_a(t)$, then the transformation from potential at the soma $v_s(t)$ to $v_a(t)$ is time varying and nonlinear. If, however, the axon output is defined as a mean pulse rate $\hat{p}_a(t)$ over some specified time interval, then in some experimental conditions the transformation can be approximated by a set of linear *describing functions*. That is, for limited domains of $v_s(t)$ and t there is a range of output $\hat{p}_a(t)$ in which both additivity and proportionality hold, and the function $G_s(v, t)$ is replaced by a family of straight lines, one for each value of t.

Example A. A microelectrode is placed in the soma of a large neuron, and depolarizing current is passed across the membrane in steps of varying size $Iu(t)$. The mean rate of firing of the neuron $\hat{p}_a(t)$ is determined as a function of the input. For many neurons, there is a range for $\hat{p}_a(t)$ for which the steady state firing rate is linearly dependent on $Iu(t)$, this demonstrates proportionality (Fig. 2.21a) (Granit, Kernell & Shortess, 1963). □

Example B. Two afferent subsets of axons that deliver input to a motor-neuron in the spinal cord are isolated. Electrical stimulation in the form of a high-frequency pulse train is given to each subset. One input causes sustained excitation (depolarization) and the other input causes sustained inhibition. Both inputs are smoothed by dispersive, synaptic, and cable delays. The neuron is induced to fire at a steady low mean rate $\hat{p}_a(t)$ by the depolarizing input at a certain low level. The inhibitory input is then added at a level sufficient to reduce $\hat{p}_a(t)$ to a lower but nonzero level, by an amount $\Delta\hat{p}_a(t)$. On each subsequent trial the level of depolarizing input is raised, so that $\hat{p}_a(t)$ is higher. The same inhibitory input causes the same change $\Delta\hat{p}_a(t)$ irrespective of the value of $\hat{p}_a(t)$. This experiment (Fig. 2.21b) demonstrates the property of additivity (Granit & Renkin, 1961). □

Many experiments have been done to demonstrate limited domains of proportionality and additivity in the relations between transmembrane potential or current and pulse rate of different types of neurons, when the output is a pulse train having constant interspike intervals. The same principle can be shown to hold for pulse trains having randomly varying interspike intervals. We are not yet ready, however, to consider this aspect and will take it up in Chapter 3.

For the present we define an operator $G_a(v)$ that has the dimensions of pulses per second (pps) divided by a unit of transmembrane potential

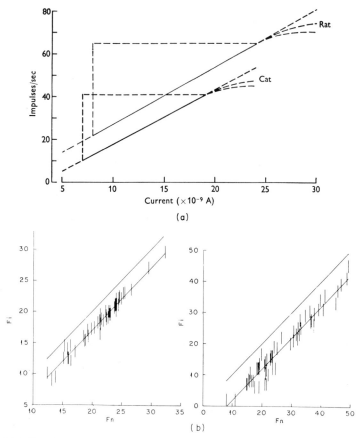

Fig. 2.21. Experimental demonstration by superposition of a linear range for wave to pulse conversion by single neurons. (a) Proportionality (Granit *et al.*, 1963); (b) Additivity (Granit, 1963).

such as microvolts (μV) and that is a nonlinear function between transmembrane potential $v_s(t)$ and pulse output $p_a(t, v)$:

$$p_a(t, v) = G_a(v) v_s(t). \tag{176}$$

There is a domain for v in which the function $G_a(v)$ can be replaced by a fixed coefficient g_a. Then with this substitution into Eq. (176) the Laplace transform is

$$P_a(s, v) = g_a V_s(s). \tag{177}$$

From Eq. (168) the transfer function for the neuron model is

$$P_a(s, v) = g_a \, abe^{-sT_c}/(s+a)(s+b). \tag{178}$$

For small values of T_c we can use a rational approximation for the term e^{-sT_c} (see Section 2.3.5)

$$P_a(s,v) = g_a ab(c-s)/(s+a)(s+b)(s+c), \qquad (179)$$

where $c = 2/T_c$.

The corresponding differential equation (assuming impulse input) is

$$\frac{d^3 p_a(t)}{dt^3} + a_1 \frac{d^2 p_a(t)}{dt^2} + a_2 \frac{dp_a(t)}{dt} + a_3 p_a(t) = a_3 \delta(t) - a_4 \frac{d}{dt}\delta(t), \quad (180)$$

$$a_1 = a + b + c, \qquad a_2 = ab + bc + ac, \qquad a_3 = abc, \qquad a_4 = ab.$$

Equation (180) provides a crucial element in the analysis of KII sets in Chapter 6.

2.5.   Linear Models for Neural Masses

2.5.1.   USE OF NONLINEAR REGRESSION

Measurement of input and output of a neural mass implies the expression of particular events as functions, which are ordered pairs of real numbers, representing a domain t such as time and a range v such as potential difference. The first step is measurement at a set of points in time and space with the digitizing basis function (Section 2.1.1). The analysis of a digitized event $v'(t)$ or of an ensemble average over a set of digitized events $\hat{v}\,T) = \mathscr{E}[v'(t)]$ requires a measurement by a theoretical basis or set of basis functions $w_y(t), y = 1, 2, \ldots, Y$, a set of units in the dimensions of the measuring space, and a procedure for evaluating the parameters of the basis functions (Section 2.1.1). That procedure consists in fitting the curve for the sum of the basis functions to the digitized event

$$v(t) = \sum_{y=1}^{Y} w_y(t), \qquad (181)$$

$$v'(t) = v(t) + \varepsilon(t), \qquad (182)$$

where $\varepsilon(t)$ is an error term.

Measurement of responses of membranes and single neurons seems seldom to require more complicated techniques than linear regression, as when a PSP is fitted with a straight line in semilogarithmic coordinates to determine a rate parameter, or trial and error variation of one or two parameters in an equation, as for example in the Hodgkin–Huxley equations (Section 3.1.4), when the value for axonal conduction velocity is introduced. The forms of neural mass responses are in general complex, and multiple parameters must be simultaneously evaluated. A more sophisticated technique is needed (see Chapter X in Simon, 1972; Freeman, 1964a).

In the usual case a set of single-shock electrical stimuli is given to a nerve or tract, and a potential difference in a neural mass is digitized at N points over time T and averaged over the set of trials to give an AEP $\hat{v}(T)$. The basis is the sum of a set of exponential terms with parameters, c_j and c_{j+1}:

$$v(T) = \sum_{j=1,3,\ldots}^{J} c_{j+1} e^{-c_j T}, \tag{183}$$

$$\hat{v}(T) = v(T) + \varepsilon(T), \tag{184}$$

where c_{j+1} and c_j are real or complex numbers. A measure of the error term is found by squaring the difference between each pair of calculated and observed values and summing over the N points in time

$$D = \sum_{n=1}^{N} [\hat{v}(T_n) - v(T_n)]^2. \tag{185}$$

The object of the curve fitting is to find values for the parameters $c_1, c_2, \ldots, c_J$ which minimize D. Those values are called *optimal* with respect to the criterion of least squares deviation.

It is essential that all the parameters be optimized simultaneously and not seriatim. If the basis functions are straight lines, or are power functions that can be reduced to straight lines, linear regression is the procedure of choice. Equation (183), however, is the sum of at least two exponential terms for which there is no linearizing transformation. Therefore the technique of nonlinear regression is used by means of a computer.

A set of values is assigned to the basis functions as initial guesses. These are chosen by fitting an exponential curve on a damped sine wave by hand to a graph of an AEP, subtracting the two curves, fitting another curve by hand to the residue, subtracting, and so forth, until the residue approaches the form of white noise, and the initial guesses are obtained for all the parameters $c_1, c_2, \ldots, c_J$.

A new set of "improved" coefficients is desired for the parameters, $c_1', c_2', \ldots, c_J'$, which require that the initial guesses be changed by the increments, $\Delta c_1 = c_1' - c_1, \Delta c_2 = c_2' - c_2$, etc. The assumption is made that the value of the initial function $v_1(T_n)$ at each digitizing time $T_n, n = 1, 2, \ldots, N$, is a continuous function of every parameter

$$v_1(T_n) = f(T_n, c_1, c_2, \ldots, c_J), \qquad n = 1, \ldots, N. \tag{186}$$

For the new parameters,

$$v_2(T_n) = f(T_n, c_1', c_2', \ldots, c_J') \qquad n = 1, \ldots, N. \tag{187}$$

By a first-order Taylor series expansion of the initial curve in the parameters,

$$v_2(T_n) = v_1(T_n) + \Delta c_1 \frac{\partial v(T_n)}{\partial c_1} + \cdots + \Delta c_J \frac{\partial v(T_n)}{\partial c_J}, \qquad n = 1, \ldots, N. \quad (188)$$

The values for the partial derivatives are estimated numerically and are set equal to constants, $k_{1n}, k_{2n}, \ldots, k_{Jn}$

$$v_2(T_n) - v_1(T_n) = k_{1n} \Delta c_n + \cdots + k_{Jn} \Delta c_J,, \qquad n = 1, \ldots, N. \quad (189)$$

The differences $v_2(T_n) - v_1(T_n), n = 1, \ldots, N$, are set equal to zero. This yields a set of N linear equations in J unknowns. The equations are solved by linear regression to determine values for $\Delta c_j, j = 1, \ldots, J$, which are added to c_j to give a new set of coefficients c_j'.

A new curve $v_2(T)$ is generated with the new parameters, and a new value is calculated for D_2 by Eq. (185). If $D_2 > D_1$, the corrections Δc_j are reduced by a fraction $\alpha \Delta c_j, \alpha < 1$, and D_3 is calculated. The procedure is repeated until $D_j < D_1$ or until a preset number of iterations is reached. If $D_2 < D_1$, the procedure beginning with Eq. (186) is repeated. Iterations are continued until D fails to decrease significantly or until a preset number of iterations is reached.

If the generated curve fails to converge onto the observed data, a new set of initial guesses is supplied. If there is failure with one or more sets of initial guesses, the basis may be rejected, and a new set of basis functions is constructed. This of course means that a certain class of differential equations has been rejected, and a new class is considered for describing the dynamics of the neural mass generating the AEP.

There are two limitations to the use of nonlinear regression or related algorithms for parameter optimization. (1) The calculations require the use of a large general purpose computer and an appropriate computer program. (Such programs are available through any computer center.) (2) The optimized values for the coefficients have no confidence intervals, which with the results of linear regression provide. However, confidence intervals can be established by measuring several AEPs from the same set of experimental conditions and determining the means and distributions of the values for the optimized c_j. This adds to the cost of measurement. However, there is no realistic alternative if proposed explanatory models are to be tested against electrophysiological data.

Minimal values for D are necessary but not sufficient for acceptance of fitted curves $v(T)$. If the set of basis functions subsequently is proved to be inadmissible on anatomical or physiological grounds, or if the parameters take meaningless values, or if the variation of the parameters is too great in a set of AEPs, the fitted curves are rejected.

The use of a large number of variable parameters does not necessarily make the curve-fitting process easier. On the contrary if the parameters are not carefully defined to extract as much information as possible from each AEP and to represent independent aspects of a complex neural system, the regression process fails. The matrix of coefficients for the normal equations (189) Δc_j may be singular. Whereas curve-fitting is usually judged best done with the least number of parameters, the best result in fitting AEPs is the most physiological information irrespective of the number of parameters. A basis with 9 parameters having physiological meaning is preferable to a basis with 5 parameters having no meaning, if both yield the same value for D. Economy of representation is not the aim of measurement of AEPs.

The severest test of a proposed basis is that it must hold for a neural mass over a suitably wide range of experimental conditions, and it must hold in those conditions for all animals of the same or similar species (see Section 7.1.2). This is not a trivial requirement. Fitting an AEP with a generated curve often seems more difficult than fitting it barehanded with a steel rod.

2.5.2. THE KO NEURAL SET

The KO set consists of a set of neurons having a common source of input, a common sign of output, and no interaction. We select a set that is normally an interactive excitatory set KI_e and suppress pulse formation by the neurons in the set with an appropriate general or local anesthetic, to produce a KO_e set. The source of input is an afferent tract that is electrically stimulated with single shocks $\delta(t)$ at an input amplitude I. The afferent volley arrives at the KO_e set with a delay T_a which is specified by the arrival of a compound action potential $p_d(t)$. There is a brief synaptic delay T_c and the dendrites of neurons in the set undergo depolarization which, in each activated neuron, is manifested by an EPSP. The EPSPs are subthreshold.

The EPSP for each neuron is the extracellular manifestation of loop current with emf in the dendritic membranes. The passage of the current across the resistance in the common extracellular compartment is manifested by and extracellular field of potential. The fields of potential sum for the set of activated neurons. Under certain geometric conditions to be discussed in Chapter 4, the amplitude of potential difference $v_e(t)$ between a selected point extracellularly located in the set to a far distant point is proportional to the ensemble average of transmembrane potential $\mathscr{E}[\hat{v}_s(t)]$ at the somas of the neurons in the set. Over repeated single-shock trials an ensemble average is taken to give an AEP that is designated $\hat{v}_e(T)$. We take $\hat{v}_e(T)$ as an output of the KO_e mass.

We now have a topology consisting of an axon tract, a set of synapses, a set of dendrites, an input state variable $G_d(I)\delta(T)$, which is an impulse, and an output state variable $\hat{v}_e(T)$, which is an impulse response. We collect a set of input–output pairs for fixed I at one level to demonstrate that the KO set is time invariant. We then fix I at a set of different amplitudes and collect another set of input–output pairs to demonstrate the existence of a domain of I and a range of v_e in which proportionality holds. By giving two stimuli at the same amplitude I, but separated by a short time interval, we collect a set of input–output pairs to demonstrate additivity. These procedures establish a linear domain and range for the function relating cortical input to output (Biedenbach & Freeman, 1965).

We measure the impulse response for a value of I in the linear domain by means of the digitizing basis function. An example is shown in Fig. 2.22 as the dotted curve. The time of onset $T = 0$ is set at the second zero crossing of the compound action potential (not shown). The impulse response consists of a concave upward initial deflection, a rise to a crest, a decay, and an overshoot. We choose a set of basis functions consisting of the sum of J exponentials with real coefficients and fit the AEP:

$$v_e(T) = \sum_{j=1}^{J} B_j e^{-a_j T}, \tag{190}$$

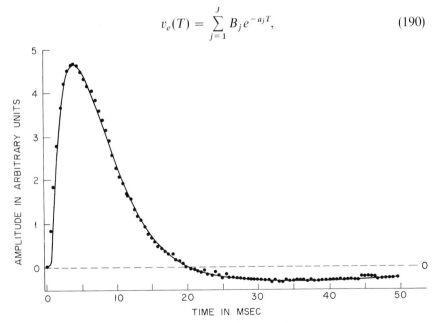

FIG. 2.22. Impulse response of prepyriform cortex in the open loop state. Curve from Eq. (190): calculated values; points: observed values. See Figs. 2.19 and 2.23 (Freeman, 1964b).

where the B_j are real numbers depending on input and output amplitudes, and where a_1 is the lowest rate constant and a_J is the highest.

The number of basis functions J is found by trial and error. We have two criteria. First, for a set of AEPs from the same and different animals, there must be close conformance of $\hat{v}_e(T)$ to each AEP. Second, the values for the coefficients, B_j and a_j, must be consistent across the set of AEPs. That is, the values for each a_j and B_j should cluster near the means for a_j and B_j. Experimentally the criteria are met for $J \geq 4$.

The transfer function of the cortex is found by taking the Laplace transform of Eq. (190). It is found to be

$$V_e(s) = K_f(s+z) \prod_{j=1}^{4} a_j/(s+a_j). \tag{191}$$

The four poles at $s = -a_j$ are self-explanatory but the existence of a zero at $s = -z$ is not so obvious. Its existence is shown by the fact that B_1 must be negative, because it is the amplitude coefficient for the exponential term with the lowest rate constant in Eq. (190). In fact, the term represents the long-lasting overshoot of the AEP in Fig. 2.22.

This happens as follows. Suppose that the transfer function for a system is given by

$$V(s) = 200 \cdot 700/(s+200)(s+700). \tag{192}$$

The impulse response by partial fraction expansion is

$$v(t) = 280\,e^{-200t} - 280\,e^{-700t}, \tag{193}$$

as shown in Fig. 2.23a. The response increases from zero at $t = 0$ to a crest and decays without overshoot. Suppose, however, that the transfer function is given by

$$V(s) = 200 \cdot 700s/(s+10)(s+200)(s+700). \tag{194}$$

That is, there is a zero at $s = 0$ and an additional pole at $s = 10$. Then the impulse response is

$$v(t) = -11\,e^{-10t} + 295\,e^{-200t} - 284\,e^{-700t}. \tag{195}$$

In the second case (Fig. 2.23b) the overshoot is represented by the term $-11\,e^{-10t}$ which has the smallest rate constant. In general we can infer that the presence of a long-lasting overshoot of an impulse response means that there is an odd number of zeros on or very near the real axis that have real values less than that of the smallest rate constant. In the simplest case there is only one zero with the value $z < a_1$.

The value for z is determined experimentally by taking the inverse transform of Eq. (191) such that the B_j in Eq. (190) are functions of the

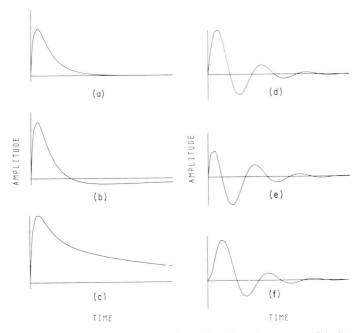

FIG. 2.23. Demonstration of the effects on the predicted impulse response of the introduction of a single real zero into the transfer function.

a_j, and fitting the curve to the AEPs. When this is done, the value for z is 0.6 ± 3.6/sec (SE, $N = 8$). The rate constant for the overshoot is $a_1 = 92 \pm 20$/sec, which is equivalent to a time constant of 10.8 msec. The higher rate constants are $a_2 = 223 \pm 18$/sec, $a_3 = 716 \pm 89$/sec, and $a_4 = 3164 \pm 452$/sec. When equations (190) and (191) are evaluated by the means they become

$$v(t) = -182 e^{-92T} + 576 e^{-223T} - 466 e^{-716T} + 72 e^{-3164T}, \quad (196)$$

$$V_e(s) = k_f (s + 0.6)/(s + 92)(s + 223)(s + 716)(s + 3164). \quad (197)$$

Equation (197) implies that the dynamical system in the KO set can be described by a set of four first-order differential equations. We interpret Eq. (197) in terms of the parts of the neurons in the set by assuming that the rate coefficients a_j are equivalent to the means for the rate coefficients of the neurons in the set. The transfer function is separated into three parts,

$$V_1(s) = a_1 k_f \frac{(s + z)}{(s + a_1)}, \quad V_2(s) = \frac{a_2}{(s + a_2)}, \quad V_3(s) = \frac{a_3 a_4}{(s + a_3)(s + a_4)},$$

$$(198)$$

where

$$V_e(s)/I(s) = V_1(s) V_2(s) V_3(s). \tag{199}$$

The topology of the KO set is given by

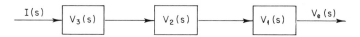

We infer that $V_2(s)$ represents the passive membrane property, because the decay rate $a_2 = 223/\text{sec}$ gives a time constant $1/a_2 = 4.5\,\text{msec}$, which is similar to that found for many neurons. (Time constants measured intracellularly are often shorter for reasons discussed in Section 2.3.4). We infer that $V_1(s)$ represents a restorative process reflected in a dendritic afterpotential. On experimental grounds (the mean of z is less than the standard error) and for reasons given in Section 3.2.3 we infer that $z = 0$, and

$$V_1(s) = a_1 k_f s/(s+a_1). \tag{200}$$

$V_3(s)$ is a second-order rational approximation for the set of distributed delays in the afferent tract, synapses, and dendritic cables of the neurons in the KO mass. The similarity of the term for $V_3(s)$ is Eq. (198) to the approximating term for $z \gg s$ in Eq. (164) should be noted.

Additional zeros can be inferred to exist in the open loop transfer function on other grounds. Suppose, for example, the transfer function has the form

$$V(s) = 200 \cdot 700(s+100)/(s+10)(s+200)(s+700). \tag{201}$$

The inverse transform (Fig. 2.23c) gives

$$v(t) = 96\,e^{-10t} + 147\,e^{-200t} - 243\,e^{-700t}. \tag{202}$$

The impulse response rises to a crest and then decays to the baseline without overshoot, but the decay is not that of a single exponential. The initial decay is at e^{-200t}, and the terminal decay is at e^{-10t}. That is, the amplitude coefficients of two adjacent terms have the same sign. An example and its physiological significance are described in Chapter 5.

2.5.3. OSCILLATORY RESPONSES FROM A KII SET

The AEP in Fig. 2.24 from a KII set is fitted by means of nonlinear regression with two basis functions in the following equation:

$$v(T) = V_1\left[\sin(\omega_1 T + \varphi_1)e^{-\alpha_1 t} - \sin\varphi_1\,e^{-\beta T}\right]$$
$$+ V_2\left[\sin(\omega_2 T + \varphi_2)e^{-\alpha_2 T} - \sin\varphi_2\,e^{-\beta T}\right], \tag{203}$$

where V is initial amplitude in microvolts, ω is frequency in radians per

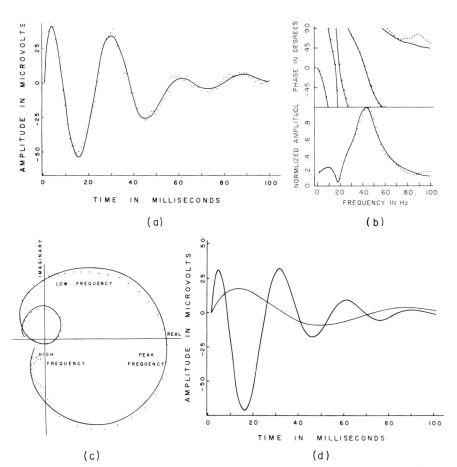

FIG. 2.24. Impulse response of the prepyriform cortex in the closed loop state. (a) AEP (●) and fitted curve from Eq. (203). (b) Phase and amplitude using Eqs. (206) and (207). (c) Fourier transform by numerical integration using Eqs. (204) and (205). (d) Dominant and subsidiary components of the AEP, of which the sum is the curve in part (a) (Freeman, 1970).

second, α is decay rate in radians, β is rise time of the initial peak[†] in reciprocal seconds, φ is phase in degrees or radians, and 1 and 2 denote, respectively, the dominant and subsidiary or minor of the two damped sinusoids.

The digitized data representing the AEP from the prepyriform cortex of

[†] The subtractive terms in Eq. (203), $\sin \varphi_x e^{-\beta T}$, are used to shape the rising part of N^1 of the AEP. When the foot of N^1 is concave upwards, an alternative subtractive term is used, $\sin \varphi_x \cos \omega_x T e^{-\beta T}$. The value assigned to ω_x is that of ω_d or ω_m on the basis of analysis of the KII sets generating the wave forms (see Section 5.3.3).

a cat is shown in Fig. 2.24a as a row of dots. The sum of basis functions in Eq. (203) fitted to the dots is shown as a continuous curve. The basis functions are shown at part (d). In part (c) the dots represent the Fourier transform of the AEP in the complex plane, computed numerically by

$$\text{Re}(\omega) = \sum_{n=1}^{100} \text{AEP}(T_n)\cos(\omega T_n)\,\Delta T, \tag{204}$$

$$\text{Im}(\omega) = -\sum_{n=1}^{100} \text{AEP}(T_n)\sin(\omega T_n)\,\Delta T, \tag{205}$$

where $\Delta t = .00125\,\text{sec}$ (the digitizing interval), $f = \omega/2\pi$ (frequency in hertz) is changed in steps of 2 Hz from 0 to 100 Hz/sec, and at each value of f the sums are computed. This simple form of the Fourier transform is used because the AEP amplitude is zero for $T \le 0$ and usually approaches zero as $T \to 100\Delta T$. Time T_n ranges in 100 steps from 0 to 123.75 msec. The curve is the polar plot of the transformed sum of basis functions. Each dot corresponding to one test frequency represents the tip of a vector extending from the origin to that point. Separate plots for phase $\Phi(\omega)$ and vector length $B(\omega)$ as functions of frequency are shown in part (b):

$$B(\omega) = [\text{Re}(\omega)^2 + \text{Im}(\omega)^2]^{.5}, \tag{206}$$

$$\Phi(\omega) = \tan^{-1}[\text{Im}(\omega)/\text{Re}(\omega)]. \tag{207}$$

These together constitute the spectrum for the AEP.

The examples in Figs. 2.24 and 2.25 illustrate the decomposition of the AEP into two damped sinusoids [part (d)], the dominant one accounting for the peak in the spectral energy distribution near 40 Hz. A sharp minimum in spectral energy occurs in the low-frequency region of the spectrum. In the polar plots the vector locus passes very near to the origin. Additional minor cusps and loops are present at both low- and high-frequency ends of the observed loci (dots) as distinct from the calculated loci (curves).

The calculated loci may be described in terms of the location in the s plane of sets of poles and zero. The maximum in the amplitude spectrum clearly manifests a complex pair of poles near the imaginary axis at about $\pm j250\,\text{rad/sec}$, whereas the minimum is the manifestation of a pair of complex zeros at a somewhat lower frequency. The method for locating these zeros is exemplified for the case in Fig. 2.24.

The minimal model required to describe the patterns is a set of two parallel band-pass filters, each represented by a complex pair of poles and each cascaded into a lead-lag filter represented by a pole and a zero on the real axis. Each filter generates a damped sine wave in response to impulse driving. Let the transference for the dominant filter be denoted $C_1(s)$ and

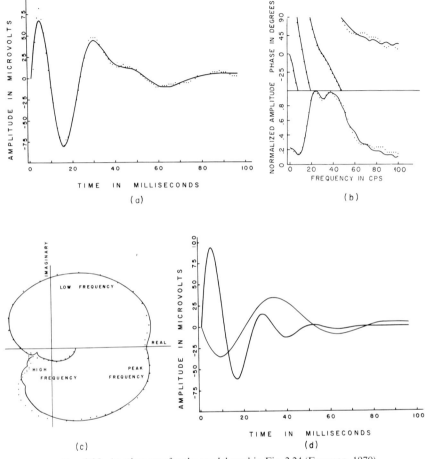

FIG. 2.25. Another case for the model used in Fig. 2.24 (Freeman, 1970).

that for the minor filter by $C_2(s)$. For a given input $\delta(T)$, the output $c(T)$ is given by

$$c(T) = c_1(T) + c_2(T) \qquad (208)$$

for the filters in parallel combination. In accordance with the minimal hypothesis

$$C_j(s) = K_j(s + \gamma_d)/(s + \alpha_j + j\omega_j)(s + \alpha_j - j\omega_j)(s + \beta), \qquad j = 1, 2. \quad (209)$$

The gain constants K_1, K_2, and the frequencies ω_1, ω_2, are different for the two systems, but the rise times β are the same.

The pairs of conjugate complex poles in Eqs. (209) represent the damped sine wave components in the fitted curve and are self-explanatory, but the introduction of the real pole and real zero in each component needs clarification. Suppose that in either of the components the values for γ_j and β are equal. Then there is pole–zero cancellation, and the transfer function is reduced to the complex poles. The inverse transform gives

$$v(T) = V_0 \sin(\omega T) e^{-\alpha T}, \tag{210}$$

a damped sine wave (Fig. 2.23d). If the value for β (the pole) exceeds the value for γ_j (the zero), the sine wave is shifted earlier in time (phase lead, Fig. 2.23e). The rate of rise in response amplitude from $c_1(T) = 0$ or $c_2(T) = 0$ at $T = 0$ depends on the value of β. If the value for β is less than the value for γ, the sine wave is shifted later in time (phase lag, Fig. 2.23f). Again, the rate of change to the first response minimum is determined by the value for β. Thus the value for γ_j is the determinant of the phase, once β has been fixed by the rate of change of the initial peak, and ω and α have been fixed by the frequency and decay rate of the component in the AEP.

Each of these is treated by partial fraction expansion (Section 2.2.3):

$$C_1(s) = \frac{C_{11}}{s + \alpha_1 + j\omega_1} + \frac{C_{12}}{s + \alpha_1 - j\omega_1} + \frac{C_{13}}{s + \beta}, \tag{211}$$

and similarly for $M(s)$, where

$$C_{11} = \frac{K_1}{2\omega_1} \cdot \frac{\alpha_1 - \gamma_1 + j\omega_1}{\omega_1 - j(\alpha_1 - \beta)}, \tag{212}$$

$$C_{12} = \frac{K_1}{2\omega_1} \cdot \frac{\alpha_1 - \gamma_d - j\omega_1}{\omega_1 - j(\alpha_1 - \beta)}, \tag{213}$$

$$C_{13} = K_1 \cdot \frac{\gamma_1 - \beta}{\omega_1^2 + (\alpha_1 - \beta)^2}. \tag{214}$$

Upon separation into gain and phase,

$$C_1(s) = \frac{K_1}{\omega_1} \left[\frac{\omega_1^2 + (\gamma_1 - \alpha_1)^2}{\omega_1^2 + (\beta - \alpha_1)^2} \right]^{.5} \left[\frac{\frac{1}{2} e^{j\theta_1}}{s + \alpha_1 + j\omega_1} + \frac{\frac{1}{2} e^{-j\theta_1}}{s + \alpha_1 - j\omega_1} \right. $$
$$\left. + \frac{\omega_1(\gamma_1 - \beta)}{[\omega_1^2 + (\beta - \alpha_1)^2]^{.5} [\omega_1^2 + (\gamma_1 - \alpha_1)^2]^{.5} (s + \beta)} \right]. \tag{215}$$

The same holds for $C_2(s)$.

The sum of basis functions used to approximate the experimental AEPs is denoted by $v(T)$ in Eq. (203). The approximate combinations of basis functions can be taken as the output of the hypothesized minimal model so that

$$v(T) = c(T) = c_1(T) + c_2(T).\tag{216}$$

By use of Euler's theorem, Eq. (203) may be combined with Eq. (216) to yield

$$c_1(T) = \tfrac{1}{2}V_1 \exp\left[-(\alpha_1 + j\omega_1)T + j(\varphi_1 - \tfrac{1}{2}\pi)\right]$$
$$+ \tfrac{1}{2}V_1 \exp\left[-(\alpha_1 - j\omega_1)T - j(\varphi_1 - \tfrac{1}{2}\pi)\right]$$
$$- V_1 \sin\varphi_1 \exp[-\beta T],\tag{217}$$

and similarly for $c_2(T)$.

Where, as in the present case, the input to the filters is a single impulse, the Laplace transform of the input $\delta(T)$ and output $c(T)$ yield the relation

$$V(s) = C(s) = C_1(s) + C_2(s).\tag{218}$$

In expanded form this becomes

$$C_1(s) = V_1\left[\frac{\tfrac{1}{2}\exp[j(\varphi_1 - \tfrac{1}{2}\pi)]}{s + \alpha_1 + j\omega_1} + \frac{\tfrac{1}{2}\exp[-j(\varphi_1 - \tfrac{1}{2}\pi)]}{s + \alpha_1 - j\omega_1} - \frac{\sin\varphi_1}{s + \beta}\right],\tag{219}$$

and similarly for $C_2(s)$. By comparison of Eqs. (215) and (219) it follows that

$$K_1 = V_1\omega_1\left[\frac{\omega_1^2 + (\beta - \alpha_1)^2}{\omega_1^2 + (\gamma_1 - \alpha_1)^2}\right]^{.5},\tag{220}$$

$$\sin\varphi_1 = -\omega_1(\gamma_1 - \beta)[\omega_1^2 + (\beta - \alpha_1)^2]^{-.5}[\omega_1^2 + (\gamma_1 - \alpha_1)^2]^{-.5},\tag{221}$$

$$\theta_1 = \varphi_1 - \tfrac{1}{2}\pi.\tag{222}$$

Parallel equations hold for K_2 and θ_2.

Evaluation of V, ω, α, φ, and β from AEP is by means of Eqs. (203) and (216). The values for the real zeros γ_j can be obtained graphically by plotting poles at $s = -\alpha_j \pm j\omega_j$ and at $s = -\beta$. The location of each zero at $s = -\gamma_j$ is specified by the phase φ_j. Equation (221) is easily verified from elementary trigonometric relationships. The calculated value for φ_j then serves as a check on the validity of the graphic evaluation of γ_j.

The next step is the combination of the transfer functions for the two parallel channels in order to evaluate the closed loop zeros. From Eq. (209), (210), and (218)

$$C(s) = \sum_{j=1}^{2}\frac{K_j(s + \gamma_j)}{(s + \alpha_j + j\omega_j)(s + \alpha_d - j\omega_j)(s + \beta)}.\tag{223}$$

When reduced to the least common denominator

$$C(s) = \frac{K_1 + K_2}{s + \beta}\left[\frac{s^3 + B_1 s^2 + B_2 s + B_3}{(s + \alpha_1 + j\omega_1)(s + \alpha_1 - j\omega_1)(s + \alpha_2 + j\omega_2)(s + \alpha_2 - j\omega_2)}\right],\tag{224}$$

wherein

$$B_1 = \frac{K_1(2\alpha_2 + \gamma_1) + (2\alpha_1 + \gamma_2)}{K_1 + K_2}, \tag{225}$$

$$B_2 = \frac{K_2(2\alpha_2\gamma_1 + \alpha_2^2 + \omega_2^2) + K_2(2\alpha_1\gamma_2 + \alpha_1^2 + \omega_1^2)}{K_1 + K_2}, \tag{226}$$

$$B_3 = \frac{K_1(\alpha_2^2\gamma_1 + \omega_2^2\gamma_1) + K_2(\alpha_1^2\gamma_2 + \omega_1^2\gamma_2)}{K_1 + K_2}. \tag{227}$$

The solution for the roots of the third-order polynomial in s contained in the numerator of Eq. (224) yields the desired values for the locations of a pair of complex zeros and one zero on the real axis in the s plane. Two

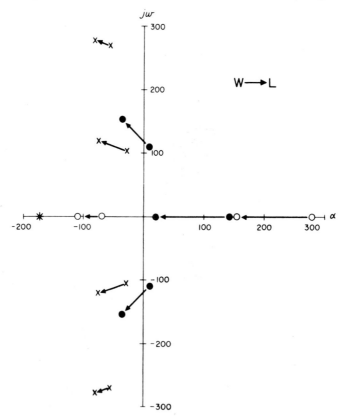

FIG. 2.26. Demonstration of the validity of the parallel topology implied in Eq. (203). Locations in the s plane for the poles ($\times$), open loop zeros ($\bigcirc$), and closed loop zeros ($\bullet$) derived from two AEPs (Table 2.1), showing the changes accompanying a change in behavioral state (waiting, W, to lapping, L) (Freeman, 1970).

TABLE 2.1

POLES AND ZEROS[a] IN FIG. 2.26

State	Component	V (μV)	ω (rad/sec)	α (1/sec)	φ (deg)	γ (1/sec)	β (1/sec)	z_1 (1/sec)	z_2 (1/sec)	z_3 (rad/sec)
W	Dominant	123	271	55	74	-280				
							173	-145	-10	$\pm j108$
W	Minor	26	104	27	31	70				
L	Dominant	131	277	80	58	-155				
							173	-21	36	$\pm j152$
L	Minor	53	121	74	23	110				

[a] z_1, z_2, and z_3 are closed loop zeros.

sets of solutions are shown in Fig. 2.26 and in Table 2.1, the first taken during the behavioral state of the cat working for food (W) and the second during food consumption (L). It is noteworthy that the pairs of complex poles move to the left in characteristic fashion, and that as they do so the single pair of complex zeros moves to the left across the imaginary axis. This change is also manifested in an upward shift of the minor loop in Fig. 2.24c in such fashion that it no longer encloses the origin.

This pattern of change is commonly observed for AEPS from individual cats during random variation or unsystematically with changes in behavioral state or in stimulus intensity. It is equivalent to the casual addition or subtraction of 360° of phase lag at the high-frequency end of the spectrum. It provides definitive evidence that the two linear band-pass filters postulated in the minimum must be parallel.

An additional problem to be considered is whether the peaks in the amplitude spectrum (Figs. 2.24, 2.25, and 2.27b accurately reflect the characteristic frequencies of the two linear filters. Figure 2.28 shows the result in $B(\omega)$ of adding two damped sinusoids differing by a factor of two in their frequencies (40 and 20 Hz) and amplitudes (2:1) but having the same decay rate. The phase of the larger component is fixed at 70°, whereas the phase of the smaller component is changed in steps of 60° from 0° to 300°. The amplitude spectra calculated using Eqs. (204)–(207) display the resulting variability of peak frequency, i.e., that frequency at which $B(\omega)$ reaches a maximum. Owing to the existence of the closed loop zeros, two parallel modes may given one or two spectral peaks, neither of which coincide with values for either of the two component frequencies. Characteristic frequencies can be derived best from measurements of AEP in the time domain using Eq. (203).

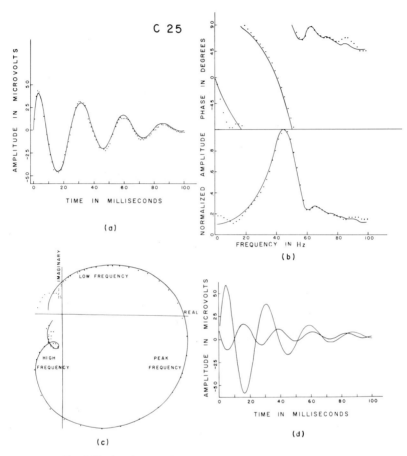

FIG. 2.27. Another case for the model of Fig. 2.24 (Freeman, 1970).

Two linear filters in parallel are necessary for a linear approximation for the prepyriform dynamics. The question is now considered whether these two are sufficient. They prepyriform AEP is a brief and relatively simple wave form, and especially in the presence of noise there is a limit to the number of independent parameters it serves to evaluate. Use of an ensemble average AEP (AAEP) reduces the noise, and it is always possible to fit two damped sinusoids to the AAEP but never three simultaneously.

An equivocal circumstance arises. The AEP in Fig. 2.25 is fitted with two damped sinusoidal basis functions having frequencies of 40.8 and 15.0 Hz. It can be fitted equally well with two basis functions having frequencies of 39.7 and 62.1 Hz. In the first case the calculated phase and amplitude spectra deviate slightly from the observed spectra at the high-

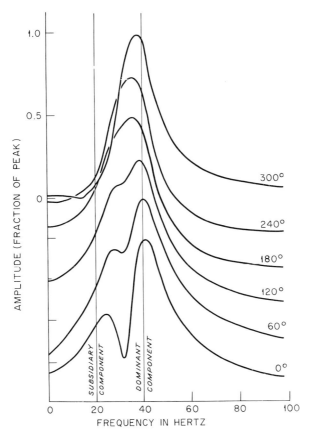

FIG. 2.28. Effect on the spectral distribution $B(\omega)$ of varying the phase of the subsidiary component φ_s. The precise frequencies of the impulse response cannot be identified from $B(\omega)$ (Freeman, 1970).

frequency end as shown, whereas in the second case they deviate at the low-frequency end (not shown). The same result occurs in Fig. 2.27 in which optimal fit in the time domain is found with two components at frequencies of 44.5 and 21.7 Hz and slightly closer conformation with two at 42.0 and 49.2 Hz with deviation of calculated and observed spectra at the high end in the first case and at the low end in the second (as shown). Mean values for frequency for eight cats in which two pairs of frequencies were determined are 40.5 ± 1.0 (SE) and 20.9 ± 2.9 Hz, or 37.5 ± 2.3 and 52.5 ± 3.5 Hz.

Clearly there are at least three components in these AEP, but there is sufficient information in the AEP to define only two basis functions numerically. The parameters for those two are altered from their presumed true values by $\pm 5\%$ to give the closest fit of generated and observed wave forms in a least squares sense. Figure 2.28 shows how small changes in the phases of two wave forms might produce widespread changes in their combined spectrum. It is the near interchangeability of the subsidiary basis functions that causes singularity in the attempt to solve the normal equations, when both are included in the regression equation, yet exclusion of one necessarily causes distortion of values for the other two.

CHAPTER 3

Amplitude-Dependent Properties

3.1. Nonlinear Models for Neural Membranes

The neural phenomena thus far considered have been treated solely in terms of potential, current, and equivalent networks or topologies of lumped or distributed resistances and capacitances. Certain difficulties have been avoided by restricting consideration to those phenomena that can be described by sets of linear equations. This constraint must now be set aside as we examine nonlinear phenomena in terms of the chemical basis of neural activity, both for axon potentials and dendritic potentials.

The basis for this examination is the recognition that neural currents are carried by moving ions, not electrons. A net current is heterogeneous, because there are many different ions dissolved in and between nerve cells, all moving in response to electrical and other energy gradients. The main seat of the forces that move and oppose the movement of ions lies in or on the nerve cell membrane. This is where the energy transformations take place as is manifested by the establishment of electrical, chemical, and thermal gradients in the surround. The basis for neural events is the movement of ions across membranes. The basis for description must be a model for membrane function. Such a model is embodied in the ionic hypothesis of nerve activity (Katz, 1966).

3.1.1. THE IONIC HYPOTHESIS

The molecular structure of the membrane is not yet fully understood, nor are the chemical processes by which ions are moved across it. In the absence of such knowledge the main source of information about the membrane is the measurement of concentration and electrical gradients across it, and the densities of ionic currents j in response to the forces implied by those gradients. The ratio of current density j to force f driving each ion species y defines a specific conductance (conductance/unit area of membrane) for that ion in respect to that force

$$g_y = j_y/f_y. \tag{1}$$

This is, of course, the ionic equivalent to Ohm's law and reduces the description of membrane function to sets of coupling coefficients between current density and force. The coefficients themselves are then interpreted in terms of the existence of certain types of molecular events in membrane, e.g., diffusion of ions through aqueous pores in a lipid barrier, transport of ions across membranes by carrier molecules, exchange of ions by selective adsorption to fixed charges in the membrane, etc., but in the description of common neuronal events such exploratory proposals are speculative overlay that might confuse understanding rather than aid it.

As an example, suppose that a membrane is given that separates the aqueous compartments comprising an idealized neuron and its medium. For each ion there is a current density j_y across the membrane in response to multiple driving forces $f_{y'y}$, such as its own concentration gradient, the electrical and thermal gradients across the membrane, the concentration gradient for the solute (osmotic pressure), the hydrostatic pressure, the forces exerted by other ions in the medium, etc. Each force acts on the ion to induce movement so that the net flux density is expressed by the sum of several forces, each with its appropriate coefficient:

$$j_y = g_{1y}f_{1y} + g_{2y}f_{2y} + \cdots + g_{ny}f_{ny}. \tag{2}$$

For r ions and nr forces the current of the membrane can be expressed as a set of equations at any instant in time

$$j_1 = g_{11}f_{11} + g_{21}f_{21} + \cdots + g_{n1}f_{n1}$$
$$j_2 = g_{12}f_{12} + g_{22}f_{22} + \cdots + g_{n2}f_{n2}$$
$$\vdots \tag{3}$$
$$j_r = g_{1r}f_{1r} + g_{2r}f_{2r} + \cdots + g_{nr}f_{nr}.$$

The coefficients represent the functional properties of the membrane, and subsidiary statements about them embody any assumptions and additional evidence available for the analysis.

The concentration forces f_{cy} and electrical forces f_{zy} acting across the membrane are much more prominent in their actions on ion movements than are other known forces. Thus in Eq. (3), n is set equal to 2. In the Bernstein model for the membrane the conductances for potassium, g_{cK^+}, and g_{zK^+}, are assumed to be much larger than those for any other ion, so that all others are set equal to zero. Thus the membrane function is described by

$$j_{K^+} = g_{cK^+} f_{cK^+} + g_{zK^+} f_{zK^+}. \tag{4}$$

In respect to the chemical force the conductance is the same as the mobility μ_y. In respect to the electrical force it is the product of mobility and concentration, because the ease of flow depends on the number of ions available:

$$g_{zK^+} = \mu_{K^+} c_{K^+}, \qquad g_{cK^+} = \mu_{K^+}. \tag{5}$$

The electrical force acting on each ion is

$$f_{zK^+} = -Z_{K^+} F \, dv/dx, \tag{6}$$

where dv/dx is the gradient of potential in the membrane, Z_y is the valence, and F is the Faraday constant (96,500 C/equivalent). The chemical force is

$$f_{cK^+} = -RT \, dc_{K^+}/dx, \tag{7}$$

where dc/dx is the concentration gradient, T is the absolute temperature (degrees Kelvin), and R is the universal gas constant (8.31 J/mole °K). From Eqs. (4)–(7),

$$j_{K^+} = -\mu_{K^+} c_{K^+} [Z_{K^+} F \, dv/dx + (RT/c_{K^+})(dc_{K^+}/dx)]. \tag{8}$$

In the steady state it is assumed that the inward and outward currents in response to these two forces are equal and opposite, so that the net flux is zero

$$j_{K^+} = 0. \tag{9}$$

From Eqs. (8) and (9),

$$Z_{K^+} F \, dv = -RT \, dc_{K^+}/c_{K^+}. \tag{10}$$

By integration across the membrane,

$$v_m = (RT/Z_{K^+} F) \ln([K^+]_o/[K^+]_i), \tag{11}$$

where v_m is the membrane potential in volts inside with respect to zero outside, $[K^+]_o$ the K^+ concentration outside, and $[K^+]_i$ the concentration inside the membrane. The typical neuron has an internal negative potential that manifests an inward force on K^+ ions. The internal K^+ concentration (e.g., 110 milliequivalents/liter) is higher than the external K^+ concentration (4.3 milliequivalents/liter), so the chemical force is outwardly directed. For zero flow these forces must be equal and opposite [Eq. (10)]. Equation (11), the Nernst equation, predicts that at body temperature ($37°$C or $310°$K) the inward electrical force required to give zero current (at the given typical concentration difference) is -87 mV. Further, the transmembrane potential is predicted to change with the logarithm of the ionic concentration ratio (Fig. 3.1).

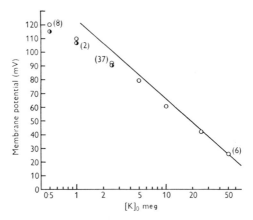

FIG. 3.1. Relation between external potassium concentration $[K^+]_o$ and transmembrane potential difference (negative inward) of the sartorius muscle using Eq. (11) (Adrian, 1956).

There is substantial evidence that this prediction holds for a variety of types of membranes over a rather wide range of external concentrations, but that this range does not include the range of normal extracellular concentration for potassium (Fig. 3.1). In this range v_m is consistently less negative than predicted from the inner and outer concentrations.

This deviation from the expected relation implies that the membrane is permeable to other ions besides potassium. The use of radioactive tracers over the past three decades has demonstrated that all ions in inner and outer solutions of nerve membranes are in continuous flow across the membrane. Hence the assumption that all μ_y other than μ_{K+} are zero is not valid.

The Bernstein model breaks down in another way. The model is based on the additional postulate that during the active state of nerve, there is an increase in conductance to all ions. This leads to the prediction that membrane potential should approach zero during the action potential. In fact, it is reversed in polarity at the crest, rendering this postulate untenable. Despite these shortcomings the Bernstein model (in modified form) persists as the basis for interpretation of neural electrical activity. In brief, the membrane is selectively permeable to some ions more than to others, and the essential processes on which nerve activity is based occur through changes in membrane conductances.

3.1.2. METABOLIC FORCES

As potassium is the major intracellular cation, so is sodium the dominant extracellular cation. At rest there is continuous inward and outward flow of sodium so that $\mu_{Na^+} \neq 0$. The Na^+ concentration difference (using typical values for squid nerve) is 145 milliequivalents/liter outside less 14 milli-equivalents/liter inside, so that there is a strong tendency for Na^+ to diffuse into the cell. The internal negative potential implies an electrostatic force acting inwardly. The sum of these two forces cannot be zero, so that

$$\mu_{Na^+}(c_{Na^+} f_{zNa^+} + f_{cNa^+}) \neq 0. \tag{12}$$

In the steady state however, it is certain that

$$j_{Na^+} = 0. \tag{13}$$

From Eqs. (3), which hold also for Na^+, it must be concluded that the limitation to two forces, $n = 2$, is not valid. It is generally accepted that energy derived ultimately from oxidative metabolism in the neuron supplies the requisite force, and that Na^+ is forced outwardly across the membrane as fast as it diffuses inwardly along the concentration and electrical gradients. Thus in the steady state

$$j_{Na^+} = \mu_{Na^+}(c_{Na^+} f_{zNa^+} + f_{cNa^+}) + g_{mNa^+} f_{mNa^+}, \tag{14}$$

where f_{mNa^+} represents the sum of unknown forces and g_{mNa^+} the unknown transport processes.

There is evidence that the outward movement of Na^+ is partially coupled with the inward movement of K^+, for when the external K^+ is removed entirely, the rate of outward movement of Na^+ falls to one-third its normal value. It is likely that potassium is also affected by forces other than those of concentration and electrical gradients, some of which are derived from metabolic energy. A similar situation occurs for chloride and most other (if not all) ions. It has become the custom to represent these unknown forces on each ion by a single mechanism known as the membrane "pump" or battery for that ion species. Thus the equations for the membrane can be written as

$$\begin{aligned} j_{K^+} &= \mu_{K^+}(c_{K^+} f_{zK^+} + f_{cK^+}) + g_{mK^+} f_{mK^+} \\ j_{Na^+} &= \mu_{Na^+}(c_{Na^+} f_{zNa^+} + f_{cNa^+}) + g_{mNa^+} g_{mNa^+} \\ j_{Cl^-} &= \mu_{Cl^-}(c_{Cl^-} f_{zCl^-} + f_{cCl^-}) + g_{mCl^-} f_{mCl^-} \\ &\vdots \end{aligned} \tag{15}$$

For purposes of describing transient neural activity in terms of ionic currents it is permissible to assume that the μ_y and their associated forces are independent of the g_{my} and f_{my}, because the rate constants of the μ_y are far faster than those of the g_{my}. Furthermore, the active, transactional, information-bearing events (including action potentials and PSPs) are attributed to changes in the μ_y whereas the restorative, nutritive, anabolic functions are attributed to the g_{my}. This separation is based on demonstrations that metabolic inhibitors that block oxidative metabolism (fluoride, cyanide, etc.) or that depolarize the nerve membrane (e.g., excess external potassium) do not prevent the formation of the action potential, provided membrane potential is restored to normal by anodal polarization (using an external battery). On the other hand local anesthetics (cocaine, procaine, etc.) or sodium-deficient solutions applied externally to the membrane prevent conduction without significant effect on membrane potential or resting ion exchanges.

Obviously there is a link between the active states and the restorative processes, as implied by Eq. (15), because on the average over periods of quiescence or normal activity, the total ionic transport currents in response to metabolic forces must be equal but opposite to those in response to known forces. The nature of this link is also unknown, so that the separation of transactional and restorative events is imposed as much by lack of knowledge as by convenience in describing nerve function.

It is widely believed that the fluctuations in membrane potential following the action potential (depolarizing and hyperpolarizing afterpotentials) are manifestations of these metabolic forces, but proof for this is not yet at hand. One of the main reasons for believing this is that the afterpotentials and the metabolic forces are much slower to develop and decay than the transactional potentials and forces. Afterpotentials are usually identified with axons, but they are also found to follow dendritic events, when they are looked for. The reason is simple: The transactional events are the result of brief ion-specific changes in membrane conductance, and the energy is supplied by ion concentrations previously accumulated at metabolic cost. Following each transactional event, the concentrations are restored to their initial values. This is done by moving ions in the reverse of their directions of flow during the transactional event. In the appropriate geometric conditions, the restorative ionic flows are accompanied by detectable fields of potential, the afterpotentials of axons and dendrites (see Fig. 2.19 and 2.22).

3.1.3. The Concept of Equilibrium Potential

The ionic hypothesis states that the basis for neural action currents is the occurrence of conductance changes in the membrane specific to certain ions or groups of ions. The currents can be measured in equivalents per second or in amperes. The conductance changes are expressed as variable conductances measured in mhos. The electrical energy is measured in volts. The energy of concentration must also be expressed in volts, in order that the sum of forces be calculated. This is done by use of the Nernst equation [Eq. (11)], which expresses a concentration difference for a given ion as an equivalent potential difference or equilibrium potential for that ion. For each ion the net driving force is the difference between v_m and the equilibrium potential v_y, for that ion. There is reason to doubt the quantitative validity of this step, because the Nernst equation applies to reversible systems in which a true equilibrium has been achieved and in which there is zero current. Across the membrane there is at best a steady state for sets of irreversible reactions, including the steady outflow of heat and hydrogen ions. Further, the concept is applied also to active states in which net ion currents do flow. Like the core conductor and the membrane capacitance, it is a useful concept that can be misused but not readily replaced.

The relationships between transmembrane potential and the conductances and concentration gradients for the major ions are expressed by means of the so-called "constant field equation," which will now be derived. Let a neuron have an outside a and an inside b separated by a single differentially permeable membrane of thickness d. In each compartment there are differing concentrations of cations c_y^+, and anions c_y^-. The total current across the membrane J is the sum of the independent ionic currents j_y. It is assumed that the conductances across the membrane are constant for each ion but not necessarily equal in the two directions. Then using the superscript $+$ to denote the direction from outside to inside (a to b),

$$j_y^+ = \mu_y^+ f_{cy} + \mu_y^+ c_y^+ f_{zy}, \qquad j_y^- = \mu_y^- f_{cy} + \mu_y^- c_y^- f_{zy}. \qquad (16)$$

From Eq. (8)

$$j^+ = \mu_y^+ c_y^+ \left(F \frac{\partial v}{\partial x} + \frac{RT}{c_y^+} \frac{\partial c_y^+}{\partial x} \right), \qquad j^- = \mu_y^- c_y^- \left(F \frac{\partial v}{\partial x} + \frac{RT}{c_y^-} \frac{\partial c_y^-}{\partial x} \right), \qquad (17)$$

where $Z_y = 1$, which restricts consideration to univalent ions.

It is assumed that the ionic currents for the differing species are independent (equivalent to Dalton's law for a mixture of gases), and that the μ are constant over time and thickness of the membrane. A solution to this equation is obtained by assuming that $\partial v/\partial x$ is constant over the thickness of the membrane d. This is justified mainly on the basis that there are presumed to be both bound and unbound charges in the membrane, which will distribute themselves so as to minimize local deviations from a uniform gradient. Let

v_m be the transmembrane potential, so that

$$\partial v/\partial x = v_m/d. \tag{18}$$

When the electric gradient is linearized by this assumption, Eqs. (17) become ordinary first-order linear differential equations. The solutions are

$$j_y^+ = \frac{\mu_y^+ F v_m}{d(e^{-\beta}-1)}[c_{ya}^+ e^{-\beta} - c_{yb}^+], \qquad j_y^- = \frac{\mu_y^- F v_m}{d(e^{-\beta}-1)}[c_{yb}^- e^{-\beta} - c_{ya}^-], \tag{19}$$

where $\beta = F v_m/RT$. The net membrane current is the sum of cations c_y^+ moving from a to b and of anions c_y^- moving from b to a:

$$J = \sum_y (j_y^+ - j_y^-). \tag{20}$$

From Eqs. (19) and (20),

$$J = \frac{F v_m}{d(e^{-\beta}-1)}[e^{-\beta}\sum_y(\mu_y^+ c_{ya}^+ + \mu_y^- c_{yb}^-) - \sum_y(\mu_y^+ c_{yb}^+ + \mu_y^- c_{ya}^-)]. \tag{21}$$

In the steady state, $J = 0$. Equation (21) is then solved for v_m,

$$v_m = \frac{RT}{F} \ln\left[\frac{\sum_y(\mu_y^+ c_{ya}^+ + \mu_y^- c_{yb}^-)}{\sum_y(\mu_y^+ c_{yb}^+ + \mu_y^- c_{ya}^-)}\right]. \tag{22}$$

This equation states that the membrane potential in the steady state is determined by the concentration ratios of all the ion species, which are weighted by the relative mobilities of the ions across the membrane.

Consideration is commonly restricted to the concentrations of three ions. These are $[Na^+]$, $[K^+]$, and $[Cl^-]$. The mobilities across the membrane often are expressed as specific membrane permeabilities, p_{Na^+}, p_{K^+} and p_{Cl^-}. Using the subscript $e = a$ to denote outside concentration and $i = b$ to denote inside concentration, we obtain

$$v_m = \frac{RT}{F} \ln\left[\frac{p_{Na^+}[Na^+]_e + p_{K^+}[K^+]_e + p_{Cl^-}[Cl^-]_i}{p_{Na^+}[Na^+]_i + p_{Na^+}[K^+]_i + p_{Cl^-}[Cl^-]_e}\right]. \tag{23}$$

This is known as the Goldman (1943) *constant field equation*. If any one of these ionic permeabilities should become much larger than all of the others, then Eq. (23) reduces to the Nernst equation. The transmembrane potential v_m approaches the equilibrium potential for that ion species.

This is the conceptual basis for the ionic hypothesis. At rest in the normal neuron p_{K^+} is very much larger than p_{Na^+}, but it does not occlude the presence of p_{Cl^-}. In the presence of excess external potassium p_{K^+} increases and becomes dominant, so that the membrane potential can be predicted by the Nernst equation from the concentration ratio for K^+. During the nerve action potential p_{Na^+} rises 1000-fold to become dominant, and v_m approaches the equilibrium potential for Na$^+$ (Fig. 3.2). Membrane potential is therefore dependent on selective permeabilities to particular ions in the presence of concentration gradients determined by metabolic processes. The ionic analysis of neural events requires the measurement of these permeabilities (usually as conductances) and of their functional determinants.

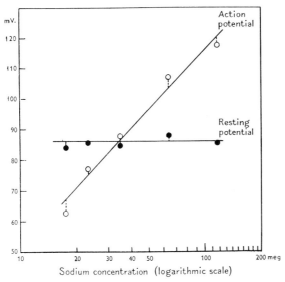

FIG. 3.2. Relation between external sodium concentration [Na$^+$]$_o$ and transmembrane potential difference (negative inward) in the resting and active states (Nastuk & Hodgkin, 1950).

3.1.4. THE SODIUM PERMEABILITY MODEL

The system for measurement devised by Hodgkin & Huxley (1952) is not derived from the constant field equation but requires use of Eqs. (15) and the concept of the equilibrium potential as an energy source expressed in volts. The ionic mobilities are replaced by equivalent specific ionic conductances expressed in mhos per centimeter squared and the current densities expressed in amperes per centimeter squared. Across a given area of membrane, the total current density j is the sum of a capacitative and a resistive (ionic) fraction

$$j = C_m \, dv_m/dt + j_{Na^+} + j_{K^+} + \cdots + j_r. \tag{24}$$

Let us restrict consideration to Na$^+$ and K$^+$. Each ion moves along its path in accordance with the sum of two forces. The electrical force is proportional to the transmembrane potential v_m in volts. The concentration force is given by the Nernst equation also in volts, v_y. The specific conductance for each ion is defined by the ratio (Section 2.2.1),

$$g_y = j_y/(v_y - v_m), \tag{25}$$

and is measured in mhos per centimeter squared. The conductance defined in this way (see footnote in Section 2.3.4) differs from the concepts of mobility or permeability, in that it includes both the properties of the membrane and the ion and the concentration of the ion in the membrane into a single term. There is no allowance (or need) for separating these attributes in the Hodgkin–Huxley system. It should be recalled that mobility is defined as the ratio of current to voltage (a conductance) in an ionic solution, divided by the concentration of the solution. In the membrane the intramembrane concentration cannot be defined (the membrane is not a homogeneous solvent) or measured. In squid nerve it is found empirically that the g_y are instantaneous linear functions of v_m, which reinforces the usefulness of Eq. (25). In nodes of Ranvier the definition for conductance is more conveniently made using the constant field equation (Hodgkin, 1964).

Substituting Eq. (25) into (24) after solving for j_y,

$$j_m = C_m \, dv_m/dt + g_{Na^+}(v_{Na^+} - v_m) + g_{K^+}(v_{K^+} - v_m). \tag{26}$$

The conductances have been calculated as functions of time and of v_m by fixing v_m at each of a series of values from resting v_m and measuring j_m. During short periods of current the inner and outer concentrations do not change significantly, so that v_{Na^+} and v_{K^+} remain constant. Then v_m is fixed by means of a high-gain negative-feedback amplifier (voltage clamp) with a very short time constant. Two long wire electrodes are inserted the full length of a giant axon (to give uniform current density over the axon), one for measuring v_m and the other for delivering whatever current is required to maintain v_m constant. Within the first 30 μsec of changing v_m from its resting value to some new level there is a very brief current charging membrane capacitance, the time course of which is dependent mainly on the characteristics of the amplifier. Thereafter the current changes in direct proportion to the membrane conductance.

The circuit diagram for the lumped membrane is shown in Fig. 3.3a. Three variable resistors are in parallel with a fixed capacitance C_m and are each in series with an ionic "battery." The voltage is maintained constant by the current source $I\mu(t)$ and the output is the current required to do this as shown by curve A in Fig. 3.3b.

Sudden depolarization of the membrane to zero volts requires a very brief outward current pulse to discharge the membrane capacitance. Thereafter, for a period of about 1 msec an inward current is required in order to maintain depolarization, followed by a sustained outward current (Fig. 3.3b,

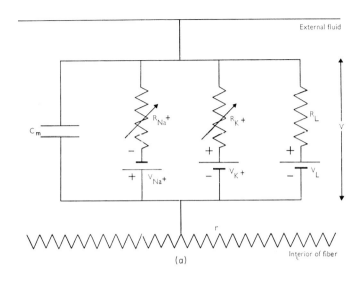

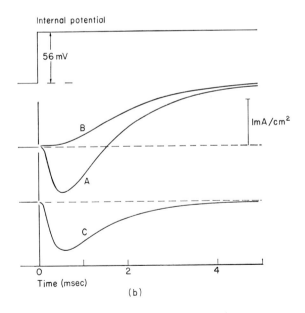

FIG. 3.3. (a) Equivalent circuit for an element of membrane to represent specific ionic currents. (b) Separation of Na^+ and K^+ currents by use of the voltage clamp on axon in external solutions with and without Na^+, respectively, A and B. Na^+ current is $C = A - B$ (Hodgkin, 1964).

curve A). This ionic current is separated into its two components by (R_L is ignored) repeating the experiment using an external fluid in which the Na^+ is replaced by choline. The current in the second case (curve B) is that carried by K^+ ions. The Na^+ current is obtained by subtracting the second curve from the first (Fig. 3.3b, curve C).

The specific conductances are directly proportional to these currents:

$$g_{Na^+} = j_{Na^+}/(v_{Na^+} - v_m), \qquad g_{K^+} = j_{K^+}/(v_{K^+} - v_m), \qquad (27)$$

because v_{Na^+}, v_{K^+}, and v_m are all fixed. There is a rapid early increase in g_{Na^+} followed by a return to baseline. The g_{K^+} increases more slowly but remains elevated for the duration of the depolarization. Repolarization terminates both increases in conductance, g_{Na^+} returning more rapidly than g_{K^+}. However, g_{Na^+} is self-limited in time.

The interpretation is that upon depolarization the large increase in g_{Na^+} causes the membrane potential calculated by Eq. (23) to shift toward the equilibrium potential for Na^+. Since this is approximately $+40$ mV, an inward current is required to neutralize membrane potential with a super-imposed IR drop. At the termination of the increase in g_{Na^+}, the sustained increase in g_{K^+} causes v_m to shift toward the equilibrium potential for K^+ (-80 mV). To neutralize the inwardly negative potential setup by the K^+ concentration difference, a strong outward current is required.

By setting membrane potential to differing levels it is found that both g_{Na^+} and g_{K^+} are dependent on membrane potential (Fig. 3.4). This is the key property of the Hodgkin–Huxley system as it accounts for the major nonlinear property of the nerve, its threshold. Following depolarization of a region of membrane by an outward current both g_{Na^+} and g_{K^+} increase. The former causes Na^+ ions to move inwardly with still further depolarization; the latter causes K^+ ions to move outwardly leading to repolarization. The resting g_{Na^+} is far lower than resting g_{K^+}, and must be greatly increased before it becomes dominant, but it increases far more rapidly follow-ing a step change in v_m than does g_{K^+}, so that a regenerative increase in g_{Na^+} can take place well before the restorative effect of the increase of g_{K^+} occurs.

A major unanswered question concerns the nature of the mechanism that limits the duration of the increase in g_{Na^+}. This process is called *sodium inactivation* on the basis of the macroscopic model proposed by Hodgkin & Huxley (1952). The transport of a sodium ion is assumed to require the simultaneous occurrence of three events (e.g., the arrival of a carrier molecule at the surface of the membrane, the occurrence of the first steps of a three-stage chemical reaction, the opening of a "pore" in a three-layer barrier, etc.), each of probability **m** ranging from 0 to 1.0 and the absence of a fourth event of probability **h**. The total probability that transport will occur is then m^3h.

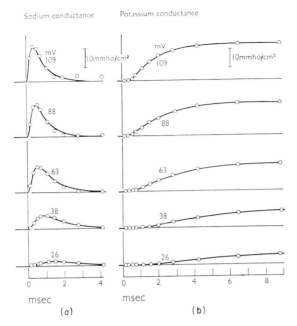

FIG. 3.4. (a) Time and (b) voltage dependencies of g_{Na^+} and g_{K^+} (Hodgkin, 1964).

Therefore $g_{Na^+} = \bar{g}_{Na^+} \mathbf{m}^3 \mathbf{h}$, where $\bar{g}_{Na^+}$ is the maximum value for g_{Na^+}. The probabilities are given by

$$d\mathbf{m}/dt = \alpha_m (1 - \mathbf{m}) - \beta_m \mathbf{m}, \tag{28}$$

$$d\mathbf{h}/dt = \alpha_h (1 - \mathbf{h}) - \beta_h \mathbf{h}, \tag{29}$$

where the α and β are rate constants dependent only on membrane potential at given temperature and external calcium concentration. Depolarization increases α_m and β_h and decreases α_h and β_m.

The transport of K^+ requires the simultaneous occurrence of four events, each of probability $\mathbf{n}$, so that $g_{K^+} = \bar{g}_{K^+} \mathbf{n}^4$, where $\bar{g}_{K^+}$ is the maximum of g_{K^+}. The probability is given by

$$d\mathbf{n}/dt = \alpha_n (1 - \mathbf{n}) - \beta_n \mathbf{n} \tag{30}$$

in which α_n increases and β_n decreases with depolarization.

At fixed voltages the α and β are constant, so that Eqs. (28)–(30) are easily solved. The experimental data are fitted with these results to evaluate the dependence of the rate constant and the probabilities, $\mathbf{m}$, $\mathbf{h}$, and $\mathbf{n}$ on membrane potential.

The expression for membrane current density (omitting a minor term for leakage conductance) is now

$$j_m = C_m dv_m/dt + (v_{Na^+} - v_m)\bar{g}_{Na^+} \mathbf{m}^3\mathbf{h} + (v_{K^+} - v_m)\bar{g}_{K^+} \mathbf{n}^4. \qquad (31)$$

Equations (28)–(31) constitute a system of nonlinear equations in which the coefficients are dependent on only one parameter, the transmembrane voltage. This simplification, in itself a remarkable achievement, has provided a means for quantitative evaluation of the action potential and of the local circuit theory of propagation.

Some common misconceptions may be avoided by emphasizing the fact that in some axons the transmembrane potential during the action potential is determined entirely by the change in transmembrane sodium conductance [Eq. (23)]. Depolarization is due to an increase in g_{Na^+} and not to the turning off of the sodium pump or to an increase in internal sodium concentration. Repolarization is due to the decrease in g_{Na^+} and not to the delayed potassium conductance increase or to potassium outflow. The absence of action potentials in most dendrites is due to the lack of the voltage-dependent sodium conductance in the membrane, but there are other conductances that depend on transmitter substances and not on membrane voltage. In all cases the membrane system at rest consists of a dynamic balance of many forces including several important concentration gradients and a set of ionic currents adding to zero for each ion. A conductance change in an active state represents an unbalancing of the forces leading to a new set of ionic currents. The membrane then becomes a current generator with high internal impedance, provided the conductance change is in part of the neural membrane and not over the entire neural surface. The energy source for the electromotive forces (emf) is the preexisting concentration gradients, which are built from metabolic energy. The current is the sole basis for transmission within the neuron in the active states being considered here.

3.2. Nonlinear Models for Neurons and Parts of Neurons

3.2.1. ACTION POTENTIALS IN AXONS

According to the Hodgkin–Huxley model local depolarization of the axonal membrane by a sufficient amount (the threshold) and for a minimal time leads to a voltage-dependent regenerative increase in g_{Na^+} (Fig. 3.4a). According to Eq. (23) the membrane potential in that region shifts toward v_{Na^+}, the sodium equilibrium potential. Differential polarization of the membrane establishes a longitudinal flow of current that must be in the form of a closed loop crossing the membrane twice. The inward current in the active segment must equal the outward current in the passive segment. The resistive drop across the passive membrane is subtracted from the resting membrane potential. The reduction in electrical field strength across the passive membrane by itself is sufficient to increase g_{Na^+} there, causing local membrane potential to approach v_{Na^+}. Thus the process repeats itself for the length of the fiber. The increase in g_{Na^+} is self-limited, which leads to the return of membrane potential toward rest. The delayed increase in g_{K^+} (Fig. 3.4b) causes hyperpolarization as membrane potential shifts toward v_{K^+}. During these changes in g_{Na^+} and g_{K^+} there is some net entry of Na^+ ions and loss of K^+ ions across the membrane, which are subsequently exchanged at a slow rate by metabolic processes, long after repolarization has been effected. The amounts exchanged for each impulse are about one-millionth part of the total Na^+ and K^+ ions that are present in the axoplasm.

There are four main lines of evidence in support of this model. First, Eq. (31) has been used to calculate the forms of the transmembrane potential and impedance changes during the propagated action potential (Fig. 3.5).

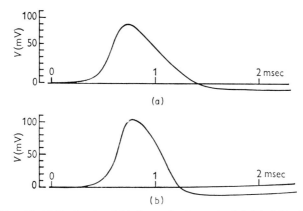

FIG. 3.5. (a) Predicted and (b) observed action potentials (Hodgkin, 1964).

From Section 2.3.3 the transmembrane current density j_m is proportional to the second derivative of transmembrane potential along the axon. If a is the diameter of the fiber and r_i is the specific resistance of the axoplasm, then

$$j_m = (a/2r_i)\partial^2 v_m/\partial x^2. \tag{32}$$

If the velocity of propagation θ is constant, then $x = -\theta t$ and

$$j_m = (a/2r_i\theta^2)d^2 v_m/dt^2. \tag{33}$$

Equation (33) combined with Eq. (31) gives an ordinary second-order non-linear differential equation in potential with respect to time:

$$\frac{a}{2r_i\theta^2}\frac{d^2v_m}{dt^2} = C_m\frac{dv_m}{dt} + \bar{g}_{Na^+}\mathbf{m}^3\mathbf{h}(v_{Na^+} - v_m) + \bar{g}_{K^+}\mathbf{n}^4(v_{K^+} - v_m). \quad (34)$$

For a specified initial condition of v_m Eq. (34) can be solved for v_m as a function of time by numerical or analog techniques. The value for θ for which v_m returns to zero as t goes to infinity must be found by iterative guess work. Recorded and computed action potentials are shown in Fig. 3.5 (Hodgkin & Huxley, 1952). The theoretical curves for g_{Na^+} and g_{K^+} are shown in Fig. 3.6. Their sum gives a curve for transmembrane conductance (Fig. 3.7) that

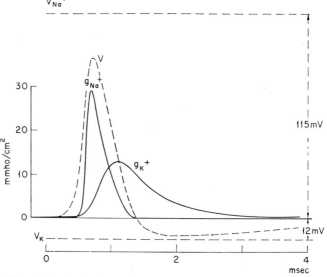

FIG. 3.6. Theoretical solutions for propagated action potential and conductances (Hodgkin, 1964).

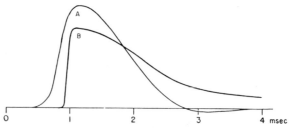

FIG. 3.7. Action potential (curve A) and membrane conductance (curve B) measured with an alternating current bridge (Cole & Curtis, 1939).

parallels that measured during the action potential with an alternating current bridge (Cole & Curtis, 1939).

A second line of evidence is comparison of predicted and measured Na^+ gain and K^+ loss from an active fiber. The instantaneous value for Na^+ and K^+ current densities can be calculated using the data in Fig. 3.6 and Eq. (27). The area enclosed by the curves for j_{Na^+} and j_{K^+} gives the total ionic charge exchanged per unit area of membrane, which on conversion using F (Faraday's constant) gives $q_{Na^+} = 4.33$ pmole/cm^2 and $q_{K^+} = 4.26$ pmole/cm^2 surface of membrane. These values agree well with measurements of Na^+ gain (3–4 pmole/cm^2) and K^+ loss (3–4 pmole/cm^2) per impulse in squid axon using tracers or flame photometry. The amount of charge required to change the potential on membrane capacitance (1 μF/cm^2) by 100 mV is 10^{-7} C/cm^2, which is equivalent to 1 pmole/cm^2 of Na^+, so that the observed and calculated exchanges are well in excess of the minimum required.

A third line of evidence is the relation between spike amplitude and the concentration gradient for Na^+. External concentration can be varied by replacing part or all of the Na^+ with choline in the bathing solution. Internal concentration in giant fibers is varied by injecting artificial solutions with micropipettes or by removing the axoplasm by squeezing (like toothpaste from a tube) and replacing it with known solutions (Hodgkin, 1964). With some exceptions the peak amplitude of the action potential is found to vary in accordance with the Nernst equation (Fig. 3.2). Also, when the membrane is clamped at the calculated value for v_{Na^+}, the initial inward current disappears, and if v_m is made more positive than v_{Na^+}, the initial current is outward.

The fourth line of evidence stems from the study of saltatory conduction. Extracellular recording has shown that inward current occurs only at nodes of Ranvier in myelinated fibers, and that such blocking agents as cold, ultraviolet radiation and chemical inhibitors act only at the nodes. This implies that a cylinder of membrane perhaps .03 μm long and 10 μm in diameter can induce a regenerative permeability change in the same axon at a distance of 1 to 3 internodal lengths (up to 6 mm or 6000 μm). There is no other possibility in the neuron for action at such relatively immense distances than an electrical field of force. The point is crucial, because the greater part of contemporary neurophysiology is based on the concept of the loop current as the sole basis for intraneuronal transmission at high speed.

It should now be clear why conduction velocity is proportional to axon diameter. The membrane capacitance must be discharged in order to change membrane potential, and the time constant τ_1 for this is given by the product of longitudinal (mainly internal) resistance R_1 and membrane capacitance C_m (the initial outward current of the action potential is mainly capacitative). With increasing diameter R_1 decreases with the square and C_m in linear proportion, so that τ_1 decreases in proportion to diameter. The conductance changes are so rapid that τ_1 is the limiting constant and determines θ. (Note $\tau_1 \neq \tau_m$).

Large fibers have low R_1 and high action currents, with relatively large energy losses per action potential. In myelinated fibers τ_1 is reduced by the successive layers of membrane-like material; the capacitances of these layers are in series, so that the net capacitance is the reciprocal of the sum of the reciprocals, i.e., it is far less than the capacitance of a single layer. The action current and energy per action potential are much reduced. In the internodal segments the total voltage drop is distributed across the multiple layers, whereas in the node it lies mainly across the axon membrane.

The Hodgkin–Huxley equations explain the axon properties of accommodation and adaptation (see Section 1.2.5). They can also serve to account for the linear relationship (Dodge, 1972) between the amplitude of a steady depolarizing transmembrane current and the rate of firing of a neuron (see Section 2.4.4).[†] However, acceptance of the ionic hypothesis has not been universal, mainly because of the simplifying assumptions required to use the Nernst equation, which limit the scope of the theory, e.g., the omission of consideration of thermal and hydrostatic gradients (particularly transients), the assumption of equilibrium when at best the steady state can be attained, the still unsatisfactory treatment of the role of divalent ions, and the failure to extend the theory to the analysis of afterpotentials. It is likely that major advances in understanding of the molecular structure of the membrane will be required before the ionic hypothesis is superceded. Meanwhile the concepts of equilibrium potential, of the control of membrane potential by specific ionic conductances, and of the voltage and time dependencies of the selective sodium and potassium conductances together constitute a model that suffices to organize most of the available data on the properties of axon membrane.

3.2.2. THRESHOLD UNCERTAINTY IN AXONS

Threshold is defined with reference to an amplitude of stimulation below which an axon does not fire, and at or above which it does. In the vicinity of threshold there is uncertainty of what value threshold amplitude has, because on repeated trials at some fixed stimulus level firing occurs on some trials and not on others. Let us suppose that a range of stimulus intensity is broken into a set of levels, and that for each level N trials are made. The response of the axon is measured in the usual way, and it is observed that at each level of intensity there are n responses. The results can

[†] However, whether this or some other ionic mechanism accounts for the relationship is still unknown.

be expressed as the fraction n/N of successful firings. For stimuli well below threshold there are no responses, and the relative frequency is zero. Well above threshold the axon responds every time and the relative frequency is 1.0. Somewhere between the nerve responds on the average of half of the trials, giving a relative frequency of .50. This level of intensity is taken as threshold.

Provided the trials are made sufficiently far apart (e.g., 1.0 sec), the occurrence or not of a response on a preceding trial does not affect the tendency for a response to occur on the next trial. By appropriate statistical testing it can be shown that the outcomes of successive trials are independent of each other. There is, furthermore, no way to predict before a given trial whether a response will occur or not on that trial. We have, therefore, a collection of random events, the relative frequency of which depends on stimulus intensity and ranges between zero and unity.

The results can be presented in tabular or graphic form giving a probability distribution. This increases from 0 to 1 monotonically over a specified range of stimulus intensity. Empirically it is found that the probability distribution for axon firings can be closely fitted with a cumulative Gaussian or normal distribution function, i.e., the integral of the normal density function. Let $P(v)$ be the probability of firing in response to a particular input v. Then

$$P(v) = 1/(2\pi)^{1/2}\sigma \int_0^v \exp[-(v-v_0)^2/2\sigma^2]\,dv \qquad (35)$$

where v_0 is the intensity at which $P(v) = .50$ and σ is the standard deviation. Values can be taken from a table for the area enclosed by the normal density function for specified values of the independent variable.

The source of this variability lies in the axon and not in the stimulus source or electrodes, for when two parallel axons are excited by the same stimulus the probability of occurrence of response is independent for each axon. Either the threshold v_{thr}, the resting transmembrane potential v_r, the penetrating fraction of stimulus current density j_m, or the membrane specific resistance r_m, or some combination is undergoing spontaneous fluctuation. From measurements of v_r using intracellular electrodes in large axons it is known that v_r is very stable (unlike v_r in the somata of central neurons undergoing continuous synaptic bombardment). Both v_{thr} and j_m depend on the levels of the ionic conductances, which also determine r_m, so that the internal state of the membrane is presumed to undergo random fluctuations. The Hodgkin–Huxley system is based on the concept of randomly occurring events, the probabilities of which are dependent on v_m, so that the unpredictable behavior of axon near threshold is intuitively expected. This behavior, however, is not explicitly represented in their equations by a parameter equivalent to the standard deviation of v_{thr}, σ, or to the coefficient of variation or "relative spread" [defined by Ten Hoopen & Verveen (1963) as σ/v_{thr}] as in Fig. 3.8.

Uncertainty is not a prominent feature of isolated axonal transmission, because the currents generated by active membrane cause changes in v_m at an adjacent sensitive membrane far outside the range of uncertainty of v_{thr} or v_r. It introduces, however, a statistical characteristic of nerve function that is exceedingly important for the function of neurons in their neural masses.

3.2.3. POSTSYNAPTIC POTENTIALS IN DENDRITES

As described in Section 2.4.2, the transmembrane potential of a neuron v_m is briefly changed by a monosynaptic impulse input on a presynaptic set of axons. If the axons are excitatory, v_m increases rapidly to a maximal deviation or crest and then returns more slowly to the rest level, with a small but long lasting overshoot. If the axons are inhibitory, v_m decreases and then decays to rest in much the same way. These dendritic impulse responses, called, respectively, excitatory and inhibitory postsynaptic potentials (EPSPs and IPSPs), are basically different from the output of axons. They are nonpropagated; apparent delays within the neuron are due to the cable properties of dendrites. They are "graded" rather than all-or-none; their amplitudes are roughly proportional to the input amplitude, and there is no threshold. They have no refractory periods and can be added.

The mechanism of PSPs is the formation of loop current by the release of emf at synaptic sites in the dendritic membrane, which results in the flow

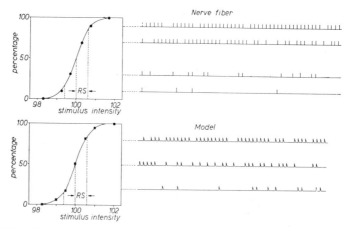

FIG. 3.8. Relation between probability of response and stimulus intensity in percentage of threshold (Ten Hoopen & Verveen, 1963).

of ions across the passive part of the dendritic membrane and the initial segment of the axon. There are two classes of mechanism for the release of emf. In electrical synapses, the loop currents generated by presynaptic axons pass across the postsynaptic membrane through special channels. The resulting changes in v_m alter g_{Na^+} and g_{K^+}. We are not concerned with this class. In chemical synapses the presynaptic axon terminals release a specialized transmitter substance that crosses to the postsynaptic membrane by diffusion, attaches to it, and alters its state.

In terms of the ionic hypothesis the alteration is described as a change in transmembrane conductance g_{PSP} that is selective for certain ions. In accordance with Eq. (23) the level of v_m in the subsynaptic dendrite changes toward the equilibrium potential for those ions v_{PSP}. The difference between the local level of v_m and the resting level of v_m elsewhere in the neuron causes current to flow. The current density j_m is given by

$$j_m = g_{PSP}(v_{PSP} - v_m). \tag{36}$$

The increase in conductance occurs mainly during the phase of the PSP before its crest. The rate of change toward the equilibrium potential is rapid because the conductance is raised. After the crest, the rate of return toward the resting level of v_m is determined mainly by the passive membrane conductance, which is relatively low.

The applicability of Eq. (23) has been tested in two ways. First the intracellular ionic concentrations have been changed by electrophoretic injection of various ions through a microelectrode (Eccles, 1957). This changes the value for v_{PSP} in Eq. (36). Second, the resting level of v_m has been changed by passing a step current across the membrane with a microelectrode prior to the onset of the testing impulse. Examples of results of the second procedure are shown in Figs. 3.9 and 3.10. If v_m is biased beyond the equilibrium potential for the PSP, $v_m < v_{PSP}$ the PSP should invert. The EPSP vanishes as v_m approaches the junctional potential between the intracellular and extracellular ionic solutions, which is not far from 0 mV (Fig. 3.9). It is inferred that the conductance increase is for all ions, but significantly for Na^+, K^+, and Cl^-, which are the predominantly available ions. The IPSP vanishes at different values of v_m, which are usually more negative than v_m (Fig. 3.10). From this evidence and from the effects of ionic electrophoresis, it is inferred that v_{IPSP} is determined by v_{K^+} or v_{Cl^-}, or by both. That is, the conductance increase is selective for K^+ or Cl^- or both.

The sources of energy for PSPs (as in the action potential) are the transmembrane concentration gradients of the relevant ions. The energy is dissipated as heat and the ionic concentrations are restored by energy from metabolic sources. The replacement gives rise to afterpotentials (see Fig.

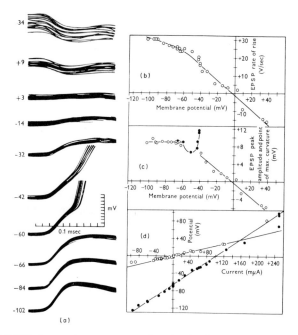

Fig. 3.9. (a) EPSPs in a motorneuron at various levels of transmembrane potential set by passing current across the membrane with an intracellular electrode. (b) Maximal rate of rise of EPSP against pre-set level of transmembrane potential. (c) EPSP peak amplitude, also against preset level of transmembrane potential. (d) Relations between applied current and recorded steady potential with electrode inside (●) and outside (○) the motorneuron (Coombs et al., 1955).

2.19, Fig. 2.22, and Section 3.1.2). For example, during an EPSP positive charge moves inwardly across the active membrane, chiefly because Na^+ ions move in and Cl^- ions move out. Positive charge moves outwardly across the passive membrane, chiefly because K^+ ions move out and Cl^- ions move in. These movements are local, because there is not sufficient time for Na^+ ions to move longitudinally in the dendrites. During the replacement phase, the metabolically derived emf are distributed over the previously active and passive membranes, but the net flow of charge is in the reverse direction. When the neuron is in the steady state, the total exchange of charge is zero. For this reason, the areas under the curves of the PSP and its afterpotential should be equal (see Section 2.5.2 and Fig. 2.22).

The synaptic conductance changes can be detected by use of the voltage clamp technique and by transmembrane current steps, but precise measurements of the time courses and spatial distributions are prevented by the complexities of dendritic geometry. Despite this limitation the conductance

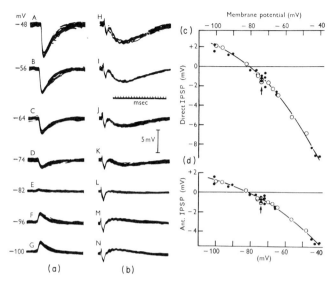

FIG. 3.10. (a) Direct (orthodromic) and (b) antidromic IPSPs in a motorneuron at various levels of transmembrane potential set by passing polarizing current across the membrane with an intracellular microelectrode. (c) Direct IPSP peak amplitude against preset level of transmembrane potential. (d) Same for antidromic IPSPs. Arrows show resting transmembrane potentials (Coombs *et al.*, 1955).

changes, and the PSPs as well, are inferred to be nonpropagating because unlike g_{Na^+} and g_{K^+} in axon membrane, the synaptic conductances g_{EPSP} and g_{IPSP} are independent of v_m. Transmission delays are attributed to the cable properties of dendrites (see Fig. 2.16). Similarly, the amplitudes of PSPs are proportional to input, because there is no v_m dependent regenerative increase in conductance. They are additive because there is no inactivation process, as for g_{Na^+}; however, proportionality and additivity are limited to a narrow range of output near a median resting level of v_m. This is because the PSP amplitudes are determined by the synaptic current j_m, which is given by Eq. (36). For each increment in v_m as a response to a previous input, the available driving force $v_{PSP} - v_m$ for another response is reduced. Moreover, there is evidence that the synaptic conductance increase in response to one input can change the membrane time constant for the response to a second input. That is, if the amplitude of the first input is large enough, the synaptic conductance channel established by the first input may shunt the passive membrane resistance, across which the current of the second response flows. This type of nonlinearity is assumed not to occur at the amplitudes occurring in the EEG and evoked activity described in this book.

3.2.4. AMPLITUDE-DEPENDENT INPUT–OUTPUT RELATIONS

In general, we know that the transmembrane potential at the soma of a neuron $v_s(t)$ increases with the total rate of pulses on excitatory afferent axons, less the total rate of pulses of inhibitory afferent axons $p_d(t)$. The pulse rate on the efferent axon $p_a(t)$ increases with $v_s(t)$. It is very difficult, however, to construct input–output functions for $v_s = G_d(p_d, t)$ and $p_a = G_s(v_s, t)$ because in most instances the functions are nonlinear and time varying, and because $p_d(t)$ cannot be precisely measured (Section 2.4.4).

A nonlinearity in pulse to wave conversion, $v_s = G_d(p_d, t)$ due to the ionic mechanism of PSPs is described in Section 3.2.3. There is another non-linearity in the relation between the crest amplitude of the presynaptic action potential v_{pre} and the crest amplitude of the PSP v_{post}. The function $v_{post} = G_d(v_{pre}, t)$ is exponential in pairs of neurons large enough to permit simultaneous intracellular recording from the pre- and postsynaptic sides of a synapse, there being an e-fold ($e = 2.73$, the natural logarithm base) increase in v_{post} for each 5-mV increase in v_{pre} (Fig. 3.11). Indirect observations suggest that the same or a similar function holds for many synapses and may be part of the mechanism for presynaptic inhibition (Section 1.2.5).

Time variance is seen when the input pulse rate $p_d(t)$ is changed from a low steady rate to a high steady rate and then back again to the low rate. During the high rate of input, successive PSPs may increase in crest amplitude (facilitation), decrease (defacilitation), or wax and wane (recruit-

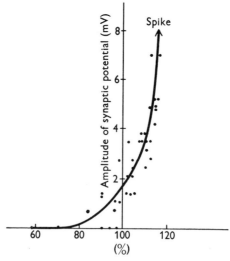

FIG. 3.11. Relation between amplitude of presynaptic action potential (varied by preliminary electrical polarization) and the size of the postsynaptic potential (Hagiwara & Tasaki, 1958).

ment). If the rate is so high that successive PSPs fuse into sustained depolarization or hyperpolarization, the input is called *tetanic*. Following
several seconds of tetanic input the successive PSPs on stimulation at a low
rate are commonly facilitated or defacilitated for several minutes. These
changes are called posttetanic potentiation and depression (see Section 1.2.5).
Depression may result from accumulation of K^+ ions outside the membranes
of the tetanized presynaptic axons, which decreases their resting v_m. If v_m is
increased above the threshold transmembrane potential, the axons undergo
what is called *cathodal block* and cannot conduct action potentials, or
depression may result from depletion of transmitter substance in the axon
terminals. Potentiation may result from fusion of hyperpolarizing afterpotentials attributable to elevation of g_{K^+}, which results in increased resting
v_m, increased amplitude of presynaptic action potentials v_{pre}, and an increase
in v_{post}, or it may be due to increased availability of transmitter substance.

The nonlinearities in wave to pulse conversion, $p_a = G_s(v_s, t)$ have been
described in terms of thresholds and refractory periods (Sections 1.2.5 and
2.1.3). Time variance has been described in terms of accommodation and
adaptation (Section 1.2.5) and threshold variation (Section 3.2.2). Linear,
time-variant approximations are described in Section 2.4.4. The location of
the trigger zone at which an impulse is initiated may vary. Large dendritic
trees may have multiple trigger zones, so that the relation between $v_s(t)$ and
$p_a(t)$ may depend on which segment of the dendritic tree receives input.

It is commonly assumed that the soma, the large proximal dendrites and
the initial segment of the axon are isopotential, so that the measured
$v'_s(t)$ is equal to $v_s(t)$ at the trigger zone, but there is evidence that the
assumption is not generally valid. Granit, Kellerth & Williams (1964) present
four criteria, by which to measure the amplitude of a sustained inhibitory input to a motorneuron. The inhibitory input is induced by
sustained stretch of muscle which is antagonistic to the muscle innervated
by the motorneuron under observation with an intracellular microelectrode.
The four criteria are; (a) reduction in magnitude of a monosynaptic EPSP
in response to single-shock stimulation of an afferent nerve; (b) reduction in
tonic firing rate evoked by sustained cathodal current delivered through an
intracellular electrode; (c) an increase in "synaptic noise," i.e., rapid random
fluctuations in background membrane potential, indicative of mixed E and
I input leading to an overall increase in g_m without change in average
v_m, and (d) sustained hyperpolarization of the neuron. Of these criteria, (b)
proves to be most sensitive, but its magnitude is not well correlated with
the magnitudes of the others.

The description in this section includes only the more common types of
amplitude-dependent nonlinearity and time variance that hold for most
neurons. The task of describing the properties of networks of 10 to 100 or

more neurons appears to be formidable. The difficulties for the most part evaporate when we consider the properties of masses of neurons, but we would be unwise to proceed without some understanding of a wide range of neural input–output relations.

3.3. Nonlinear Models for Neural Masses

Events in neural masses occur in the wave mode o_v and in the pulse mode o_p. We are chiefly concerned with waves as a time-invariant function of pulses, which is pulse to wave conversion $o_v(t) = G_1[o_p(t)]$, and with pulses as a function of waves, which is wave to pulse conversion $o_p(t) = G_2[o_v(t)]$. These nonlinear functions are to be used to define the amplitude-dependent forward gain of a neural mass.

The data on which the analysis rests consist of digitized trains of pulses from single neurons and unit clusters in an interactive mass $p'(t)$, which are treated as representative of the states of neuron subsets in the mass, and digitized segments of EEG waves $v'(t)$, which are treated as representative of the dendritic currents of the neurons in the mass. We will not seek to justify these representations at present and will defer the problems involved to later chapters. The nonlinear functions to be described are designated $v'(t) = G_1[p'(t)]$ and $p'(t) = G_2[v'(t)]$ or simply $v = G(p)$ and $p = G(v)$.

In the study of amplitude-dependent input–output relations of single neurons, the most common background state is the zero equilibrium state (Section 1.3.5). Interactive masses cannot exist unless they have background activity. When their background or "spontaneous" activity is suppressed, the masses are reduced to the KO level. Therefore, we must begin the study of amplitude-dependent input–output relations for masses by describing the background active states in the wave and pulse modes. Description is restricted to neural masses in the olfactory system, because the required data have been obtained only for these masses.

3.3.1. BACKGROUND ACTIVITY IN THE WAVE MODE

Within interactive masses intracellular recordings of potential from single neurons commonly show irregular fluctuations in the baseline between action potentials, which are referred to as "synaptic noise." This activity results from repeated bombardment of the neuron by excitatory and inhibitory impulses, and is abolished by deep anesthesia or isolation of the local region of recording from other parts of the nervous system, particularly from afferent tracts. Recognizable patterns of voltage with time commonly recur as wave forms embedded in the continuing signal that resemble EPSPs and IPSPs, but for the most part future values of potential cannot be reliably predicted from past measurements.

Extracellular recordings display the same type of fluctuations in base-line, constituting what is referred to most generally as the "electroen-cephalogram" or EEG. The most prominent, though not the only source of this activity, is the passage of synaptic currents from innumerable neurons across the fixed resistance of the extracellular medium. The EEG is an indispensible source of information about the properties of neuron popu-lations, though the extraction of relevant information is a difficult task. Recurrent patterns of waveforms can be observed (Fig. 3.12) such as spikes, spindles, slow wave complexes, and slow baseline shifts, but irregularity is an outstanding feature of the EEG.

Both synaptic noise and EEG can be treated as random time series. With the application of appropriate behavioral controls on the animals from which the recordings are made, the neural generators can be regarded as stationary, in the sense that the statistical properties of the signals remain constant over intervals of measurement lasting from several seconds to several minutes. Repeated measurement of voltage at a regular rate over a desired interval yields an ensemble of values of a random variable as a function of time. Numerous statistical procedures can be used to extract use-ful information about the processes generating these random signals, of which two are particularly relevant in the present context.

The first of these procedures is the amplitude histogram. The range of variation is divided into J equal intervals of voltage Δv, each assigned the

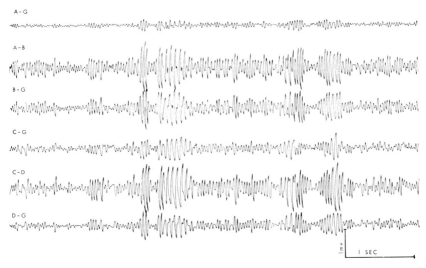

FIG. 3.12. EEG waves recorded from the prepyriform cortex of a waking cat with implanted electrodes. A and C are surface points about 6 mm apart. B and D are points deeper than A and C by 1.5 mm. G is a reference point over the frontal sinus.

bin number $m = 1, ..., J$. Each value of the random variable $v'(t)$ lies within the range of one of the bins for $v(m)$, and for each such correspondence one count is added to the bin. The amplitude histogram is normalized to an empirical probability density function by dividing the sample number in each bin by the total number in the set N, and by multiplying this ratio by the ratio of the standard deviation of the sample σ to the bin width Δv:

$$P(v) = [v(m)/N] \cdot (\sigma/\Delta v). \tag{37}$$

The probability density function of the EEG resembles a Gaussian probability density function (Fig. 3.13), though it often deviates slightly, but

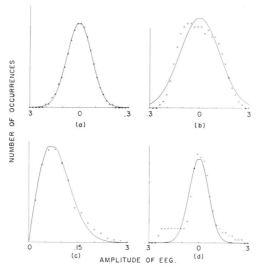

FIG. 3.13. Histograms of prepyriform EEG amplitudes. (a) Normal density, characteristic of most recording periods; $N = 21,200$. (b) Platykurtic distribution with skew to left, seen during prolonged sinusoidal oscillation $N = 256,000$. (c) Rayleigh distribution of the envelope of the EEG (successive upward and downward crests); $N = 7811$. (d) Leptokurtic distribution, seen during barbiturate spikes under moderately deep anaesthesia; $N = 134,400$. The curves in parts (a), (b), and (d) are from the normal density equation. The Rayleigh curve is given by $f(v) = \sigma^{-2}v\exp(-v^2/2\sigma^2)$, $v \geq 0$. This distribution is predicted for the output of a narrow bandpass filter with white noise input.

significantly, in being too sharply peaked (leptokurtosis) or in being skewed.

The second approach is based on autocorrelation and is aimed at disclosure of sinusoidal periodicities buried in the random background activity. The underlying assumption is required that the system be linear, or that it respond in a linear range of function to some random input. The auto-correlation function is defined as the normalized ensemble average of the product of the signal with itself displaced in time,

$$\hat{a}(\tau) = \int_0^\infty v'(t)\,v'(t+\tau)\,dt \bigg/ \int_0^\infty [v'(t)]^2\,dt. \tag{38}$$

It is a form of convolution (Section 2.3.1). For use with sampled data, this is converted to a summation, using Eq. (34) in Chapter 2:

$$\hat{a}(\tau_m) = \sum_{n=1}^N v'(t_n)\,v'(t_n+\tau_m)\,\Delta t \bigg/ \sum_{n=1}^N [v'(t_n)]^2. \tag{39}$$

Examples are shown in Fig. 3.14. The resultant autocorrelation function $\hat{a}(\tau)$ is converted by the Fourier transform to an empirical power spectrum (Fig. 3.15):

$$A(\omega) = \int_{-\infty}^\infty \hat{a}(\tau)\,e^{j\omega t}\,d\tau. \tag{40}$$

The computational steps, restrictions, and precautions have been described in many previous works (see Matoušek, 1973) and need not be recounted here. The end result is a set of estimates of the spectral distribution of energy in the currents generated by single neurons or by neural masses.

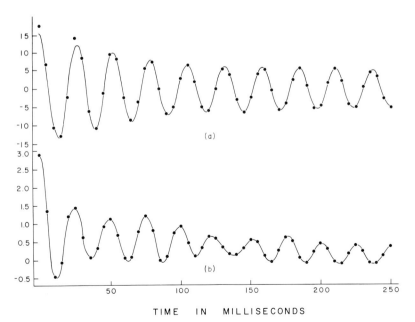

FIG. 3.14. Autocovariances from prepyriform EEGs of two cats (Freeman, 1962d).

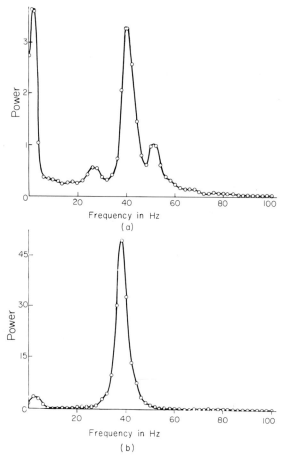

FIG. 3.15. Power spectra computed from autocovariances in Fig. 3.14 for two cats (adapted from Boudreau & Freeman, 1963).

3.3.2. BACKGROUND ACTIVITY IN THE PULSE MODE

Except when isolated or depressed by drugs single neurons in interactive masses characteristically discharge repeatedly in the absence of deliberate and controlled stimulation. Although this activity is commonly called "spontaneous" or "maintained" to distinguish it from "induced" or "evoked" activity, it will be referred to here as the "background state" or "reference level," partly because it has determinants that may vary with time and partly because the causal factors may be subject to change by deliberate intervention.

Occasional neurons are found to fire at regular intervals, so that the pulse train is adequately described by its frequency. More commonly, the intervals are not regular, nor can the future time of occurrence of a pulse be predicted reliably from knowledge of the times of occurrence of pulses in the past, as is the case with regular firing rates.

The time of occurrence of each pulse is completely independent of all others, if the pulse train manifests what is known as a "Poisson process," which can be completely described by use of the mean firing rate, n pulses/sec, assuming that n remains constant in time, i.e., that the random process is stationary. Two assumptions are required. First, it is assumed that in an arbitrarily short interval of time having the duration $\Delta\tau$ the joint probability of occurrence of a single pulse $P(1 \cap \Delta\tau)$ is uniform throughout the duration and is proportional to the product of the mean firing rate and the duration

$$P(1 \cap \Delta\tau) = n\,\Delta\tau. \tag{41}$$

For sufficiently short intervals the probability that more than one pulse will occur in $\Delta\tau$ becomes negligibly small. Either one pulse will occur, $P(1 \cap \Delta\tau)$, or no pulse will occur, $P(0 \cap \Delta\tau)$, and the sum of these two probabilities is unity

$$P(0 \cap \Delta\tau) + P(1 \cap \Delta\tau) = 1. \tag{42}$$

The second assumption is that the occurrence of a pulse in any interval τ preceding $\Delta\tau$ does not alter the probability of occurrence of a pulse in $\Delta\tau$. Therefore the joint probability that no pulse will occur in τ and $\tau + \Delta\tau$, $P(0 \cap \tau + \Delta\tau)$, is equal to the product of the probabilities that no pulse will occur in either interval

$$P(0 \cap \tau + \Delta\tau) = P(0 \cap \tau)\,P(0 \cap \Delta\tau). \tag{43}$$

Substitution of Eqs. (41) and (42) into (43) yields

$$P(0 \cap \tau + \Delta\tau) = P(0 \cap \tau) - nP(0 \cap \tau)\,\Delta\tau. \tag{44}$$

Rearrangement of terms gives

$$P(0 \cap \tau + \Delta\tau) - P(0 \cap \tau)/\Delta\tau = -nP(0 \cap \tau). \tag{45}$$

As $\Delta\tau$ is allowed to become vanishingly small, Eq. (45) becomes a simple first-order differential equation

$$dP(0 \cap \tau)/dt = nP(0 \cap \tau). \tag{46}$$

The solution is

$$P(0 \cap \tau) = e^{-n\tau}. \tag{47}$$

In the limiting case where $\Delta\tau$ approaches zero, $P(1 \cap \Delta\tau)$ also approaches zero

$$P(0 \cap 0) = \lim_{\Delta\tau \to 0} P(0 \cap \Delta\tau) = 1. \tag{48}$$

The probability that no pulse will occur diminishes from one exponentially in time following the occurrence of the last preceding pulse.

One test of whether a neural pulse train conforms to this property of a random pulse train is done by forming a histogram of the intervals between successive pulses. The time axis of the pulse train t is divided into a set of equal segments $\Delta t = \Delta\tau$, which are at least an order of magnitude shorter than the mean pulse frequency n. The intervals between a set of $N+1$ pulses are measured in units of $\Delta\tau$ and the N intervals are assigned to the appropriate bin on the time axis of the histogram τ adding one count for each interval. The empirical distribution is normalized by dividing the counts $\tilde{f}(\tau)$ by the total number of intervals N and multiplying by the ratio of the standard deviation of the distribution of intervals σ, which is equal to the mean pulse rate n, to the segment $\Delta\tau \neq 0$:

$$\hat{P}(1 \cap \tau) = [\tilde{f}(\tau)/N](\sigma/\Delta\tau) \tag{49}$$

and $P(1 \cap \tau) = \hat{P}(1 \cap \tau) + \varepsilon(1, \tau)$, where ε is an error term, P and $\hat{P}$ are the predicted and observed probabilities, and $P(1 \cap \tau) = n\tau e^{-n\tau}$ (Parzen, 1960).

Interval histograms derived from most "spontaneously" active neurons in the central nervous system resemble the form predicted for a Poisson process, but they differ in two crucial ways, reflecting violation of the two assumptions underlying the description of a Poisson process. First, the probability of the occurrence of one pulse following another is not uniform, owing to the presence of depolarizing and/or hyperpolarizing afterpotentials, associated with delayed conductance changes, absolute and relative refractory periods, or "recovery" processes involving metabolic forces. Typically the normalized interval histogram is zero for some msec after $\tau =$ zero and then rises to a maximum with increasing τ (Fig. 3.16a).

Second, the interval histograms of many interactive neurons show more than one maximum. This reflects the fact that most neurons are embedded in feedback loops in neural masses and the occurrence of a pulse at some time t is not independent of the occurrence of a pulse at some earlier or later time. For example, a mass action that imposes an inhibitory event back onto the neuron that generated a pulse decreases the probability of firing at an interval corresponding to the loop delay. The failure to fire results in subsequent disinhibition, so that the probability of firing increases at τ equal to twice the loop delay. In the interval histogram a peak occurs at τ equal to twice the loop delay.

These periodicities may be revealed by application of the technique of

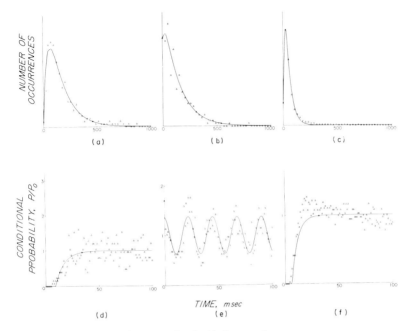

FIG. 3.16. (a)–(c) Interval histograms fitted with the equation

$$p(T) = p_0(e^{-T/\alpha} - p_f e^{-T/\beta}).$$

(d)–(f) Expectation densities fitted with the equations

$$p(T) = p_0(1 - e^{-\alpha(T-T_0)}) \qquad \text{or} \qquad p(T) = p_0[1 + p_f \cos(\omega T + \varphi)].$$

The values of the constants have no importance here. (a, d) Single bulbar unit. (b, e) Multiple bulbar units. (c, f) Single prepyriform cortical unit. $N = 80{,}000$ pulses for each frame.

autocorrelation to neural pulse trains. Eq. (89) in Chapter 2 is written as

$$p(\tau_m) = (1/N) \sum_{n=1}^{N} p'(t_n)p'(t_n + \tau_m) \Big/ \sum_{n=1}^{N} [p'(t_n)]^2. \tag{50}$$

For convenience this may be transformed (Gerstein & Kiang, 1960) to a series of sums as

$$\hat{p}(\tau_m) = Np'(\tau_m) + \sum_{n=2}^{N} p'(t_n - t_{n-1} - \tau_m) + \sum_{n=3}^{N} p'(t_n - t_{n-2} - \tau_m) + \cdots. \tag{51}$$

This corresponds to translating the origin to each successive pulse in turn and adding the pulse trains, one unit for the occurrence of a pulse in each successive bin. The resulting set of values is an expectation density function that yields two kinds of information. The empirical curves from neural pulse trains are $\hat{p}(\tau_m) = 0$ for $\tau_m = 0$ and rise to some level corresponding to the mean probability of firing. This rising curve, generally corresponding to an exponential, represents the recovery process of the neuron following a discharge, e.g., it corresponds to a relative refractory period, a hyper-polarizing afterpotential, or to inhibitory feedback (Fig. 3.16d). If after this initial recovery period the pulse-generating process is random, the probability of firing is uniform and the expectation density is nonoscillatory. The Fourier transform can be used to show the presence or absence of spectral peaks.

The interval histogram and expectation density function are useful for limited purposes. If the frequency of firing $\hat{p}(\tau)$ is zero for the first few milliseconds in both functions, the pulse train is most likely to have been generated by a single neuron. If $\hat{p}(\tau)$ is not zero in that interval, the pulse train must have been generated by two or more neurons. If the decay phase of the interval histogram is Poisson and if the expectation density is constant following an asymptotic rise in $\hat{p}(\tau)$ from zero, the pulse train can be treated as random. If these conditions are not met, the pulse train is not random. Some degree of order and predictability must exist, although those two techniques are not usually optimal for describing the order.

3.3.3. RELATIONS OF WAVES AND PULSES

The EEG of an interactive neural mass and the pulse trains of the neurons in the mass are manifestations of the active state of the mass. When appropriate averages are taken of measurements on these modes of activity, the averaged measurements are estimates of two of its state variables, namely the active states in the pulse mode or in the wave mode for one or another KI set in the neural mass. The pulse and wave functions may be generated by the same KI set or by different KI sets.

We proceed now to construct a function that relates activity in the pulse mode to activity in the wave mode. We know that the neurons in the KI sets, comprising the interactive mass, transform waves to pulses and pulses to waves, and that the output pulses of each neuron are input pulses for many other neurons. It is not necessary at the outset to know which KI sets generate the observed activities, nor do we need to know what the topology of connections is or what the level of complexity is. We must know, however, that the EEG being recorded is generated by only one KI set, and that it is not a mixture of potential differences generated by two or more KI sets in the mass. The pulse train must be generated by one neuron, or by a small number of neurons that are close together and are members of the same KI set. The momentary values of the EEG, which are $v'(t)$, and the instantaneous rate (reciprocals of the intervals) of the pulse trains $p'(t)$ vary, but their statistical properties may be constant. These are the means and standard deviations of the measured properties, such as amplitude, rate, etc., such that the mass is in a stationary state.

The location of the recording site for the EEG must be chosen carefully, so that the values for $v'(t)$ can be treated (Sections 4.3.3 and 4.4.3) as proportional to the mean for transmembrane potential $v_s(t)$ in some subset of a KI set. The pulse train must be generated by neurons in close spatial proximity to the subset of neurons generating the EEG. This is because the activity density functions are in general not uniform across neural masses. The neuron or small subset of neurons generating the pulse train must belong to a subset that is a part of the mass and not a subset of an afferent KO or KI mass.

If these conditions are met, we construct a function relating pulse values to wave values in the following way. We collect an adequate sample of from 10^4 to 10^5 pairs of measurements on simultaneous observations of $v'(t)$ and $p'(t)$ at intervals of time of 1 msec (the approximate duration of each pulse). The pulse measure is 0 or 1 depending on whether a pulse is absent or present. The wave measure is in microvolts. Let v denote the digitized amplitude and let the range be divided into W intervals of amplitude Δv.

An amplitude histogram is constructed in the standard way. The set of wave–pulse pairs is examined seriatim. For each occurrence of a value of amplitude in a given interval, a count of one is added to the designated interval. A second histogram is constructed concurrently that has one interval corresponding to each amplitude interval. If a pulse occurs in the same wave–pulse pair, a count of one is added to the second histogram. If there is no pulse, a count of zero is added.

When the total number of pairs N has been examined and classified, the number of amplitude occurrences in each interval $n_v(v)$, is divided by the total number of pairs. This gives the probability density for amplitude $\hat{P}(v)$:

$$\hat{P}(v) = n_v(v)/N. \tag{52}$$

The number of occurrences of a pulse in each amplitude interval $n_p(p, v)$, is divided by the total number of pairs to give the joint pulse–amplitude probability density

$$\hat{P}(p \cap v) = n_p(p, v)/N. \tag{53}$$

The pulse probability density is then divided by the amplitude probability density to give the pulse probability conditional on amplitude

$$\hat{P}(p|v) = \hat{P}(p \cap v)/\hat{P}(v). \tag{54}$$

This function $\hat{P}(p|v)$ is not useful because it describes the conditional pulse probability only for simultaneous occurrences. From Chapter 2 we know that there are time delays in transmission in neural masses. The active state in the wave mode leads or lags the active state in the pulse mode by a time lag T determined by the linear properties of the masses. We describe the time dependency in the following way. For each occurrence of a value for amplitude in a wave–pulse pair $v'(t)$, we ask whether a pulse $p'(t+T)$ occurred at the same time $T = 0$ as above, and then we ask whether a pulse occurred in any of the preceding k pairs, $T = -k$ (msec), and whether a pulse occurred in any of the following k pairs, $T = +k$ (msec). A two-dimensional histogram is constructed for $n_p(T, v)$. At the conclusion of the classification of observations we divide the number of pulse occurrences for each time interval and amplitude interval by the total number of pairs

$$\hat{P}(p \cap T \cap v) = n_p(p, T, v)/N. \tag{55}$$

The pulse probability density in time and amplitude is divided by the amplitude probability density

$$\hat{P}(p|T \cap v) = \hat{P}(p \cap T \cap v)/\hat{P}(v). \tag{56}$$

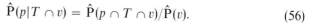

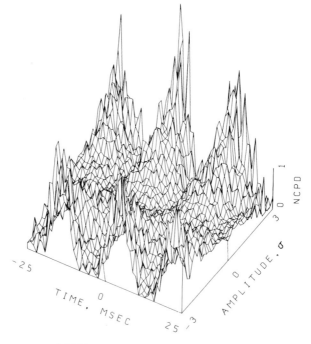

NORMALIZED CONDITIONAL
PROBABILITY SURFACE
(a)

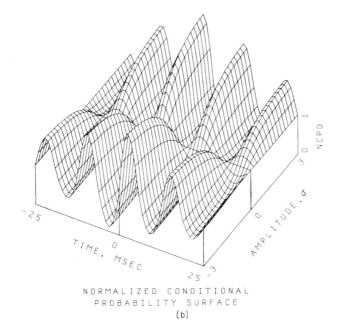

NORMALIZED CONDITIONAL
PROBABILITY SURFACE
(b)

FIG. 3.17. (a) Experimental normalized conditional probability density (NCPD) for a single mitral-tufted cell in the olfactory bulb, $\hat{P}_M(p|T \cap v \cap \omega)$. (b) Theoretical NCPD from Eqs. (69), $P_M(p|T \cap v \cap \omega)$.

This yields the pulse probability conditional on time and amplitude (Fig. 3.17). For $T = 0$, Eq. (56) predicts the same result as Eq. (54).

The limits on a table of conditional probability are set as follows. The mean $\hat{v}$ and standard deviation σ are calculated for v', and the table is truncated at $\pm 3\sigma$. This is because the number of occurrences of values of amplitude outside these limits is too few to give reliable estimates for $\hat{P}(p|T \cap v)$. The limits on time are set at $k = \pm 25$ (msec) as a compromise between the range of time needed to define $\hat{P}(p|T \cap v)$ and the cost of computation. For convenience, $\hat{P}(p|T \cap v)$ is divided by the mean pulse probability for the entire set of pairs $\hat{P}_0$ to give the normalized conditional pulse probability:

$$\hat{P}_0 = \sum_w n_p(p, 0, v)/N, \qquad \hat{P}_n(p|T \cap v) = \hat{P}(p|T \cap v)/\hat{P}_0, \qquad (57)$$

where w is the number of amplitude intervals from -3σ to $+3\sigma$. For most EEG recordings, including those described here, the mean for $\hat{v}$ is zero; at the center of the amplitude range, $v = 0$, and of course, $T = 0$ is at the center of the lag time range. An illustration of a table of the experimental normalized conditional pulse probability density $\hat{P}_n(p|T \cap v)$ is shown in Fig. 3.17a. For assistance in visualization, a table of predicted probability density $P_n(p|T \cap v)$ is shown in Fig. 3.17b. (The function is derived in Section 3.3.4.) The values of $\hat{P}(p|T \cap 0)$ and the values for $\hat{P}(p|0 \cap v)$ often tend to the value of $\hat{P}_0$. The values for $\hat{P}(p|T \cap +3\sigma)$ and $\hat{P}(p|T \cap -3\sigma)$ vary between zero and a maximum well in excess of $\hat{P}_0$. For any time $T = T_+$ at which $\hat{P}(p|T \cap +3\sigma)$ is maximal, $\hat{P}(p|T \cap -3\sigma)$ is minimal, and for any time $T = T_-$, the reverse holds.

The principal information to be found in the table is the time–dependence of the functions $\hat{P}_n(p|T \cap v)$ for $v < 0$ and $v > 0$, and the amplitude dependence of the functions $\hat{P}_n(p|T_+ \cap v)$ and $\hat{P}_n(p|T_- \cap v)$. These functions are obscured by random variations in $\hat{P}_n(p|T \cap v)$. An estimate for $\hat{P}_n(p|T \cap v)$ is obtained by averaging across the upper third of the range for $v > 0$.

$$\hat{P}_+(T) = (1/w)\sum_w \hat{P}_n(p|T \cap v_w), \qquad +\sigma \leqq v_w \leqq +3\sigma. \qquad (58)$$

Similarly for $v < 0$,

$$\hat{P}_-(T) = (1/w)\sum_w \hat{P}_n(p|T \cap v_w), \qquad -3\sigma \leqq v_w \leqq -\sigma.$$

These are usually oscillatory functions of $\hat{P}$ on T, which often tend to be sinusoidal (plotting symbols in Fig. 3.18d–f). They have the frequency of

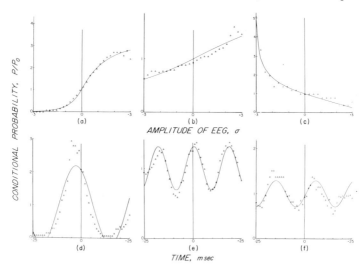

FIG. 3.18. (a)–(c) Pulse probability sigmoid curves, predicted $P_\mu(v)$ and experimental $\hat{P}_\mu(v)$. (d)–(f) Pulse probability waves, predicted $P_\mu(T)$ and experimental $\hat{P}_\mu(T)$. Reproduced with permission from W. J. Freeman, Linear analysis of the dynamics of neural masses, *Annual Review of Biophysics and Bioengineering*, **1**, 232. Copyright 1972 by Annual Reviews Inc. All rights reserved.

the concomitantly recorded EEG (see Figs. 3.12–3.15). They are approximately mirror images. The difference of the two functions divided by two,

$$\hat{P}(T) = [\hat{P}_+(T) - \hat{P}_-(T)]/2, \tag{59}$$

is called an *experimental pulse probability wave*. It is measured by a sinusoidal basis function. (Section 2.1.1) to give the predicted pulse probability wave $P(T)$

$$P(T) = P_0[1 + \tilde{p}\cos(\omega T + \varphi)e^{-\alpha|T|}], \qquad \hat{P}(T) = P(T) + \varepsilon(T), \quad (60)$$

where $\tilde{p}$ is modulation amplitude, ω is frequency in radians per second, φ is phase in radians, α is decay rate in reciprocal seconds, and $\varepsilon(T)$ is the least squares error. The value for φ is the difference between the phase of $P(T)$ and the phase of the autocorrelation function $\hat{a}(\tau)$ (Fig. 3.14) of the EEG, $v'(t)$, which is zero. Representative functions for $P(T)$ are shown in Fig. 3.18d–f.

The pulse probability conditional on EEG amplitude is called the *pulse probability sigmoid curve* and is estimated by averaging $\hat{P}_n(p|T \cap v)$ over a selected number of lag times T_k, $k = 6\text{–}12$, near which $\hat{P}(T_+, v)$ is maximal:

$$\hat{P}_+(v) = (1/k)\sum_k \hat{P}_n(p|T_k \cap v), \qquad \hat{P}_+(T_k) \gg \hat{P}_0. \tag{61}$$

Similarly, for times when $P_n(T_+, v)$ is nearly minimal,

$$\hat{P}_-(v) = (1/k)\sum_k \hat{P}_n(p|T_k \cap v), \qquad \hat{P}_-(T_k) \gg \hat{P}_0.$$

Examples are shown by the plotting symbols in Figs. 3.18a–c. The mean sigmoid curve is the average of the two functions, after reversal of the amplitude domain of $\hat{P}_-(v)$ about $v = 0$:

$$\hat{P}(v) = [P_+(v) + P_-(-v)]/2. \tag{62}$$

This is the desired function that relates probability values in the pulse mode $p(t)$ to amplitude values in the wave mode $v(t)$ for the neural mass.

3.3.4. WAVE TO PULSE CONVERSION IN THE KI SET

The next step is the derivation of theoretical functions for $p(v)$ and $v(p)$ for wave to pulse conversion and and pulse to wave conversion in the mass, which can be evaluated by fitting the functions to the empirical conditional pulse probability.

We assume the existence of a stationary background state in the KI set in which the values for wave activity are randomly distributed with zero mean and unit standard deviation, and the pulse trains of neurons in the set have constant mean rate and randomly distributed interpulse intervals, except that there is an exponential rise in pulse probability from zero to the mean probability P_0 following each occurrence of a pulse. Because for each neuron the intervals vary at random above a minimal value but with constant mean and variance, the set is time invariant, and the phenomena of adaptation and accommodation need not be considered. We assume that at any time there is a value for pulse density p_d on input axons, a value for pulse density p_a on output axons, and a value for the wave density v at each point in the set (see Section 1.3.2).

From studies of variation of threshold in neurons (Section 3.1.7) and across neurons in KO sets (Rall, 1955; Rall & Hunt, 1956), we know that the thresholds in the KI set are distributed with respect to wave amplitude v. If an increment of change Δv occurs in the direction of inhibition $v < 0$, the number of neurons below threshold must increase, so that p_a decreases by Δp_a. But p_a cannot decrease indefinitely, because when all the neurons are below threshold, p_a is zero and cannot be negative. Moreover, the decrement Δp_a must decrease as p_a diminishes. Because we do not know a priori the nature of the distribution of thresholds, we assume as an approximation that the ratio $\Delta p / \Delta v$ is proportional to p_a times a constant γ_i. In the limit as $\Delta v \to 0$,

$$dp_a / dv = \gamma_i p_a, \qquad v \leqq 0. \tag{63}$$

If an increment of change Δv occurs in the direction of excitation $v > 0$, then the density of pulse output p_a must increase by an increment Δp_a. As p_a increases, neurons in the set are more likely to be in a relative refractory period, or undergoing a hyperpolarizing afterpotential based on a delayed increase in g_{K^+} such that they are less likely to fire. We assume that a limiting value p_{max} exists in the KI set as a whole for p_a, and that the increment in Δp_a for an excitatory increment Δv is equal to the difference $p_{max} - p_a$ time a constant. In the limit as $\Delta v \to 0$,

$$dp_a / dv = \gamma_e (p_{max} - p_a), \qquad v > 0. \tag{64}$$

The limiting pulse density p_{max} for the set is not the same as the maximal rate for any one neuron. Rather it represents an average over both periods of high firing rate and subsequent periods, which neurons require before firing once again at a high rate.

The solutions to the differential equations are

$$p_a = \begin{cases} p_o \exp(\gamma_i v), & v \leqq 0, \\ p_{max} - (p_{max} - p_o) \exp(-\gamma_e v), & v \geqq 0. \end{cases} \tag{65}$$

The value for p_{max} is determined from the condition that p_a has a continuous derivative with respect to $v = 0$, and p_o is mean pulse rate.

$$dp_a/dv. = \begin{cases} \gamma_i p_o \exp(\gamma_i v), & v \le 0, \\ \gamma_e (p_{max} - p_o (\exp(-\gamma_e v))), & v \ge 0. \end{cases} \quad (66)$$

$$p_{max} = p_o [(\gamma_i/\gamma_e) + 1].$$

Therefore,

$$p_a = \begin{cases} p_o \exp(\gamma_i v), & v \le 0, \\ p_o [1 + (\gamma_i/\gamma_e)(1 - \exp(-\gamma_e v))], & v \ge 0. \end{cases} \quad (67)$$

Equation (67) predicts that as $v \to \pm \infty$, p_a asymptotically approaches $p_a = 0$ and $p_a = p_o(1 + \gamma_i/\gamma_e)$. The pattern of a sigmoid curve with horizontal asymptotes is commonly observed (Fig. 3.18a and d) for $\hat{p}(v)$. The value for the ratio is found empirically to be $\gamma_i/\gamma_e = 2$. Therefore, γ_e is set equal to γ, and

$$p_a = \begin{cases} p_o e^{2\gamma v}, & v \le 0, \\ p_o(3 - 2e^{-\gamma v}), & v \ge 0, \end{cases} \quad (68)$$

$$G(v) = p_a \quad \text{for all } v.$$

Equations (68) are used to infer the function for wave to pulse conversion in the KI mass, because the limits apply to values for pulse density and not wave density.

The results are listed in Table 3.1 for fitting Eqs. (68) and Eqs. (60) to the pulse probability gradients and waves from mitral–tufted (KI_M) cell pulse trains of anesthetized cats and rabbits (see Section 4.3.1), with N the number of pulse–wave samples at 1000/sec; σ the standard deviation of EEG amplitude; p_x the total number of pulses divided by $N/1000$; p_o, ω, φ, and $\tilde{p}_m$ the values obtained following nonlinear regression of Eqs. (60) onto the pulse probability waves; and γ is obtained by fitting Eq. (68) to pulse probability sigmoid curves. EEG frequency is the average peak frequency from the power spectra of selected short segments (5 sec) of the wave train. Additional values in Table 3.2 are from pulse trains of Type A neurons in the prepyriform cortex of anesthetized cats and rabbits (see Section 4.4.1).

A curve from Eqs. (68) is fitted to $\hat{P}_+(v)$ in parts (a) and (b) of Fig. 3.18. The surface shown in Fig. 3.17b is generated by Eqs. (68) and (60), modified to fit $P_+(T)$ as follows:

$$P_+(T) = 1 + \cos(\omega T + \varphi)e^{-\alpha|T|},$$

$$P(p|T \cap v) = \begin{cases} P_+(T)e^{2\gamma v}, & vP_+(T) \le 0, \\ P_+(T)(3 - 2e^{-\gamma v}), & vP_+(T) \ge 0. \end{cases} \quad (69)$$

In most sets of data, the power spectrum of the EEG displays two prominent peaks, one at the respiratory rate near $\omega = 6$ rad/sec (1 Hz) and

TABLE 3.1

MEASUREMENTS ON CONDITIONAL PULSE PROBABILITIES OF PULSE TRAINS FROM NEURONS IN THE KI_M (MITRAL-TUFTED) SET IN THE BULB $P_M(p|T \cap v \cap \omega)$

Sample[a]	N ($\times 1000$)	σ (μV)	p_x (pps)	p_o (pps)	ω (rad/sec)	EEG (rad/sec)	φ (rad)	$\tilde{p}$	γ (1/mV)
1	64	35	27.3	27.6	484	490	1.62	.24	2.0
2	99	23	9.3	9.6	436	427	1.79	.34	2.7
3	320	23	9.2	9.4	356	346	1.26	.32	3.9
4	256	79	15.3	14.1	168	170	.41	1.22	9.8
5	304	62	2.3	2.5	192	188	.43	.90	5.6
6	234	31	30.8	29.2	455	465	2.11	.64	7.4
7	262	34	3.7	3.5	441	427	2.48	.40	4.2
8	234	33	13.4	12.8	481	458	2.52	.39	1.6
9	121	66	12.6	16.7	237	226	1.14	.35	1.9
10	304	23	15.2	14.5	415	396	2.37	.29	2.5
11	96	36	30.6	31.4	377	377	1.83	.33	2.0
12	253	39	17.4	17.6	321	320	1.40	1.13	14.5
13	96	37	18.8	18.2	286	283	.88	.81	5.3
14	80	46	6.9	4.2	282	289	.39	.85	9.7
15	109	32	13.9	15.5	281	290	.23	.67	7.0
16	83	28	16.9	16.2	311	302	1.62	.51	3.4
17	80	44	10.4	11.4	288	288	2.29	.32	1.9
18	80	53	23.2	22.4	295	295	1.10	.78	5.7
19	80	49	12.1	12.3	289	283	.96	.73	5.2
20	80	56	17.1	18.3	275	289	1.19	1.04	7.6
21	80	29	10.8	10.5	263	270	1.40	.40	3.3
Mean:		41	15.1	15.1	330	328	1.40	.60	5.1
SD:		15	7.8	7.8	91	89	.71	.30	3.3

[a] Includes multiple units (mean = 21.2 pps) and single units (mean = 9.5 pps).

the other at a characteristic frequency near $\omega = 250$ rad/sec (40 Hz) (Fig. 3.15a). The pulse probability wave $\hat{P}(T)$ oscillates at corresponding frequencies. Measurement requires a set of two basis functions,

$$P(T) = \sum_{j=1}^{2} P_j \cos(\omega_j T + \varphi_j) e^{-\alpha_j |T|}, \qquad \hat{P}(T) = P(T) + \varepsilon(T). \quad (70)$$

Alternatively, activities at the two frequencies are separated by filtering prior to construction of a table $\hat{P}(p|T \cap v)$ for each frequency band. The function $P(T)$ varies with the frequency ω or frequency range $\Delta\omega$ over which the conditional pulse probability is determined. Therefore another dimension ω is introduced, $\hat{P}(p|T \cap v \cap \omega)$ and $P(p|T \cap v \cap \omega)$. Figure 3.17a

TABLE 3.2

MEASUREMENTS ON CONDITIONAL PULSE PROBABILITIES OF PULSE TRAINS IN THE KI_A
(SUPERFICIAL PYRAMIDAL) SET IN THE PREPYRIFORM CORTEX $P_A(p|T \cap v \cap \omega)$

Sample	N ($\times 100$)	σ (μV)	p_x (pps)	p_o (pps)	ω (rad/sec)	EEG (rad/sec)	φ (rad)	$\tilde{p}$	γ (1/mV)
1	144	44	28.4	40.3	345	364	$-.16$	.31	1.78
2	144	52	22.6	23.2	298	339	$-.03$	.08	.44
3	54	57	8.8	49.2	437	398	.01	.08	.44
4	144	46	5.9	5.6	292	314	.63	.24	2.21
5	144	42	6.5	6.7	298	302	$-.07$	.27	1.49
6	128	53	2.2	2.2	313	333	$-.23$	.16	3.79
7	96	33	7.4	7.3	259	248	$-.17$	.22	1.62
8	96	49	27.3	28.1	284	279	$-.39$	.13	2.84
9	120	54	13.2	13.5	271	282	.42	.29	.72
10	80	44	4.5	4.4	302	306	.27	.24	1.09
Mean:		47	12.7	18.0	310	316	.03	.20	1.64
SD:		± 7	± 12.4	± 16.5	± 50	± 44	$\pm .32$	$\pm .08$	± 1.08

displays $P_+(T)$, for a frequency range fixed by filters with half-amplitude
frequencies near 60 rad/sec (10 Hz) and 500 rad/sec (125 Hz). The evidence
available at present indicates that $\hat{P}(v)$ is not dependent on frequency.

3.3.5. PULSE TO WAVE CONVERSION IN THE KI SET

The chief nonlinearities in the conversion of input pulse density p_d to
wave density v occur in the presynaptic terminals (Fig. 3.11) and in the
ionic mechanism of the dendritic PSPs. The presynaptic nonlinearity depends
on pulse amplitude, which in turn depends either on synaptic mechanisms
for presynaptic inhibition (Sections 1.2.5 and 3.2.4) or on after potentials
or other changes established by preceding pulses. We assume that the input
pulse trains are random occurrences at an invariant mean rate, so that
accommodation and adaptation need not be considered (Section 1.2.5).

We assume that the spatial density of synaptic activity is sufficiently low
during background activity of neural masses that the conductance change
for each PSP does not affect any other PSP. The remaining nonlinearity is
imposed by the nature of the ionic emf of the PSPs. According to the ionic
hypothesis (Sections 3.1.1–3.1.3) the emf for each PSP asymptotically approaches zero as the wave amplitude approaches the equilibrium potential
for the PSP. We can represent the equilibrium potential for the EPSP by
$\tilde{v}_e$, which is the potential difference between v_{EPSP} and $v = v_o = 0$, and the

equilibrium potential for the IPSP by $\tilde{v}_i$, which is the potential difference $v_{\mathrm{IPSP}} - v_o$.

We infer that for an increment Δp_d in excitatory input pulse density $p_d > p_o$ there is an increment in wave density Δv. From Section 3.2.3 and Eq. (36) we infer that

$$\Delta v = \zeta_e(\tilde{v}_e - v)\,\Delta p_d, \qquad v \geqq 0, \tag{71}$$

where $\tilde{v}_e > 0$ is the average equilibrium potential for the EPSP of neurons in the KI set, and ζ_e is a constant. In the limit as $\Delta p_d \to p_o$,

$$dv/dp_d = \zeta_e(\tilde{v}_e - v), \qquad p_d \geqq p_o, \quad v \geqq 0. \tag{72}$$

Similarly,

$$dv/dp_d = \zeta_i(\tilde{v}_i - v), \qquad p_d \leqq p_o, \quad v \leqq 0. \tag{73}$$

where $\tilde{v}_i < 0$ is the average equilibrium potential for IPSPs of neurons in the KI set, and ζ_i is a constant. From the condition that the derivatives are continuous at $v = 0, \zeta_e\,\tilde{v}_e = \zeta_i\,\tilde{v}_i$. A constant $r < 0$ is defined such that $\tilde{v}_e = r\tilde{v}_i, \zeta_i = \zeta$, and $\zeta_e = \zeta/r$. Therefore, for $\zeta > 0$ and $r < 0$,

$$dv/dp_d = \begin{cases} \zeta(v - \tilde{v}_i), & v \leqq 0, \\ \zeta\,[(v/r) - \tilde{v}_i], & v \geqq 0. \end{cases} \tag{74}$$

Equations (74) are solved for p as a function of v because v is the independent variable in experimental determination of pulse probability sigmoid curves for both wave to pulse and pulse to wave conversions. The solutions are

$$p_d = \begin{cases} p_o + (1/\zeta)\ln[1 - (v/\tilde{v}_i)], & v \leqq 0, \\ p_o + (r/\zeta)\ln[1 - (v/r\tilde{v}_i)], & v \geqq 0, \end{cases} \tag{75}$$

$$G(v) = p_d \qquad \text{for all } v.$$

Equations (75) imply that as $v \to \tilde{v}_i$, $p \to \infty$, and that as $v \to +3\sigma$, p approaches or equals zero, but not asymptotically.

A common form of $\hat{P}_+(v)$ or $\hat{P}_-(v)$ is that in which it rises to a high value as v, respectively, approaches $+3\sigma$ or -3σ (Fig. 3.18c and f). Curves from Eqs. (75), P(v), have been fitted to $\hat{P}(v)$, computed from the pulse trains of type B neurons in the prepyriform cortex (see Section 4.4.1). The average value for $\tilde{v}_i$ is -3.06σ, and the average value for r is -5.7 (Table 3.3). The vertical asymptote implies that Eqs. (74) represent the function for pulse to wave conversion because the limit applies to values for wave density and not pulse density. The experimentally derived parameter, $r = -5.7$, is consistent with intracellular measurements of v_{EPSP} and v_{IPSP}, as in Figs. 3.9 and 3.10. For example, if v_{IPSP} is equal to a junctional potential of -4 mV, and

TABLE 3.3

MEASUREMENTS ON CONDITIONAL PULSE PROBABILITIES OF PULSE TRAINS FROM NEURONS IN
THE KI_B (CORTICAL GRANULE) SET IN THE PREPYRIFORM CORTEX $P_B(p|T \cap v \cap \omega)$

Sample	N ($\times 1000$)	σ (μV)	p_x (pps)	p_o (pps)	ω (rad/sec)	EEG (rad/sec)	φ (rad)	$\tilde{p}$	ζ (1/pps)	r	$\tilde{v}_i$ $(\sigma)^b$
1	144	34.8	7.5	7.3	357	364	−1.87	.19	.49	−2.3	−3.04
2	144	37.5	5.4	6.2	331	339	−1.78	.46	.36	−9.1	−3.07
3	160	43.6	26.7	25.3	324	326	−1.72	.21	.08	−9.9	−3.15
4	144	44.6	25.5	27.2	310	303	−2.25	.48	.06	−2.6	−3.06
5	144	61.5	20.1	18.9	285	296	−2.05	.12	.66	−6.0	−3.05
6	144	38.5	5.5	5.5	326	342	−1.67	.29	.68	−4.3	−3.03
7	144	50.2	3.8	3.8	351	327	−2.11	.35	.59	−9.2	−3.02
8	112	44.7	2.2	2.0	347	312	−1.70	.37	.42	−1.9	−3.07
Mean:		44.4	12.1	12.0	329	326	−1.89	.31	.42	−5.7	−3.06
SD:		8.1	10.0	9.9	24	23	.22	.13	.24	3.4	.04
9^a	144	49.2	6.1	6.2	184	297	−1.47	.16	.67	−2.8	−3.01
						114					
10^a	144	47.2	2.8	2.7	212	322	−1.68	.29	.82	−4.8	−3.02
						136					

[a] Trimodal EEG power spectrum.
[b] Units of standard deviation of EEG amplitude, σ.

the resting potential is −70 mV, the expected value for v_{IPSP} is −81 mV
(Fig. 3.10).

3.3.6. THE FORWARD GAIN OF THE KI SET

The transfer function for a KI set has been reduced (Section 1.3.4) to a
single feedback loop between two KO subsets in the set: a transmitting
subset and a receiving subset. The transfer function for each KO subset,
which is identical to the transfer function of the other, consists of four
serial parts. The afferent path is linear $F_1(s)$ and transmits in the pulse mode
to the nonlinear pulse to wave conversion mechanism $G_1(p)$. The dendrites
operate linearly in the wave mode $F_2(s)$ and transmit to the nonlinear
wave to pulse conversion mechanism $G_2(v)$ which determines the output.
In serial order,

$$F(s,p,v) = G_2(v)\,F_2(s)\,G_1(p)\,F_1(s). \qquad (76)$$

The analysis of this system containing two nonlinear elements is simplified
by piecewise linear approximation. Both nonlinear elements have bilateral
saturation. For any bounded input domain, the nonlinear function between
input and output is approximated by a straight line segment over the

domain. The nonlinear gain is replaced by a fixed gain coefficient given by the slope of the line segment. The dependence of the slope on the input domain is now derived.

If the pulse to wave mechanism does not itself saturate but does transmit over a sufficient range to saturate the wave to pulse mechanism, the output is determined by $G_2(v)$ (Fig. 3.19b), and $G_1(p)$ can be replaced by a linear function $g_1(p_o)$. In this case the order of elements can be changed:

$$F(s, p, v) = G_2(v) g_1(p_o) F_2(s) F_1(s). \tag{77}$$

If the pulse to wave mechanism does not transmit over a sufficient range to saturate the wave to pulse mechanism, but itself undergoes saturation, the output is determined by $G_1(p)$ (Fig. 3.19a), and $G_2(v)$ is replaced by a linear function[†] $g_2(v_o)$:

$$F(s, p, v) = F_2(s) g_2(v_o) G_1(p) F_1(s). \tag{78}$$

By redefinition of the loop transfer function between the two KO subsets (see Section 2.4.1),

$$F(s, p, v) = g_2(v_o) G_1(p) F_1(s) F_2(s). \tag{79}$$

By definition,

$$
\begin{aligned}
F(s) &\triangleq F_1(s) F_2(s) = F_2(s) F_1(s), \\
G(p) &\triangleq G_1(p) \quad \text{iff} \quad G_2(v) \approx g_2(v_o), \\
G(v) &\triangleq G_2(v) \quad \text{iff} \quad G_1(p) \approx g_1(p_o), \\
g_o &\triangleq g_1(p_o) g_2(v_o).
\end{aligned}
\tag{80}
$$

The transfer function of the KO subset consists of a linear and a nonlinear element in series in one of three alternative forms.

$$
F(s, p, v) =
\begin{cases}
G_2(v) g_1(p) F(s), & p = p_o, \\
F(s) g_2(v) G_1(p), & v = v_o, \\
g_1(p) g_2(v) F(s), & v = v_o, \quad p = p_o.
\end{cases}
\tag{81}
$$

[†] With regard to notation, the sigmoid input–output curves are designated $G(v)$ and $G(p)$. The derivatives of the curves are designated $g(v)$ and $g(p)$. The fixed number that is the slope of a straight line replacing $G(v)$ or $G(p)$ is designated by a subscripted coefficient such as g_1, g_2, g_e, or g_i. The slope is given by $g(v)$ or $g(p)$ for a fixed value of v or p such as $v = v_e^*$ as in $g_e = g(v_e^*)$. Both g_e and g_i are forward gain coefficients of the KO transmitting subsets in KI_e and KI_i sets, and by assumption the square root of the feedback gain K_e or K_i is equal to the forward gain, as in $K_e^{;5} = g_e$ and $K_i^{;5} = g_i$. More generally, $G(v)$ and $G(p)$ can be viewed as operators that give the rules for converting one time function $v(t)$ to another time function $p(t)$ or vice versa, whereas $g(v)$ and $g(p)$ can be viewed as functions that give the rules for determining a fixed number such as g_e from a real number such as v_e^*. The nonlinear operators should perhaps more precisely be written as $G(p) = G[p(t)]$ and $G(v) = G[v(t)]$, but this is avoided in order to simplify the notation.

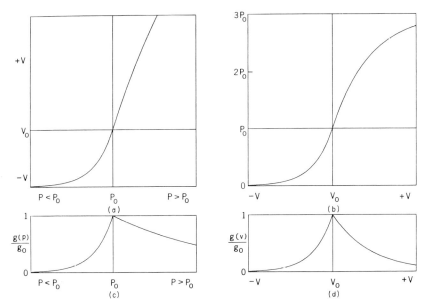

FIG. 3.19. (a, b) Input–output curves for (a) pulse to wave conversion and for (b) wave to pulse conversion. (c, d) Gradients of input–output curves, from which the forward gains are derived.

The amplitude-dependent nonlinear gains are determined by the ratios of output to input, and are designated by $g(p)$ and $g(v)$:

$$g(p) \triangleq dv/dp_a, \qquad g(v) \triangleq dp_a/dv, \tag{82}$$

where dv/dp_d is given by Eqs. (74), and dp_a/dv is derived from Eqs. (68). For v in dimensionless units of γ,

$$dp_a/dv = \begin{cases} 2p_o e^{2v}, & v \leqq 0, \\ 2p_o e^{-v}, & v \geqq 0. \end{cases} \tag{83}$$

For v and $\tilde{v}_i$ in units of ζ/γ (microvolts per pulses per second),

$$dv/dp_d = \begin{cases} v - \tilde{v}_i, & v \leqq 0, \\ v/r - \tilde{v}_i, & v \geqq 0. \end{cases} \tag{84}$$

By definition at $v_o = 0$,

$$g_o = -2p_o \tilde{v}_i. \tag{85}$$

If there is no saturation of the wave to pulse mechanism,

$$g(p) = \begin{cases} g_o [(\tilde{v}_i - v)/\tilde{v}_i], & v \leqq 0, \\ g_o [(r\tilde{v}_i - v)/r\tilde{v}_i], & v \geqq 0. \end{cases} \tag{86}$$

This is shown graphically in Fig. 3.19c. If there is no saturation of the pulse to wave mechanism,

$$g(v) = \begin{cases} g_o\, e^{2v}, & v \leqq 0, \\ g_o\, e^{-v}, & v \geqq 0. \end{cases} \tag{87}$$

This is shown in Fig. 3.19d.

Equations (85) and (87) imply that there are three sets of determinants of forward gain. First, the two empirical rate constants, γ and ζ, denote the lumped properties determining the sensitivities respectively of the trigger zones and of the synaptic mechanisms in the dendrites. In the following chapters these are treated as invariants.

Second, the forward gain depends on the background state, which is specified by the mean pulse rate p_o and the relative mean level of hyperpolarization $\tilde{v}_i$ or depolarization $\tilde{v}_e = r\tilde{v}_i$. By assumption the synaptic equilibrium potentials, v_{IPSP} and v_{EPSP}, are fixed by the electrochemical ionic concentration gradients across the membrane, and $\tilde{v}_i = v_{IPSP} - v_o$ and $\tilde{v}_e = v_{EPSP} - v_o$ change as the result of changes in the background level of polarization v_o. Intuitively we can expect p_o and v_o to increase or decrease together (Fig. 3.20a), but the form of the covariance is not known. A set of input–output curves for $G_2(v)$ is shown in Fig. 3.20a for three sets of values of p_o and v_o. The same three curves are shown in Fig. 3.20b, with two differences. The values on the ordinate are normalized by dividing p by p_o, and the values on the abscissa are scaled to give equal width of display for three ranges of wave amplitude v. The steepest sigmoid curve has the widest range of v.

Because of the way in which the experimental data are acquired and processed (Section 3.3.3), $v_o = 0$ in each determination of $p(T, v)$, and the range on the abscissa is fixed at $\pm 3\sigma$ (Fig. 3.20b). Further, the data are normalized with respect to p_o [Eq. (57)]. If v_o and p_o increase, then from Eq. 85 there is an increase in g_o, and the change in the form of the graphic display consists in an increase in the steepness of the sigmoid curve (Fig. 3.20c). However, an increase in σ for the EEG also increases the steepness. That is, in the form of Fig. 3.20c, the input–output curves are comparable to the experimental curves for pulse probability conditional on EEG amplitude (Fig. 3.21), in which the conditional probability is normalized, $\hat{P}/\hat{P}_0$, and the range of EEG amplitude is $\pm 3\sigma$ (standard deviations). Examples are shown for three conditions of recording mitral–tufted units from the olfactory bulb in an anesthetized cat. In part (a) the data are from the condition breathing through the mouth as well as the nose. For part (b) breathing is only through the nose, the variance of EEG amplitude is greater, and the value for $\hat{P}_0$ is increased. For part (c), EEG variance and $\hat{P}_0$ are diminished by a small supplemental dose of pentobarbital. The upper frames show

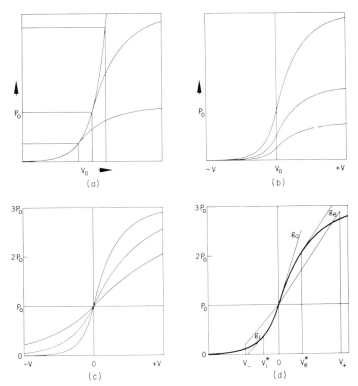

FIG. 3.20. Stages in the procedure of normalization by which the forward gain is derived for wave to pulse conversion. (a) Representation of increasing gain (slope of curve for wave to pulse conversion) with increase in both mean pulse rate p_o and mean wave amplitude v_o. (b) Effect of normalization of v_o. (c) Effect of normalization of p_o. (d) Replacement of the sigmoid function by a linear function over an operating range given by v_+ to v_-. The slope of the line segments defines a point of tangency on each limb of the sigmoid curve, and those two points define the effective operating amplitudes v_e^* and v_i^* (see Section 6.1.1).

conditional pulse probability at a lag time when the pulse probability is highest for high EEG amplitudes, and the lower three frames from the same tables show the conditional pulse probability at a lag time when the pulse probability is lowest for high EEG amplitudes (Section 3.3.3). In the following chapters, p_o and v_o are treated as constant determinants of fixed g_o over sets of AEPs within stable states and as variable (varying g_o) between stable states (Section 1.3.5) of KO, KI, and KII sets.

Third, the forward gain depends on the instantaneous wave amplitude v. In piecewise linear approximation we treat each AEP or time segment of the EEG as having a certain amplitude range v_+ and v_-, and we infer that the sigmoid input–output curve can be approximated by a straight

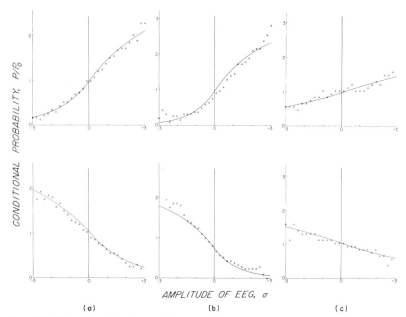

FIG. 3.21. Examples of pulse probability sigmoid curves $P_+(v)$ and $P_-(v)$ from a bulbar neuron in three conditions: (a) oral breathing, (b) nasal breathing, both under light anaesthesia and (c) under moderate anaesthesia. Curves are from Eqs. (68). Each set of triangles shows $\hat{P}_+(v)$ above and $\hat{P}_-(v)$ below (Section 3.3.3). The upper three curves should be compared with the three curves in Fig. 3.20c.

line over that range, as in Fig. 3.20d, which has a certain slope. With fixed p_o and v_o the slope is different for differing values of v_+ and v_- in differing AEPs and EEG segments. We can express the range for each event as a fixed value of v over the duration of the event. The fixed value is designated as v_e^* for a KO_e or KI_e and v_i^* for a KO_i or KI_i set. The numerical values cannot be obtained directly. Instead, a value of $g(v)$ is found by techniques to be described, and Eq. (87) is solved for v_e^* or v_i^*. In terms of Fig. 3.20 the value of $g(v^*)$ specifies the slope of a straight line, which is tangent to one of the sigmoid curves at a point, and the value for v at that point is the value for v_e^* or v_i^*. That is, in piecewise linear approximation of the dynamics of a KO set within a KI or KII set (see Section 1.3.4), the nonlinear input–output curve is replaced by a straight line segment that is tangent to the curve at the effective value for the wave amplitude of the KO set over the duration of the approximation. The slope of the line is designated g_e or g_i.

The forward gain without saturation g_o can be estimated numerically by means of Eq. (85). For this purpose, it is necessary to identify the K-sets in the mass and to determine which sets generate the wave and pulse trains. This is discussed further in Section 6.2.4, after the required topology has been described.

The requirement for a sigmoid nonlinear input–output curve of distributed neural sets is now well recognized (Wilson & Cowan, 1972; Grossberg, 1973; Zetterberg, 1973). The unique features of the curves derived from electrophysiological data are the following. The monotonically increasing curves have a single inflexion, which implies that there is a single maximum in the gain as a function of amplitude. (If the saturation at the lower end were attributed only to thresholds of the neurons, then the distribution of thresholds would be unimodal). The maximal forward gain and the maximal rate of change in gain with change in wave amplitude both occur near the central operating point. Both curves are asymmetric; the curve for pulse to wave conversion in the ratio of 6 to 1, and the curve for wave to pulse conversion in the ratio of 2 to 1. The asymptotes for the wave to pulse conversion at $p = 0$ and $p = 3p_o$ are also in the ratio of 2 to 1. This states that the theoretical maximum for pulse density in the population is directly coupled with the mean pulse density p_o so that both change together when the population changes from one stable level to another. The physiological basis for the relations between the curvatures and the asymptotes is obscure and deserves detailed exploration. These features are critical determinants of the interactive properties of KII sets which are described in Chapter 6. In particular, the near-threshold impulse responses of KI and KII sets are often exquisitely sensitive to changes in input amplitude, which reflects the maximal dependence of gain on amplitude near $v = 0$.

CHAPTER 4

Space-Dependent Properties of Neurons

4.1. Potential Fields of Single Neurons

A main source of data on the dynamics of neurons is the measurement of potential in the extracellular volume surrounding them. From measurement at n points in the volume $v'(t, x, y, z)$, we infer the existence of distributions of current $\mathbf{j}(t, x, y, z)$ in the volume. Our interest lies in learning which neurons or parts of neurons sustain the emf generating the current, and how the values for the current relate to the active states of the generating neurons. Our basic approach is to measure a given field $v'(t, x, y, z)$, postulate a time-varying distribution of emf constituting an active state $o(t, x, y)$, predict the field $v(t, x, y, z)$, and compare it to $v'(t, x, y, z)$. If the degree of fit is unacceptable, we reject the model.

There are three main difficulties. First, there is only one field v for each model, but there are many possible models for each field v'. The acceptance of a model is not based only on goodness of fit, but on whether the geometry and parameters of the model conform in detail to the anatomy and physiology of the generating neurons or neuron parts. It is more difficult to develop and justify a model than to test it.

Second, the data required for testing proposed models must consist of measurements of potential at many locations in a neural mass. The measurements are made sequentially by moving an exploring electrode to each of a predetermined set of points for sampling, or preferably by simultaneous recording at many points. Each technique has advantages and limitations, and optimally both are used for any given mass. In practice the sheer bulk of the data and the need for concise display present formidable problems.

Third, the labor of calculating predicted fields of potential by hand is prohibitive. Computers are required to perform the immense number of additions. There are several technical methods available for calculating the potential, including use of the dipole moment and *solid angle* (Woodbury, 1961); *differencing* (see footnote at the end of Section 4.1.2) to estimate source–sink density (Howland *et al.*, 1955; Haberly & Shepherd, 1973); discrete networks approximating *current vector* fields (Rall & Shepherd, 1968); and the *equivalent electrostatic* field (Lorente de Nó, 1947b, Horowitz & Freeman, 1966). The electrostatic approach is rigorous, conceptually simple, and easy to apply with computer assistance. It is described and applied in the next sections. (For more general treatments, see the work of Plonsey, 1969 and Nicholson, 1973).

4.1.1. BASIS FUNCTIONS FOR MEASUREMENT OF POTENTIAL IN SPACE

The medium of the nervous system is water, which is divided by lipid barriers (the cell membranes) into a very large number of internal closed compartments (the cells) and an external compartment extending throughout the brain (the extracellular medium). The charge in this medium is composed of ions, not electrons. Because electrical measurements of potential do not distinguish types of ions, the amount of charge in a given volume of tissue is the algebraic sum of positive and negative ions appropriately weighted for valence. Except at cell membranes the sum in any prescribed volume is everywhere equal to zero. At cell membranes a deficit of negative charge is not distinguishable from an excess of positive charge by electrical measurement and by convention is equal to a net positive charge.

If the charge is distributed in space, then the charge dq in the differential volume of space $dx\,dy\,dz$ at each point is the charge density

$$\xi(x, y, z) = dq/dx\,dy\,dz. \tag{1}$$

The presence of a fixed charge q is observed by placing a small test charge q_0 near it and measuring a force $\mathbf{F}$ acting on the test charge. For a distance η between q and q_0, by Coulomb's law,

$$\mathbf{F} = \varepsilon(qq_0/\eta^2)\,\mathbf{i}, \tag{2}$$

where ε is a proportionality constant characteristic of the medium and $\mathbf{i}$ is a unit vector. The force is a vector in the direction of the line $\mathbf{i}$ joining q and q_0. A set of measurements of $\mathbf{F}$ in the space surrounding q delineates a field of force $\mathbf{F}(x, y, z)$. The intensity of the electrical field at each point $\mathbf{E}(x, y, z)$ is given by

$$\mathbf{E}(x, y, z) = (1/q_0)\,\mathbf{F}(x, y, z). \tag{3}$$

Work is required to move the test charge along lines of force in the field. For the field of force of q an increment of work dw is given by

$$dw = -\mathbf{F}\,dr \tag{4}$$

where dr is an increment of distance along the line qq_0. From Eq. (2) and by integration from an infinite distance to a point η at q_0,

$$w = \varepsilon(qq_0/\eta). \tag{5}$$

The potential at η is

$$v = w/q_0. \tag{6}$$

If we neglect dissipative forces such as friction, the value for the potential is independent of the path on which the test charge is moved. If the test charge is moved back to its starting point, the work is recovered. The field is conservative; therefore, the potential is a scalar function. The potentials due to multiple charges q_n in a field are additive:

$$v = \varepsilon \sum_{n=1}^{N} q_n/\eta_n. \tag{7}$$

The locus of points in space having the same value of potential is an isopotential surface. Just as a field of force can be described by lines of force, a field of potential can be described by a set of isopotential surfaces. The intersection of these surfaces with a plane used for illustration gives isopotential curves or lines. The isopotentials are continuous closed curves that do not cross. Lines of force cross isopotential surfaces only perpendicularly to them.

The values of potential in a field are measured with respect to the values at some reference level of potential. There is no unique value for potential at each point, because the values depend on the potential at a selected reference point. Ordinarily this point is conceived as lying at some great distance from the field of interest, so that the reference potential is $v = 0$, and at $r = \infty$, there is a zero isopotential surface. Any other point may suffice and may be required by technical considerations. In any case, measurements are made not of potential but of potential difference.

This poses a critical problem in the measurement of neural electrical activity. The fields to be measured may or may not extend throughout the brain, so that the reference point (location of the reference electrode) should ideally be placed on some other part of the body. In so doing, however, the potential fields generated by the heart, eyes, skeletal muscles, etc. may dominate the recordings and obscure the patterns sought. Therefore, it is often necessary to record potential differences in a neural field in which the reference potential is not equal to zero, i.e., both reference and exploring electrodes are deliberately placed in the field. This is known as *bipolar recording*. In other instances the attempt is made to place the reference electrode at the margin of the field of interest, e.g., low behind the ears or over bony cavities such as the frontal sinus. By convention (not by necessity) this is known as *monopolar recording*. Only when a reference point has been chosen is the potential function defined.

From the definition of potential the intensity of the electric field is related to the rate of change of potential with distance. The rate of change is zero along isopotentials and maximal in directions perpendicular to isopotentials. The maximal rate of change of potential in the vicinity of a point is the gradient. It is designated by ∇v and is given by

$$\nabla v = \partial v/\partial x \, \mathbf{i} + \partial v/\partial y \, \mathbf{j} + \partial v/\partial z \, \mathbf{k}. \tag{8}$$

where $\mathbf{i}$, $\mathbf{j}$, and $\mathbf{k}$ are unit vectors in the x, y, and z directions. The field of force per unit charge is given by

$$\mathbf{E} = -\nabla v. \tag{9}$$

This is a vector lying opposite to the direction of maximal increase in potential with distance. The gradient is positive uphill, whereas force is positive downhill.

The rate of change of the field of force in the vicinity of a point is designated by $\nabla \mathbf{E}$ and is called the *divergence*. It is dependent on the charge density at the point. If the charge density is zero,

$$\nabla \mathbf{E} = 0. \tag{10}$$

If the charge density is not zero,

$$\nabla \mathbf{E} = \varepsilon \xi(x, y, z). \tag{11}$$

Both the charge density and the divergence are scalar quantities. In relation to potential from Eq. (9), $\nabla \mathbf{E} = -\nabla^2 v$ and

$$\nabla^2 v = \partial^2 v/\partial x^2 + \partial^2 v/\partial y^2 + \partial^2 v/\partial z^2. \tag{12}$$

At each point in an electrostatic field the divergence is proportional to the charge density (Poisson's equation)

$$\nabla^2 v = \varepsilon \xi(x, y, z). \tag{13}$$

In regions containing no charge it is equal to zero (Laplace's equation)

$$\nabla^2 v = 0. \tag{14}$$

The solutions to Eqs. (13) and (14) for any ξ and for specified boundary conditions provide the basis functions for measurement of fields of potential.

Example A. Consider two infinite planar sheets of positive and negative charge having uniform density, $\xi = \pm 1$. Let these lie parallel to the y and z axes at the values of $x = \pm c$, so that the charge density is a function of x. In this case two of the partial derivatives are zero,

$$d^2v/dy^2 = d^2v/dz^2 = 0. \tag{15}$$

For points not in the two sheets, the charge density is zero,

$$d^2v/dx^2 = 0, \qquad x \neq \pm c. \tag{16}$$

The general solution is

$$v = ax + b. \tag{17}$$

Let us take for reference the value of potential at $x = 0$ as $v_0 = 0$, and designate the potential at $x = c$ as v_c. From symmetry the potential at $x = -c$ is $-v_c$, and for the space between the planes,

$$ac + b = v_c, \qquad -ac + b = -v_c.$$

Here $b = 0$ and $a = v_c/c$, so that

$$v = (v_c/c)x. \tag{18}$$

The potential is a linear function of distance from the origin between the planes. The gradient is

$$\nabla v = (v_c/c)\mathbf{i}, \tag{19}$$

so that the field of force is uniform both in direction and magnitude between the planes. Outside the planes the boundary condition is that the potential not be infinite as x approaches infinity. Thereby $a = 0$ and $b = \pm v_c$. The potential is uniform on each side, and is equal to $+v_c$ for $x > +c$ and to $-v_c$ for $x < -c$. The gradient is everywhere zero, so there is no external field of force. □

Two infinite sheets of charge of opposite sign may be considered to form a hollow closed surface for which the radius of curvature is very large in comparison to the distance between the sheets $2c$. In this case the negative side corresponds to the interior of a neuron at rest, and the double sheet is its lining membrane. Charge separation occurs only at the membrane, and the potential is constant throughout the interior, but it differs from the exterior by an amount dependent on the charge density function. If the reference potential is chosen as $v = 0$ at $x = \infty$ outside the surface, the potential inside the surface is $v_m = -2v_c$.

4.1.2. BASIS FUNCTIONS FOR POTENTIAL IN CURRENT FIELDS

Up to this point charge has been considered as fixed in space. In the nervous system extracellular electrical fields arise only in conjunction with moving ions. By convention this current is said to flow in the direction of movement of net positive ions (cations), even if the actual flow is wholly owing to movement of negative ions (anions) in the opposite direction. In a bounded conductor the current is defined as the amount of net positive charge passing a complete cross section of the conductor per unit time

$$dq \text{ (coulombs)}/dt \text{ (seconds)} = i \text{(amperes)}.$$

In a volume conductor the magnitude of current is defined in terms of the current di flowing through a specified surface area dA which is the current density

$$di \text{(amperes)}/dA \text{(meters}^2) = \mathbf{j} \text{(amperes/meters}^2)$$

where $\mathbf{j}$ is a current vector perpendicular to dA.

Where does the moving charge come from (source) and go to (sink)? Because neurons can neither create nor destroy charge, there are no true sources and sinks in the brain. There are only two other possibilities. Either the charge is being pumped from one region to another, with changes in charge density $d\xi/dt$ in those regions, or it is moved in a closed loop. Neurons, however, cannot generate the immense electrical forces required to alter charge densities in aqueous solutions, except across membranes at which the voltage gradients are on the order of 10 million V/m. Even here the separation of charge does not change overall charge density, but only the local densities of anions and cations by separation of them. In the nervous system charge density ξ is constant at all times and places in the brain to within the smallest dimensions of a recording microelectrode. Therefore current flows only in closed loops.

The total current across any closed surface in the nervous system (such as a membrane) is always and at every instant zero. Current in must equal current out. These facts are expressed in mathematical form in terms of the spatial derivative or divergence of the current density $\nabla \mathbf{j}$. This is a scalar quantity expressing the rate of contraction or expansion of the flow at a point. The only two ways to increase the divergence are to add more charge or to decrease the density. In a source-free and sink-free volume such as the nervous system the divergence and charge density are related to each other by the equation of continuity,

$$\nabla \mathbf{j} + d\xi/dt = 0. \tag{20}$$

Because $d\xi/dt = 0$,

$$\nabla \mathbf{j} = 0. \tag{21}$$

Now we consider the relation between current, force, and potential. The movement of ions results from the application of force. As discussed in Chapter 3, electromotive forces of several kinds operate in the membranes of neurons, but in the volumes within and surrounding each neuron the only significant forces acting on ions are electrostatic and resistive. The mass of an ion is much greater than that of an electron, but in the frequency band characteristic of neural activity (0–10 kHz) there are no significant relaxation or inertial effects. Owing to the low magnetic permeability of water in comparison to its electrostatic permeability and to the low rates of change in flow, there are no significant magnetic effects. The ions do not interact viscously to produce vortices or eddy currents (such as occur in currents of water or air). All of these negatives mean that in the fields of force manifested as neural fields of potential, the ions move only in the direction of the lines of force. The rate of movement depends on the field intensity $\mathbf{E}$ and on the volume specific resistance ρ in units of ohm $\cdot$ cm^2/cm (see footnote in Section 2.3.4). For each point the function relating $\mathbf{j}$ to $\mathbf{E}$ is described by Ohm's law,

$$\mathbf{j} = \rho^{-1}\mathbf{E}. \tag{22}$$

The divergence is found by taking the spatial derivative of the current density at each point:

$$\nabla \mathbf{j} = \nabla(\rho^{-1}\mathbf{E}). \tag{23}$$

By expansion,

$$\nabla \mathbf{j} = \mathbf{E}\nabla\rho^{-1} + \rho^{-1}\nabla\mathbf{E};$$

in a homogeneous isotropic medium

$$\nabla\rho^{-1} = 0. \tag{24}$$

From Section 4.1.1,

$$\nabla\mathbf{E} = -\nabla^2 v, \tag{25}$$

so from Eqs. (23)–(25)

$$\nabla \mathbf{j} = -\rho^{-1}\nabla^2 v. \tag{26}$$

By Eq. (21), in a source-free and sink-free region,

$$\nabla^2 v = 0. \tag{27}$$

This result is formally equivalent to Laplace's equation (14). In a region containing a source, by Eq. (20),

$$\nabla^2 v = \rho \, d\xi/dt. \tag{28}$$

There is a formal equivalence of Eq. (28) to Poisson's equation (13) in which ρ is replaced by ε and $d\xi/dt$ is replaced by ξ. The equivalence means that it is permissible to represent the lines of current in a homogeneous medium by lines of force in an electrostatic field. The sources and sinks at which the current lines start and end can be represented by equivalent positive and negative charge. What is not made clear is how this can be done in a medium without sources and sinks.

Moreover, Eq. (26) depends on two simplifications regarding the medium of the nervous system, first that it is homogeneous and isotropic, and second that it is purely resistive. It is clear that every current loop associated with a neural field must twice cross a high impedance, which is the membrane of the generating cell. In the near vicinity of an active neuron there are impedances imposed by the membranes of adjacent neurons. Beyond this near range (up to .3 mm) there are differences in the specific conductances of the grey matter, white matter, and the cerebrospinal fluid. Beyond the brain there are barriers imposed by the coverings (the dura and the skull) and ultimately by the surface of the head. None of these features is entirely negligible, although not all need to be introduced into the analysis of specific fields. The requirement, however, to introduce the membrane impedance discontinuity of generating cells is inescapable. That is, $\nabla \rho^{-1}$ cannot be zero.

The solution in every case requires the separation of each current field into two parts, one inside and one outside the neuron. The membrane becomes a boundary for both the inner and outer fields. An area of current outflow is a source for the outer field and a sink for the inner field. Obviously they are equal in total absolute magnitude. The reverse holds for an area of current inflow. For both the inner and the outer fields, the sum of fictitious sources equals the negative of the sum of fictitious sinks, because the total transmembrane current adds to zero. Both the impedance discontinuity and the operation of transmembrane electromotive forces are included in the boundary conditions already specified by the distribution of fictitious sources and sinks, which we will represent by j.

The set of fictitious sources and sinks (transmembrane current) is represented by an equivalent set of positive and negative charge, which we will represent by ξ or q. The potential at each point in the inner and outer fields is predicted by means of Eq. (7).[†]

4.1.3. POTENTIAL FUNCTIONS FOR THE CORE CONDUCTOR

The core conductor (Section 2.3.4) represents a cylindrical membrane of infinite length and negligible diameter. We assume here that it has a non-uniform set of emf in its membrane at any instant of time. What are the expected functions of potential for the inner and outer fields?

The cylinder is conceived to lie along the x axis. The set of emf is given the values $E_m(x) = -1$ for all $x < 0$, $E_m(x) = 1$ for all $x > 0$, and zero for $x = 0$. The parameters are constant and homogeneous: r_m and r_i (Section 2.3.4) are the membrane and internal specific resistances, and ρ is the volume specific resistance of the external medium.

The difference in emf in the two parts of the membrane establishes a longitudinal potential difference across the internal and external conducting media, so that longitudinal current flows to the right outside the cylinder and to the left inside the cylinder. The total longitudinal resistance from $x = 0$ to $x = \pm\infty$ is infinite, so that for $x = \pm\infty$ both the longitudinal current, $i_e(x)$ and $i_i(x)$, and the transmembrane current $j_m(x)$ are zero.

The field of current is divided into an internal part and an external part.

[†] Equations (27) and (28) are the basis for the method of differencing as a means to determine the sources and sinks giving rise to a field of potential in a neural mass. Suppose that a set of measurements of potential $v(X)$ is made in a three-dimensional lattice of recording sites X in a mass either simultaneously or at fixed latency with respect to a stimulus time. Each site X is at the center of a cube formed by the adjacent six sites X_n, $n = 1, ..., 6$, lying each at the center of a face of the cube. The potential difference $v(X_k) - v(X_n)$ between the center and each of the six sites is assumed to be proportional to the current flowing into the cube through the face of that site. Then in a medium with homogeneous specific resistance the net current inflow (sink density) or outflow (source density) at the center site is proportional to $j(X_k) = \sum_{n=1}^{6} [v(X_k) - v(X_n)]$.

The method is conceptually simple, but in practice it is difficult to get measurements at sites along a number of parallel tracks sufficiently close together and in parallel planes sufficiently close together without damaging the tissue by electrode penetrations. The method tends to accentuate differences due to variation in background activity and time variance of the preparation on successive penetrations, as well as errors in the directions of successive penetrations which are never quite parallel. According to Eq. (27), the sum over all sites $\sum_{all} \kappa j(X_k)$ in the mass should be zero. Further, the results of the method must be checked by computing a potential field by means of Eq. (7) from $j(X_k)$ and comparing it with the measured field for correspondence. In the author's experience the method does not give results approaching these conditions due to the above sources of error. Therefore, differencing yields hypotheses about $j(X)$ and not definitive results. The anatomy of the mass provides an alternative source of hypotheses about $j(X)$. This is the source used in Chapter 4. Irrespective of the source, however, Eq. (7) is required to test the hypotheses regarding $j(X)$ against $v'(X)$.

For any loop current path, the total resistance along the path in the external medium is much less than the total resistance along the internal path, so when the internal current field is considered, the external specific resistance is assumed to be $\rho = 0$. Therefore the potential is taken as zero everywhere outside the membrane. The potential across the membrane at any point except $x = 0$ is

$$dv_m(x)/dx = -r_i i_i(x). \tag{29}$$

The longitudinal current $i_i(x)$ satisfies

$$di_i(x)/dx = -(1/r_m)[v_m(x) + E_m(x)] \tag{30}$$

for all x except $x = 0$. At $x = \pm \infty$, $i_i(x) = 0$. Therefore $v_m(x)$ is given by

$$v_m(x) = \begin{cases} 1 - e^{-x/\lambda}, & x \geq 0, \tag{31} \\ -(1 - e^{x/\lambda}), & x \leq 0, \tag{32} \end{cases}$$

$$\lambda = (r_m/r_i)^5. \tag{33}$$

The internal longitudinal current from Eq. (29) is

$$i_i(x) = (-1/\lambda r_i) dv_m(x)/dx$$
$$= (-1/\lambda r_i) e^{-x/\lambda} \qquad \text{for all } x. \tag{34}$$

The transmembrane current density is

$$j_m(x) = \begin{cases} (1/r_m) e^{-x/\lambda}, & x > 0, \\ (-1/r_m) e^{x/\lambda}, & x < 0, \tag{35} \\ 0, & x = 0. \end{cases}$$

These functions are illustrated in Fig. 4.1. For the internal field of current $j_m(x)$ is represented by a set of fictitious continuously distributed sources and sinks. For the external field there exists a mirror image set

$$j_e(x) = -j_m(x). \tag{36}$$

These are replaced by a set of equivalent charge densities.

$$\xi_e(x) \propto j_e(x). \tag{37}$$

For purposes of measurement, the continuous distribution of charge density is divided into N short segments of length Δx, and a value for point charge is assigned to each value of x_i:

$$q_n = \xi_e(x_n) \Delta x. \tag{38}$$

The electrostatic potential is calculated for a set of points (x, y, z), in the

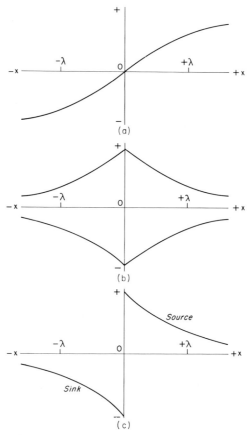

FIG. 4.1. Relations between (a) potential, (b) longitudinal current (force), and (c) trans-membrane current (source–sink density) for a core conductor in the steady state, in which the transmembrane emfs are uniform along $x > 0$ and $x < 0$ but are unequal at $x = 0$.

external medium by summation over the discrete charge:

$$v(x, y, z) = \varepsilon \sum_{n=1}^{N} q_n/\eta_n, \qquad \eta_n = [(x - x_n)^2 + y^2 + z^2]^{.5}. \qquad (39)$$

Example A. A set of isopotentials illustrating $v(x, y, z)$ from Eqs. (31)–(39) is shown in Fig. 4.2a. □

Example B. The procedure is repeated for the condition in which λ is a variable, such that $\lambda(x) = 1$ for $x \geq 0$, and $\lambda(x) = 0.33$ for $x < 0$. The resulting asymmetric function of $v(x, y, z)$ in Fig. 4.2b is commonly observed for single neurons and sets of neurons. It results when the active membrane ($E_m \neq 0$)

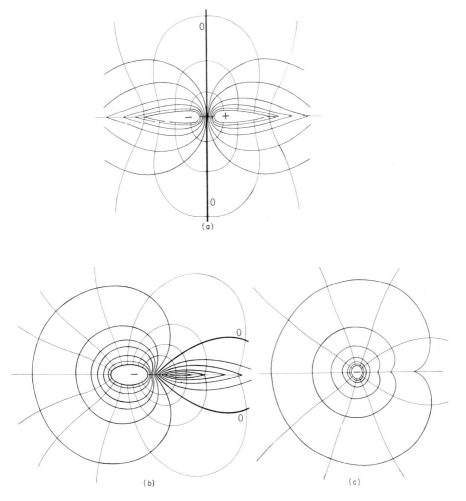

FIG. 4.2. Extracellular contours of potential (dark curves) and current lines (light curves) for a core conductor as specified in Fig. 4.1. (a) $+\lambda = -\lambda$, corresponding to the idealized case of a neuron with symmetric active and passive membranes. (b) $+\lambda = -3\lambda$, corresponding to the case of the active dendritic tree operating into the axonal tree (at left). (c) $+\lambda = -9\lambda$, showing the effect of marked disparity in λ, as in the case of the injury potential of a severed nerve, which is maximally negative at the cut end (at left).

constitutes most or all of the dendritic membrane, and the passive membrane ($E_m = 0$) is restricted to the axon, or vice versa. The dendrites have larger cross-sectional area, lower internal longitudinal resistance, and greater length constant than the axon. □

The pattern for $v(x, y, z)$ in Fig. 4.2a occurs only when the parameters of the active and passive membranes are equal, such as when one of two comparable dendritic trees of a neuron is active and the other is passive.

Example C. $\lambda(x) = 1$ for $x > 0$ and $\lambda(x) = 0.1$ for $x < 0$. This pattern for $v(x, y, z)$ in Fig. 4.2c is observed when an axon or a bundle of axons is cut at $x = 0$. For several minutes to an hour or more there is loop current due to inward diffusion of Na^+ ions through the cut end and outward active transport of Na^+ ions across the adjacent intact membrane. The potential with respect to a far distant point is known as the "injury" or "demarcation potential" and is everywhere negative. ☐

These examples illustrate a general principle. The sum of current sources and sinks across the membrane is zero, and the sum of equivalent positive and negative charge is zero. The charge density, however, in general is not uniform. If the source density is higher than the sink density, the field of potential is asymmetric, and the peak value of positive potential is greater than the negative of the peak value of negative potential, as shown in Figs. 4.2b and c. That is, total source $= -$(total sink), but in general, $v_{max} \neq -v_{min}$.

Example D. If the core conductor is surrounded by a nonconducting medium, the external conducting medium is reduced to a thin cylindrical film. This corresponds to the experimental condition, in which an axon or nerve is excised from surrounding tissue and suspended in air or oil. In this case the radial derivatives, $\partial v_m(y)/\partial y = \partial v_m(z)/\partial z$ are negligibly small and are set equal to zero, so that

$$\nabla^2 v_m = d^2 v_m(x)/dx^2. \tag{40}$$

The solution for $v_e(x)$ in the external field is identical to the function of potential $v_m(x)$, except that the sign is reversed and there is a difference in reference potential

$$v_e(x) = -\varepsilon[v_m(x) + v_o] \tag{41}$$

where ε is a positive real number and v_o is the mean transmembrane potential at rest. ☐

More generally, the external potential function is a mirror image of the internal potential function, if the lines of current in both compartments are constrained parallel to the axis of the core conductor. This principle is an important feature of certain types of neural mass (see Section 4.3.5).

Equation (23) can be solved for the more general case in which ρ is non-uniform and is a function of space $\rho(x, y, z)$ by appropriate methods (e.g.,

Nicholson, 1973). In the systems described here ρ is sufficiently uniform to be treated as a constant.

The advantage of the electrostatic equivalent model is that the potential can be evaluated at each point by scalar summation. If a computer is not available for simulation, the simplest alternative is to construct a three-dimensional network of discrete current lines to represent the vector field of current, and to solve the network equations for the potential difference between any two points.

4.1.4. POTENTIAL FIELDS OF AXONS

The core conductor model is applied to nerve axon for analysis of the distributions of both exogenous and endogenous currents, i.e., during both electrical stimulation and recording (Section 2.3.4 and 3.2.1). The analysis is simplified by suspending the nerve fiber or trunk in air or oil, which leaves only a thin sheath of conducting fluid around the nerve. This constrains the external field to a single dimension, so that the functions of potential, the gradient, and the longitudinal current outside the fiber are mirror images of those inside, except for the resting level for the potential with respect to a distant point (Example D, Section 4.1.3). For example, the action potential recorded monopolarly at the surface of an axon or nerve suspended in air is almost a mirror image of the intracellular potential except for scale and baseline. Over a straight and unbranched segment of axon or nerve the peak amplitude and velocity θ of the emf $E(t - T)$ are constant, and $T = x/\theta$. The field may be considered as stationary with respect to a set of co-ordinates undergoing translation at a velocity $-\theta$. It is a moving dc field. As the field moves past a fixed recording electrode the potential as a function of time $v_x(t)$ is directly proportional to potential as a function of distance $v_t(x)$. The time and space derivatives are related by the velocity

$$\partial v_t(x)/\partial x = (-1/\theta)\,\partial v_x(t)/\partial t. \tag{42}$$

In the frog sciatic nerve (Lorente de Nó, 1947b) a low-level stimulus is used, which activates only the largest axons having the highest conduction velocities. Higher-intensity stimulation activates smaller, slower-conducting axons, which leads to dispersion and to multiple crests in the extracellular recording. Both stimulating and recording electrodes are placed on a limited segment of nerve (e.g. 5 cm), which is twice as long as the wavelength of the compound action potential. Wavelength (28 mm) is the product of velocity (e.g., 28 m/sec) and duration (e.g., 1 msec). It is necessary to kill or inactivate the terminal end of the nerve trunk in order to avoid the appearance of two partly overlapping action potentials, the second being inverted, due to recording of the traveling wave at the terminal end with the reference electrode.

This so-called "monopolar" recording between an intact and an inactivated membrane displays the effects not only of changes in transmembrane emf but also of intramembranal longitudinal emf between the two electrodes. These secondary events called "longitudinal polarization" by Lorente de No (1947b) give rise to some of the multiple deflections (β, γ, ε) seen to follow the main spike ($A\alpha$) in the compound action potential (Example A, Section 2.3.1).

This artifact is avoided by recording bipolarly between two electrodes placed close together on the nerve in comparison to the wavelength of the action potential. This gives the difference in potential Δv between the two points separated by Δx, varying as a function of time. The bipolar record is treated as proportional to the gradient $\partial v_e/\partial x$ by Eq. (42). The potential v_e as a function of time (or distance) is obtained by graphic integration. The slope gives the divergence $\partial^2 v_e/\partial x^2$, which is proportional to transmembrane current density (Fig. 4.3).

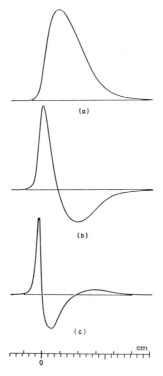

FIG. 4.3. The external compound action potential ($-v_e$) of the frog nerve (alpha fibers) and (b, c) its first two derivatives (Lorente de Nó. 1947b).

This empirical curve $\partial^2 v_e/\partial x^2$ is used to specify the values of a set of 26 point charges fixed on a line segment. From these values, the external field for the action potential is calculated using Coulomb's law (Fig. 4.4). The value of potential along each line parallel to the axon at a distance r is the potential as a function of distance and is proportional to the potential as a function of negative time. These are the basis functions to predict the waveforms recorded by electrodes spaced at a distance η from the center of the nerve trunk (Fig. 4.5).

Experimental verification is done by placing the nerve on a piece of blotting paper soaked with normal saline and recording action potentials at different distances from the nerve. Although the field is calculated (Fig. 4.5) for a volume and the measurements are made in a plane, agreement is satisfactory (Fig. 4.6).

Comparison of the extracellularly derived action potential $-v_e$ in Fig. 4.3, with the action potential recorded intracellularly (Fig. 3.5b) shows that the two observed events are similar, except for the difference in sign of potential. The similarity is explained in Example D in Section 4.1.3. Comparison of the curve $-\partial^2 v_e/\partial x^2$ in Fig. 4.3c with action potentials recorded extracellularly in a conducting medium (Figs. 2.13 and 4.7) shows similarity in waveforms with reversal of sign. Both events are triphasic. From Eq. (147) in Chapter 2 the second spatial derivative of potential is proportional to transmembrane current density. Therefore, the monopolar extracellular recording of an action potential in tissue reflects the change in transmembrane current density as the action potential travels past the recording electrode, whereas the monopolar extracellular recording in air reflects the

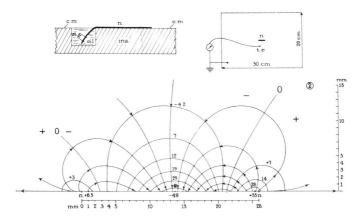

FIG. 4.4. Field of the compound action potential and lines of current in the external medium. The diagrams on top show the experimental arrangement, where n is the nerve, cm the conducting medium, and ins the insulating material (Lorente de Nó. 1947b).

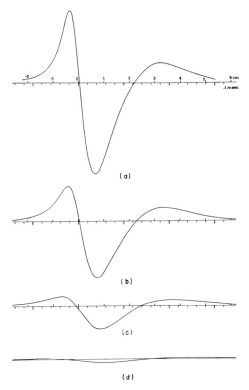

Fig. 4.5. Theoretical action potentials of nerve in a conducting medium at points (a) 2.4, (b) 4, (c) 8, and (d) 16 mm from the nerve axis (see Fig. 2.13) (Lorente de Nó. 1947b).

change in transmembrane potential. Neither of these two relations is an exact correspondence.

The triphasic wave form is seen characteristically at the midpoint of a long nerve fiber. Positivity associated with current outflow occurs at the foot and tail of the axon spike; the intervening negativity is associated with current inflow and with the region of active membrane. However, at the site of initiation of an action potential, e.g., in the initial segment, the wave form lacks the initial positive component; it is diphasic negative–positive. At the site of termination of the axon the second positive component is lacking; the wave form is again diphasic but positive–negative (Fig. 4.6). A theoretical basis for these facts is given by Lorente de Nó (1947b).

4.1.5. Nodes and Branched Fibers

The picture of the action potential as a smooth wave gliding unchanging along an endless conductor is a useful fiction that holds for large non-myelinated axons and for large bundles, but not for most neurons. They are

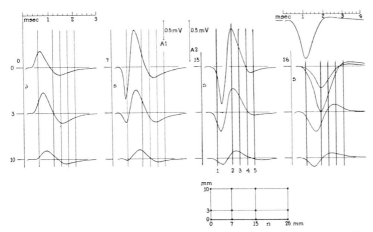

FIG. 4.6. Recorded action potentials at the indicated points in the medium. The volley enters the conducting medium at $x = 0$ and leaves it at $x = 26$. At both points the wave form is diphasic. Between them it is triphasic. The field in Fig. 4.4 corresponds to the instant labeled 2 (Lorente de Nó. 1947b).

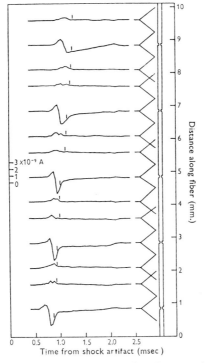

FIG. 4.7. Action currents recorded between the points shown at the right in respect to the positions of nodes of Ranvier of a single myelinated axon, demonstrating saltatory conduction (Huxley & Stämpfli, 1949).

shaped like bushes and trees, not like straws. Excitation which has begun at some section of the membrane develops and dies out with some characteristic time course. A field of current grows and collapses in a form determined by the geometry of the local cylindrical system. At the height of intensity of this field, excitation begins at one or more other parts of the tree, often relatively far distant. New, different, and partly overlapping fields of current arise. These are conditioned by differing but interconnected geometries. At the new crest, still another generation of fields begins to grow. The potential recorded in the vicinity of a neuron with respect to some distant point is the sum of all these successive and time-varying events, weighted according to distance from the active membranes.

An example of this is the sequential activity of nodes of Ranvier in single myelinated axons dissected free from nerve trunks. Active membranes during electrical activity of such axons occur only at nodes, and agents such as cocaine, sodium-free solutions, cold, ultraviolet radiation, etc., which block conduction, do so only when applied to nodes and not to internodes. The excitation of a node is achieved by an outward current across the nodal membrane, which is established either by an exogenous stimulating current or by activation of a nearby node. This is followed by an intense but brief inward flow and a secondary outward flow, when secondary activation of an adjacent node has occurred. At internodal segments there is only outward flow. The crest of the inward flow occurs at progressively later times for nodes at greater distances from the site of initial activation (Fig. 4.7 from Huxley & Stämpfli, 1949).

The nodes of Ranvier are located about 2 mm apart in each of the larger axons of the frog sciatic nerve, but they are randomly spaced with respect to nodes in other axons in the nerve. The record of activity by a single electrical stimulus applied to the nerve trunk is the smoothed average of successive activity at many nodes. The average transmembrane current density and the average transmembrane potential estimated by recording in air are consistent with each other, but they do not contain information about the local distributions and intensities of currents of single fibers.

The application of core conductor theory (Section 2.3.4) to the branched dendritic trees of central neurons is largely a problem in geometry, together with the search for neuroanatomical correlates. Rall (1959; 1968) provides an extensive set of solutions for differing types of neuron geometry, particularly for varying degrees of branching. Explicit parameters are given for the number of primary dendritic trunks (treated as cylinders) extending from the soma (treated as a sphere), the distance to the first branch point, diameter, degree of taper (if any), and length constant, the number of secondary branches and their parameters, tertiary branches, and so forth.

For a particular degree of branching, which appears to lie in an intermediate range between the extremes of paucity and profuseness of dendritic branching revealed by Golgi staining techniques, the entire tree can be described as if it were a single unbranched cylinder, in so far as its electrical relationships with the soma are concerned (Fig. 4.8). Distances x along neuron branches can be expressed in units of the length constant λ so that electrotonic length X is given by

$$X = x/\lambda. \tag{43}$$

The length X can be expected to vary with distance along a branching system, even if the specific resistivities of the membrane and of the inner medium are homogeneous, because as the branch diameter decreases, the surface area diminishes proportionately, but the cross-sectional area decreases as the square of the diameter. Rall (1962) has defined a "generalized electrotonic distance" as

$$Z = \int_0^x [1/\lambda(x)]\,dx. \tag{44}$$

For the steady state the equation for the core conductor may be written as

$$(d^2V/dZ^2) + K\,dV/dZ = V \tag{45}$$

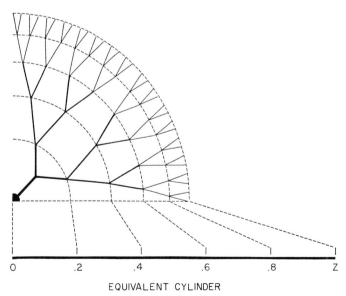

EQUIVALENT CYLINDER

FIG. 4.8. Reduction of a single branched dendritic tree ($\sum_i d_i^{3/2} = \text{const}$) to an equivalent cylindrical core conductor (Rall, 1962).

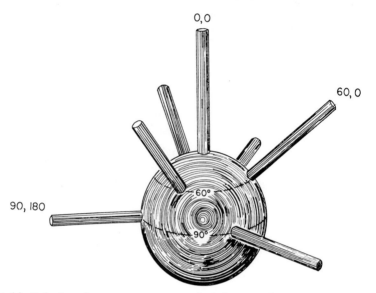

FIG. 4.9. Reduction of neuron geometry to a spherical soma and a set of radiating cylinders representing multiple dendritic trees (Rall, 1962).

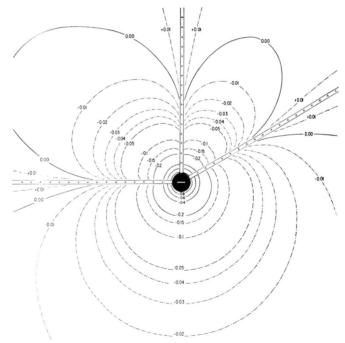

FIG. 4.10. Cross section through the field of potential of the neuron schematized in Figs. 4.8 and 4.9, in which the soma provides the sink and the dendritic trees provide the current source (see Fig. 4.2) (Rall, 1962).

for that case in which dendritic branching satisfies the relation

$$\sum_j (d_j)^{3/2} = (d_0)^{3/2} e^{KZ}. \tag{46}$$

Here the sum of the diameters d_j, each raised to the $\frac{3}{2}$ power, of all outgoing branches at the jth branch point having the electrotonic distance Z from the soma must equal the diameter of the main trunk d_0 to the $\frac{3}{2}$ power times e^{KZ}. The constant K represents the degree of branching. When $K = 0$, the system is equivalent to an unbranched cylinder of infinite length (Fig. 4.8). Negative and positive values for K denote lesser or greater profuseness of branching. For $K = \infty$ the tree is equivalent to a cut end, and for $K = -\infty$ the system is equivalent to a sealed end.

An example is shown in Fig. 4.9 of a neuron having seven main dendrites regarded as infinite cylinders extending from a spherical soma. The soma is uniformly depolarized and constitutes the sink; the dendrites provide the sources. The distribution of sources and sinks is calculated by the core conductor equation applied to the internal field. The external field of potential (Fig. 4.10) calculated from the mirror distribution resembles that in Fig. 4.2c.

4.2. Potential Fields of Neural Masses

4.2.1. MEASUREMENT OF OBSERVED FIELDS

The active states of neural masses are manifested extracellularly at various recording sites by time-varying spatial distributions of action potentials and of dendritic potential. If a microelectrode is inserted into a neural mass at a point, the amplified potential with respect to a distant site (the monopolar recording) displayed with an oscilloscope shows many action potentials on each sweep, with one or more repeated action potentials at relatively high amplitudes and many others at amplitudes diminishing to the level of thermal noise in the electrode tip. The action potentials are superimposed on relatively slowly varying potentials. The amplified potential may be passed through a high-pass filter to remove the slower waves (e.g., below 300 Hz) and a low-pass filter to remove the action potentials (e.g., potentials changing at rates above 300 Hz).

The record of action potentials is passed through a threshold comparator, which emits a 1-V 1-msec rectangular pulse each time an action potential occurs with an amplitude above a preset value. The output of the comparator is a pulse train $p'(t, x, y, z)$, which represents the time of occurrence of pulses of one neuron or a set of neurons in the mass. The distance between the active neuron or neurons is usually unknown, but the action potential of a neuron is often still detectable when the electrode tip is moved a distance of up to 100 μm from the site of maximal amplitude. The distance over which a neuron contributes to one recording $p'(t, x_1, y_1, z_1)$ is <100 μm. A set of measurements made simultaneously with multiple microelectrodes at a set of n points yields an activity distribution in the pulse mode for the mass $p'(t, x, y, z)$, which is to be used to estimate $o_{\mu p}(t, x, y)$ for the μth set in the mass.

The output of the low-pass filter represents the sum of potentials, which is established at the recording site by dendritic currents of neurons in the mass, together with possible contributions by glia and by the network of blood vessels in the tissue. The contributions of single neurons cannot be distinguished, and there is no general rule to determine over what distances neurons in the mass may contribute to the potential at any point. A set of measurements of the extracellular low-frequency potentials at a set of n points gives a neural activity distribution in the wave mode $v'(t, x, y, z)$, which is to be used as the basis for estimating $o_{\mu v}(t, x, y)$ for the μth set in the

TABLE 4.1

NOTATION FOR SPATIAL ANALYSIS OF POTENTIALS IN THE WAVE MODE

Symbol	Meaning
v	Calculated or predicted potential function
v'	Measured (digitized) potential function
$\hat{v}$	Ensemble average of observed potential function
t	Real time
T	Poststimulus time
T_n	Time delay for onset of response in a subset
$v'(t, x, y, z)$, $v'(t, X)$	Observed field of potential in real time
$v'(T, x, y, z)$, $v'(T, X)$	Observed field in poststimulus time
$\hat{v}(T, x, y, z)$, $\hat{v}(T, X)$	Ensemble average of observed fields
$v'_{x,y,z}(T)$ or $\hat{v}_X(T)$	AEP at a recording site
$\hat{v}_T(x, y, z)$ or $\hat{v}_T(X)$	Volume distribution of potential at T
$\hat{v}_{T,z}(x, y)$	Distribution in a plane parallel to a set
$\hat{v}_{T,x}(y, z)$	Distribution in a plane transecting a set
$\hat{v}_{x,y}(T, z)$	Set of AEPs along a track penetrating the set
$\hat{v}_{T,x,y}(z)$	Potential as a function of depth at fixed T, x, and y
$h_{\mu v}(x, y)$	Spatial distribution of an activity density function of KO_μ or KI_μ set in the wave mode
$q(X_n)$	$q(x_i, y_j, z_k)$ module of fixed charge
$q(X)$	$q(x, y, z)$ distribution of modular fixed charge
$H(T, X)$	$H[T_x(x), T_y(y), T_z(z), x - x_0, y - y_0, z - z_0]$ operator for input delay and translation
$f_\mu(T)$ or $f_\mu(T - T_n)$	Time dependence of charge module amplitude
$v_\mu(X)$	Component field of potential

mass. The set of n points is commonly restricted to the surface of the mass, to a plane, or a line transecting the mass, etc. The symbols used to denote restricted sets of values of potential are listed in Table 4.1.

Because of the time variance of the active state at each point, ideally the measurements at the set of n points are made simultaneously from n electrodes. In practice the technique is limited to use with arrays of electrodes at the surface of a neural mass. In depth recording the brain does not withstand placement of the large numbers of electrodes required, because the blood supply is impaired and many of the afferent and efferent axons are transected. For multichannel recording the number of electrodes is limited by the number of available amplifiers, usually $16 \leqq n \leqq 100$. The spacing of electrodes is based on the anticipated surface "grain" or maximal spatial frequency of $v'_z(t, x, y)$ and ranges from 100 μm on the cortex to several centimeters at the surface of the head. The display is in the form of a set of isopotentials in a projection plane $v'_{t,z}(x, y)$, which are found by second-order extrapolation and curve-fitting to the measured values at each successive time t of observation.

The alternative to simultaneous multichannel recording is serial penetration of the volume with a single electrode. Stable active states must exist without change in potential for the duration of the sampling procedure at n points. This holds for very slowly changing events, such as the injury current of nerve and muscle, but the potential in most fields of physiological interest changes rapidly. The solution to this problem requires the use of impulse input and the analysis of functions of potential at a set of points with poststimulus time T.

The neurons of an intact neural mass usually generate fields of potential in response to electrical stimulation of an appropriate afferent pathway. If the impulse response is invariant over a large number of trials, then the function for potential at any one point $v'(T, x, y, z)$, can be stored, the electrode moved to a new point and a new sequence recorded, stored, and so forth, at a set of points coextensive with the volume of the potential distribution.

In using this technique it is essential to place a monitor electrode at a fixed central point in the neural mass and to record at each point x, y, z and at the monitor on each trial in order to demonstrate the stability of the impulse response. If the impulse response varies from trial to trial at any one point, ensemble averages or AEPs are taken at the recording and monitor sites $\hat{v}(T, x, y, z)$. The ensemble average at the monitor site must be invariant, showing that the function of the neural mass is stationary.

The display of the depth potential function $\hat{v}_{T,x}(y, z)$ is in a set of planes for fixed values of T and x, in which isopotential curves are fitted to the data. The number of electrode tracks in the y dimension is limited by the number of penetrations the neural mass can sustain without deterioration and is commonly 5–10. The number of measuring sites on each penetration in the z direction depends on the complexity of the field and is usually ≥ 10. The number of planes in the x direction is commonly 3–5, although in conditions of axial symmetry as in the spinal cord and some areas of cortex, 1 may suffice. The number of time intervals at which potential is measured in the function $\hat{v}(T, x, y, z)$ is commonly 100, so that the number of measurements of $\hat{v}$ for each field is on the order of 10^4 times the number of planes in x.

4.2.2. Basis Functions for Potential Fields of Neural Masses

The function $\hat{v}(T, X)$, where X is x, y, z (Table 4.1), represents the potential field of the impulse response of the neural mass. The aim of analysis is to determine from the potential field one or more of the active states of the mass. Each mass is composed of one or more KO and KI sets, and the active state variables are defined only for those sets (Section 1.3.2). We must determine which KO and KI sets in a neural mass contribute to the function $\hat{v}(T, X)$. Because the fields of potential are superimposed, we infer that the potential is the sum of the fields generated by M KO and KI sets in the mass. The procedure for analysis consists in postulating M source–sink distributions, calculating $v(T, X)$, testing it against $\hat{v}(T, X)$, and inferring the set of active states from the acceptable source–sink distributions.

The current sources and sinks in a neural set μ are almost always fixed in space, because the neurons are fixed, so they are represented by an array of equivalent fixed point sources and sinks $q_\mu(X)$. The amplitudes of sources and sinks depend on time in two ways. First, when an event is initiated, such as an action potential at a node of Ranvier or a PSP at a synapse, the amplitude changes as a characteristic function of time $f(T)$. Second, when an action potential propagates along an axon, there is a succession of virtually identical events at nodes of Ranvier, but there is a delay T_a in the onset of the event at each node. The amplitude is $f(T - T_a)$, where $f(T - T_a) = 0$ for $T < T_a$. When a neural set is activated by a volley in a compound afferent nerve, each local subset is activated in a sequence. The sequence depends on the location of each subset in q_μ at X_n with respect to a reference point in the set at X_0, and the delay in each direction $T_a(X)$, with respect to stimulus time $T = 0$. That is, the afferent tract provides delay and translation. These operations can be expressed by an operator

$$T_n \triangleq H(T_a(X), X - X_0). \tag{47}$$

By this definition of T_n, the function $f_\mu(T - T_n)$ is specified in terms of post-stimulus time and location in the set, where n is a triple index, $n = i, j, k$ in the x_i, y_j, z_k coordinates.

For the source–sink density of a subset in set μ, which is $q_\mu(X_n)$, the amplitude as a function of time and location is given by the product $q_\mu(X_n) f_\mu(T - T_n)$. The predicted potential field for the set is calculated by summation

$$v_\mu(T, X) = \rho \sum_{\text{all } n} q_\mu(X_n) f_\mu(T - T_n)/\eta_n, \qquad \text{where} \quad n = i, j, k, \qquad (48)$$

$$\eta_n = [(x_i - x)^2 + (y_j - y)^2 + (z_k - z)^2]^{.5}. \qquad (49)$$

The function v_μ is a spatial basis function. The sum of basis functions over $\mu = 1, 2, ..., M$ yields the predicted potential field which is tested against the observed field by

$$\hat{v}(T, x) = \sum_{\mu = 1}^{M} v_\mu(T, X) + \varepsilon(T, X), \qquad (50)$$

where ε is an error function.

According to Eqs. (47)–(49), there are four requirements for constructing each basis function:

(a)   The source–sink distribution in a local subset of neurons in a set μ is reduced to a charge module representing the cellular architecture, such as a pair of source–sink spheres. The charge sum over the module must be zero.

(b)   The locations of the modules in space are specified by a geometry representing the set, such as a segment of a plane or cylinder, denoted $q_\mu(X)$.

(c)   The sequence of activation for the array of modules T_n, representing input delay and translation, is postulated. In most instances the input volley can be treated as having constant velocity θ in one direction. The x direction is usually chosen as the axis of input translation, so that $T_x(x) = x/\theta$, $T_x(y) = 0$, and $T_z(z) = 0$ in Eq. (47). For equal increments of Δx there are proportionate increments of ΔT_x.

(d)   A time-dependent function $f_\mu(T - T_n)$ is assigned to every subset, which differs over the set only in time of onset T_n.

It is essential to recognize that afferent delays in activation over a neural mass often give rise to the appearance of traveling waves of potential, but the waves are not propagated or conducted, nor are they reflected at the boundaries of the mass. The wave equations of classical physics are not applicable. The waves result from the finite velocity of the input channel. The delays must be accounted for in the measuring process, even though their possible functional significance is obscure.

In many cases the input delay is negligible, and the value for T_x can be set equal to zero by appropriate choice of T_n or $f_\mu(T)$. Equation (48) is then modified as

$$v_\mu(T, X) = f_\mu(T)\rho \sum_{\text{all } n} q_\mu(X_n)/\eta_n. \tag{51}$$

A new function is defined

$$v_\mu(X) \triangleq \rho \sum_{\text{all} n} q_\mu(X_n)/\eta_n. \tag{52}$$

Therefore,

$$v_\mu(T, X) = f_\mu(T)v_\mu(X), \tag{53}$$

$$v(T, X) = \sum_{\mu=1}^{M} f_\mu(T)v_\mu(X). \tag{54}$$

Each component field is represented as having a characteristic spatial distribution, and each has a characteristic weighting function to describe its amplitude over time. This formulation is used here extensively for the global description of fields of neural masses.

Example A. The choice for the local source–sink geometry depends on the typical structure of the generating neurons. If the afferent axons form synapses on one of two dendritic trees, which extend on opposite sides of the soma (often called bipolar neurons), the source and sink for each neuron can be represented as a function of distance z along the geometric axis of the neuron. Let us represent each source by a unit of charge density ξ and each sink by $-\xi$. We assume that the sources for a set of neurons form a homogeneous sphere of unit radius, $a = 1$, with its center at $x = 0$, $y = 0$, $z = 1$, and the sinks form a homogeneous sphere of unit radius centered at $x = 0$, $y = 0$, $z = -1$. We assume that $f(T)$ is constant, and that T is zero across the set.

The potential $v^+(X)$ for a spherical distribution of positive charge outside the sphere is calculated for $v(z)$

$$v_{T,x,y}^+(z) = \varepsilon\xi(a^3/3z), \qquad z > a, \qquad T = x = y = 0. \tag{55}$$

The potential inside the sphere is

$$v_{T,x,y}^+(z) = (\varepsilon\xi/2)[a^2 - (z^2/3)], \qquad z < a, \qquad T = x = y = 0. \tag{56}$$

The same functions hold for $v^-(x)$. The potential for the set is given by $v_{T,x,y}(z) = v_{T,x,y}^+(z) + v_{T,x,y}^-(z)$ and is shown in Fig. 4.11. The potential function is that of a distributed dipole field.

If the distance $z \gg 2a$, then the distributed dipole can be treated as a point dipole at $x = 0$, in which the dipole moment μ is a vector given by the product of the total charge in one pole Q and the distance of separation

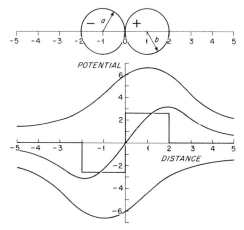

FIG. 4.11. Potential as a function of distance along a line through two homogeneous distributions of charge representing a source and a sink with equal current density. This is a form of the distributed dipole field.

$2\mathbf{a}$, where $\mathbf{a}$ is a vector. The potential is

$$v_n(\eta, \varphi) = |\mathbf{\mu}| \cos \varphi / \eta^2, \quad \eta = (x^2 + y^2 + z^2)^{1/2}, \tag{57}$$

where φ is the angle between $\mathbf{\mu}$ and the z axis and η is the distance between the origin and a point n. Use of Eq. (57) to predict the field of a neural mass requires vector summation. Scalar summation over pairs of point charges is simpler. ☐

Example B. If each neuron in the local subset has dendrites radiating in all directions from the soma (often called *stellate neurons*), all of which are activated so that the soma forms the source and the dendrites form the sink, a different field of potential results. We assume that the source for the subset is represented by a homogeneous sphere of radius $a = 1$, centered at $x = 0$. The source forms a concentric hollow sphere of outer radius $b = 3$ and inner radius $a = 1$, also centered at $x = 0$. The charge density of the source is greater than the charge density of the sink by $\xi^+ = -\xi^-(b^3 - a^3)/a^3$, so that $\xi^+ = -26\xi^-$ from the ratio of volumes. Thus $f(T)$ is constant and $T = 0$. The potential for the source $v^+(\eta)$ is given by Eqs. (55) and 56). Inside the hollow sphere of the sink,

$$v^-(\eta) = \tfrac{1}{2}\varepsilon\xi^-(b^2 - a^2), \quad \eta < a, \quad \eta = (x^2 + y^2 + z^2)^{.5}. \tag{58}$$

Between the inner and outer radii,

$$v^-(\eta) = \varepsilon\xi^-\left(\frac{b^2}{3} - \frac{a^3}{2r} - \frac{\eta^2}{b}\right), \quad a < \eta < b. \tag{59}$$

Outside the sphere,

$$v^-(\eta) = \varepsilon\xi^-\left(\frac{b^3 - a^3}{3\eta}\right), \qquad \eta > b. \tag{60}$$

The potential as a function of distance from the center is $v(\eta) = v^+(\eta) + v^-(\eta)$ as shown in Fig. 4.12 (see also Figs. 4.2c and 4.10).

This field differs in three ways from the distributed dipole field. First, the maximum and minimum values of potential are asymmetric. In the case illustrated there is virtually immeasurable negative potential even at the outer bound of the region of sink. The poles in the dipole field are equal but opposite in sign of potential. Second, the locus of reversal in sign of potential, which is the zero isopotential surface, does not have the same location as the locus of reversal in sign of charge, which is the locus for reversal of sign of transmembrane current. These two loci are identical within the distribution

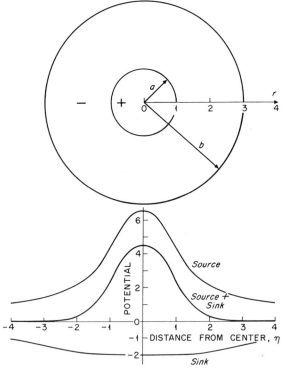

FIG. 4.12. Potential as a function of distance along a line through the center of two concentric homogeneous distributions of charges representing a source and a sink of unequal current density. This is a form of the closed field or monopole field (from Biedenbach & Freeman, 1964).

of sources and sinks for the dipole field. Third, the potential is zero everywhere outside the anatomical distribution of the filaments of the generating cells, whereas the potential of the dipole field can be recorded at great distances from the generating neurons. This feature led Lorente de Nó (1947a) to apply the descriptive label "closed field" to the field of concentric charge distributions. □

Example C. Suppose that the distributed source for a set of neurons is randomly distributed about a center at $x = 0$, with unit standard deviation, so that

$$\xi(\eta) = [1/\rho(2\pi)^{1/2}]\exp(-\eta^2/2), \qquad \eta = (x^2 + y^2 + z^2)^{.5}. \qquad (61)$$

The potential is given by

$$v(\eta) = (1/2\rho\eta)\,\mathrm{erf}(\eta/\sqrt{2}) \qquad (62)$$

and is shown as the solid curve in Fig. 4.13. Let $\xi(\eta)$ be approximated by a homogeneous sphere of charge with a radius of 2 standard deviations and centered at $x = 0$. The approximating potential from Eqs. (55) and (56) is shown by the dashed curve in Fig. 4.13. The difference between the predicted and approximating potentials is at the level of error ε in measuring $\hat{v}(T, X)$. □

Figure 4.13 in Example C demonstrates the powerful smoothing that occurs when the potentials are added across an array of distributed charge.

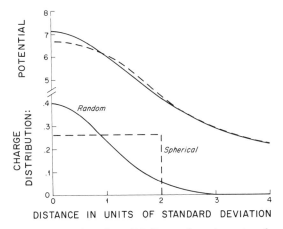

FIG. 4.13. Potential as a function of a radial distance from the center of a spherical homogeneous charge distribution, and from the center of a charge cloud decreasing in density according to the normal distribution in all directions. The potential function is insensitive to the details of the charge (source–sink) distribution. See text for discussion.

The details of source–sink distributions in local subsets are not reflected in $\hat{v}(T, X)$ so the geometric configuration of charge representing local subsets should be given the simplest form possible. This is why the dipole field and the closed field are the two most useful basis functions for describing $v(X)$. Because of the insensitivity of the potential function $v(X)$ to details in the equivalent charge distribution $q(X)$, the necessary parameters for $q(X)$ are merely the locations of the centers of each distribution of positive and negative charge, and the spread of each distribution.

Isolation and identification of each component $f_\mu(T) v_\mu(X), \mu = 1, 2, ..., M$, are based on one or more of several conditions that may hold for each given event. The delay T_μ for the onset of each component may vary. This is the basis on which the components of the compound action potential are identified. The rates of change for $f_\mu(T)$ may differ by one or more log units. On this basis the presynaptic and postsynaptic components of an evoked potential are identified. The functions $v_\mu(X)$ may be distinguished by the use of two inputs, one input being given to one of two overlapping KO or KI masses and the second input to the other or both masses. Although there is no general solution to the problem, the necessary information includes the topology and geometry of the masses and a prediction of the form of the output. This information is embodied in the set of temporal and spatial basis functions, $f_\mu(T)$ and $v_\mu(X)$.

4.2.3. COMPOUND POTENTIAL FIELDS: MODULAR ANALYSIS

On the basis of cell geometry neurons having an axial geometry (e.g., bipolar neurons, Golgi type I neurons such as cortical pyramidal cells having long apical dendrites and long axons, etc.) can be expected to generate predominantly extracellular dipole fields, whereas neurons having a radial geometry (e.g., Golgi type II neurons such as cortical granule or stellate cells or cells with short axons) should generate predominantly extracellular closed fields. Owing to the irregularities of distribution in the branches of neurons and in active sites in the membrane, neuron fields do not conform precisely to these idealized models. When the approximation fails, they can be regarded as the sum of a dipole and a closed field. This becomes important in considering the fields of KO and KI sets in neural masses. The local details of the separate fields of participating neurons are not discernible, because their branches are so densely interwoven, and the equivalent external charge density function approximates a continuous distribution over each set rather than over each neuron. The form of the resultant multicellular field depends as much on the geometry of the set as on the geometry of the single neurons.

Let us suppose that the field of each neuron can be represented by a vector quantity expressing the dipole component [Eq. (57)] and a scalar quantity expressing the closed component. Two cases arise. If the axes of the neurons in a pool are randomly directed, then the vector components cancel and leave only the scalar components. The field of the set is closed. Thus the field of reticular and nuclear structures are characteristically low in amplitude, localized, and lacking in a well-defined "turn-over" or zero isopotential surface. If the axes of the neurons lie parallel to one another, then the vector components add to produce a vector or dipole field for the set. The scalar components add also, so that the observed field may be somewhat asymmetric. The dipole field is characteristic of the laminar populations in the cortex, which generate high-amplitude fields having a well-defined zero isopotential surface in the midregion of the cortex, and which can be detected outwardly as far as the scalp and inwardly through much of the brain. The cortex also generates nondipole fields (e.g., the field of the "recruiting" response). It is never safe to assume that the locus of the "turnover" in a cortical field of potential corresponds to the locus of membrane current reversal for the neurons generating the field, even when the set of neurons is plane or nearly plane.

In most parts of the neocortex the neurons have a common orientation but are displaced vertically from one another in the laminar tissue. In the simpler and phylogenetically older parts of the cortex (paleocortex) such as the hippocampus and prepyriform cortex, the pyramidal neurons share not only an orientation but a common depth of their somas as well. This gives these structures their striking laminar appearance in histological cross sections. These and similar structures generate potential fields having the highest amplitudes to be found for spontaneous and evoked potentials anywhere in the brain, particularly in comparison to those from reticular and nuclear masses (see Section 7.3.3).

A flat sheet of axially symmetric and parallel cells generates a plane dipole field. The layers of neurons in the nervous system usually occur in the form of curved surfaces. The effects of curvature are to increase the amplitude of potential in the concavity, to decrease the amplitude over the convexity, and to shift the zero isopotential outwardly. This inequality in amplitudes is found in the fields generated by the hippocampus, the olfactory bulb, the lateral geniculate nucleus, the superior colliculus, etc., all of which are curved surfaces. The disparity becomes marked as the radius of curvature approximates the length of the component cells. In the case where the curved layer is virtually in the form of a sphere, as in several brainstem nuclei (Lorente de Nó, 1947a), a closed field results.

Example A. The superior olivary complex lies in the brainstem and is part of the auditory system. The two main structures are the S segment, which receives afferent axons from the ipsilateral cochlear nucleus and the medial segment, which receives afferent axons on the lateral side from the ipsilateral cochlear nucleus and on the medial side from the contralateral cochlear nucleus. The bipolar neurons of each segment form a single layer with dendritic branches on both sides of the layer. The medial segment is a plane, and the S segment is strongly curved. The current source and sink of each local subset for each segment are represented by an equivalent charge dipole. The medial segment is represented by a plane set of dipoles, and the S segment is represented by two spherical dipole arrays.

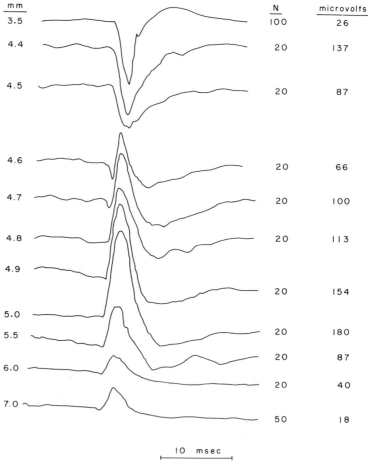

FIG. 4.14. Click-evoked potentials recorded from various points in the superior olivary complex of the cat (Biedenbach & Freeman, 1964).

A click delivered to the contralateral ear results in an evoked potential. The ensemble average $\hat{v}_{Xc}(T)$ or AEP is nonoscillatory (Fig. 4.14) and closely resembles a PSP. There is no significant delay across the sets of neurons. The potential function is evaluated only at the crest of the response. The spatial distribution of potential $\hat{v}_{Tc}(X)$ has the form of a symmetric dipole field (Fig. 4.15) with the zero isopotential surface lying at the medial edge of the medial segment and with negativity on the medial side. An ipsilateral click results also in a nonoscillatory AEP. The function $\hat{v}_{Xi}(T)$ is very similar to $\hat{v}_{Xc}(T)$. The field of potential $\hat{v}_{Ti}(X)$ is an asymmetric dipole field, negative laterally, with the zero isopotential surface at the lateral edge (Fig. 4.16). The amplitude of the negative pole is higher than the inverse amplitude of the positive pole, and its volume extends further dorsolaterally to include the S segment. The structure of the S segment implies that on activation it would produce a closed field partially overlapped by the field of the medial segment. It is known from unit recordings that its neurons are activated by clicks. It is concluded that the ipsilateral impulse response of the superior olivary complex $\hat{v}_i(T, X)$ is the sum of a closed field generated by the S segment $v_1(X)$ as in Fig. 4.12, and a dipole field generated by the medial segment $v_2(X)$ as in Fig. 4.11. Therefore, if both have the same time function $f(T) = \hat{v}_{Xi}(T)$,

$$\hat{v}_i(T, X) = f(T)v_1(X) + f(T)v_2(X) + \varepsilon(T). \quad \square \qquad (63)$$

In general the fields of potential of two or more sets contributing to the field of a neural mass overlap in the volume of the mass, and separation by use of two or more inputs is not feasible. For each of the planes of measurement, y, z, transecting the mass, the values for potential $\hat{v}_x(T, y, z)$ form a two-dimensional matrix consisting of the values in time at each point $\hat{v}_x(T)$, and the values at each time over the set of points $\hat{v}_T(X)$. We can assume that the neurons in each set μ have local and global geometries differing from those in other sets. The functions $v_\mu(X)$ must be different, and the functions $f_\mu(T)$ may or may not differ significantly. The contribution of any set $v_\mu(T, X)$ over a set of points is uniquely different from that of any other set.

If the delay in onset of an active state through the mass is negligibly small in comparison to its duration, the value for the function of amplitude with time $f_\mu(T)$ is the same for all local subsets in each set μ at each T. In this case the contributions to the potential of the nth set at any point in the mass can be treated as the product of a factor $v_\mu(T)$ and a linear coupling coefficient for the set to that point $\lambda_{n\mu}$. For any point, the sum of contributions is

$$\hat{v}_x(T, y, z) = \sum_{\mu=1}^{M} \lambda_{n\mu} f_\mu(T) + \bar{v}_n + \varepsilon_{nT} \qquad (64)$$

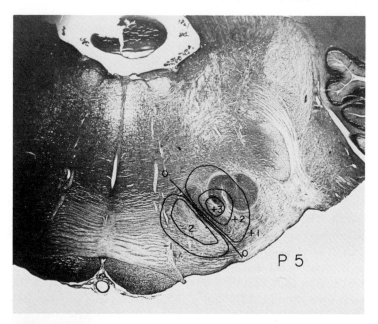

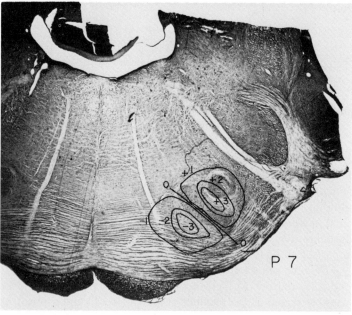

FIG. 4.15. Fields of potential at the crest of the response to contralateral click stimulation of the medial accessory nucleus of the superior olivary complex. P5 and P7 designate the distance of coronal section posterior to the midaural plane (Biedenbach & Freeman, 1964).

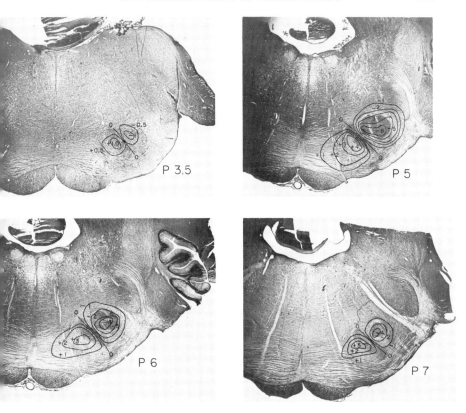

FIG. 4.16. Field of potential at the crest of the response to ipsilateral click stimulation of the S segment and medial accessory nucleus. P3.5, P5, P6, and P7 designate the distance of coronal section posterior to the midaural plane (Biedenbach & Freeman, 1964).

where $\bar{v}_n$ is the mean potential at n over time and ε_{nT} is an error term. In this way the potential function is represented by a set of n linear equations, in which the μ time functions of the sets are the factors, and the n recording sites play the role of a stratifying variable.

If the μ factors are statistically independent of each other, the appropriate procedure is factor analysis of $\hat{v}_x(T, y, z)$ to determine the principal components of the variance, which are estimates of the factors $f_\mu(T)$. The values for $\lambda_{n\mu}$ are determined by linear regression over the set of n equations in the form of Eq. (64). The values are treated as estimates for $v_\mu(X)$, from which contour maps are constructed.

The condition of statistical independence seldom holds. The time functions of different sets in the same mass may be similar, because the active states of the sets are coupled by interaction. If there is no coupling, the time

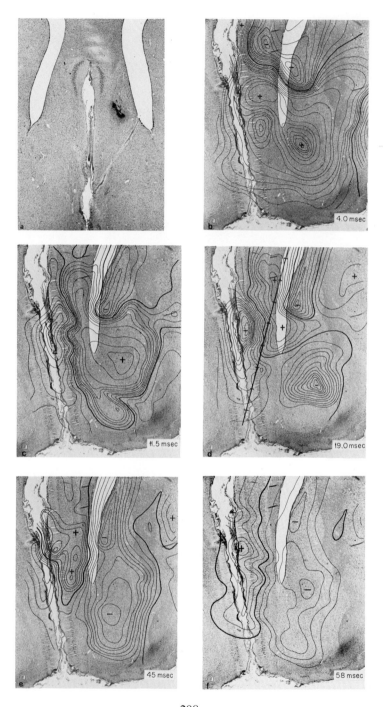

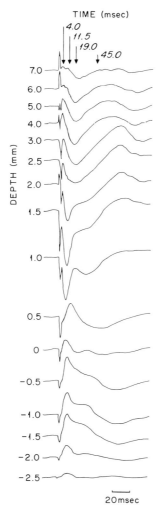

FIG. 4.18. AEPs recorded at points on the diagonal line shown in Fig. 4.17d. The arrows show the times at which the field maps were taken (Freeman & Patel, 1968).

functions may be similar because the properties of the neurons in the two sets are similar. In this case the factors $f_\mu(T)$ cannot be estimated from the principal components of the variance. By inspection of the data $\hat{v}_x(T, y, z)$, two or more subsets of points are selected at which the AEPs reflect the main features characteristic of the field of the mass. The ensemble

FIG. 4.17. Fields of potential recorded in the anterior septum and accumbens nucleus in the cat on electrical stimulation of the posterior septum (a) (Freeman & Patel, 1968).

average or AAEP over each subset is used to estimate the factors $f_\mu(T)$ and the coupling coefficients $\lambda_{n\mu}$ are determined as before.

Example B.   A single-shock electrical stimulus is given to a point in the septum of the cat (Fig. 4.17a), and a set of AEPs is taken from a coronal (vertical) plane yz, 1.5 mm anterior to the stimulus site. A representative electrode track, y = constant, is shown in Fig. 4.17e on which the crossmarks indicate the depth of recording z. A set of isopotentials $v_{T,x}(y,z)$ representing $\hat{v}_{T,x}(y,z)$ is shown in Fig. 4.17 for several times T after the onset of the event. A representative set of values for $\hat{v}_{x,y}(T,z)$ is shown in Fig. 4.18. AAEPs averaged over selected sites at maxima in the field of potential of the mass are shown in Fig. 4.19.

The analysis is based on the assumptions that resistivity ρ is constant; the number of sets μ is 2; the delay in onset T is negligible in each set; the time function for each set $f_\mu(T)$ is represented by ensemble averages of AEPs at points near the center of each set, but relatively distant from the centers of other sets; and the fields of the sets are superimposed. By linear regression using Eq. (64) two sets of $\lambda_{n\mu}$ are found from which two sets of isopotentials are constructed (Fig. 4.20).

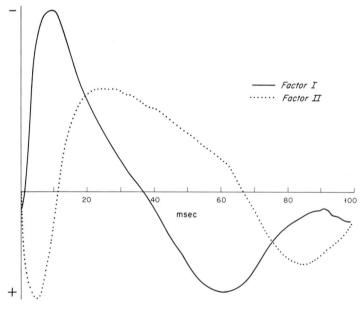

FIG. 4.19. Estimates of the time course of the active states in each of the two neural masses, based on selective averaging (Freeman & Patel, 1968).

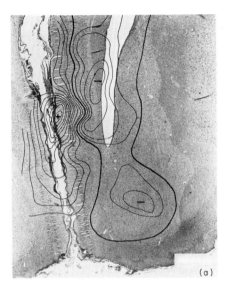
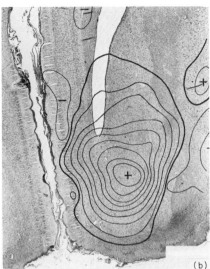

FIG. 4.20. Characterization of two overlapping fields of potential (a dipole field in the anterior septum, Factor I, and a closed field in the accumbens nucleus, Factor II) which determine the forms of the AEPs in this region (Freeman & Patel, 1968).

The results show that $\hat{v}_x(T, y, z)$ can be represented as the sum of a dipole field $v_I(X)$, and a closed field $v_{II}(X)$. For each field the amplitude, $f_I(T)$ and $f_{II}(T)$, respectively, varies with poststimulus time, as shown by Fig. 4.19. Note that the movement of the zero isopotential surface of $\hat{v}_x(T, y, z)$ shown in Fig. 4.17 is not evidence for movement of the emf in the field. According to the results the emfs of the two sets are fixed in location but variable in amplitude. They are asynchronous, although not statistically independent, in the sense that their product moment correlation coefficient is not zero. The asynchrony causes movement of the zero isopotential surface in the sum of the two component fields. □

4.3. Potential Fields in the Olfactory Bulb

Detailed analyses are given in these and the following sections of the field potentials of the olfactory bulb and prepyriform cortex. This is done in order to demonstrate some techniques for comparing observed and predicted fields, and to present some concepts and data, which are required in the next two chapters. The examples given for both bulb and cortex show the fields of AEPs. The bulbar and cortical EEG fields of potential are shown closely to resemble the evoked fields by comparing relative amplitudes of evoked and EEG activity recorded simultaneously at multiple points in the two neural masses.

4.3.1. Bulbar Geometry and Topology

Three aspects of the anatomy of a neural mass must be known. These are the global geometry of the neural sets comprising the mass, the characteristic geometry of the main cell types, and the topology of the connections, which may be lines of flow of neural activity. These anatomical properties have been studied in detail by light and electron microscopy (Ramón y Cajal, 1955; Le Gros Clark, 1957; Valverde, 1965; Rall *et al.*, 1966; Price & Powell, 1970a–d; Pinching & Powell, 1971a–d; Willey, 1973). Only the salient features are introduced here. In particular the rich variety of

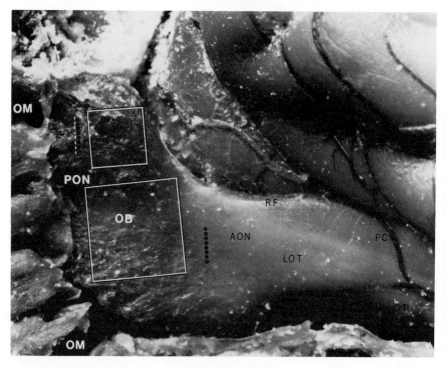

Fig. 4.21. View of the lateral aspect of the forebrain of the cat. Small square: 2 × 2 mm recording array (8 × 8 electrodes). Large square: 3.5 × 3.5 mm recording array (8 × 8 electrodes). Rows of white dots and black dots: 1 × 8 electrode arrays for stimulation, respectively, of PON and LOT. OM: olfactory mucosa; OB: olfactory bulb; AON: anterior olfactory nucleus; RF, rhinal fissure; PON: primary olfactory nerve; LOT: lateral olfactory tract; OT: olfactory tubercle; PC: prepyriform cortex; ES: entorhinal sulcus.

synapses found in the bulb by electron microscopy is not considered explicitly.

1. Global geometry.   The gross anatomy of the olfactory bulb and cortex is shown in Fig. 4.21, which is a view of the lateral aspect of the brain of the cat, after the dura, skull, and soft tissues have been removed. The bulb has the size and shape of a lima bean. The flat medial and lateral (as shown) surfaces are parallel to the sagittal (midline) plane. The olfactory or

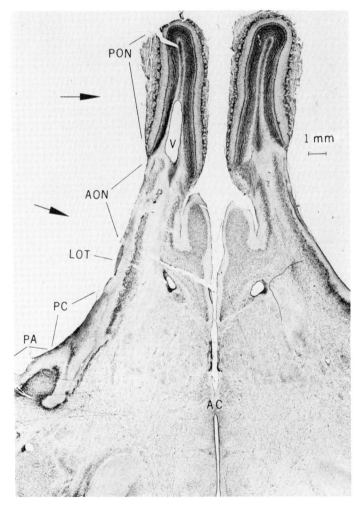

Fig. 4.22. Horizontal section through the forebrain of the cat at the level of the anterior commissure AC. Arrows show the direction of view of Figs. 4.21 (upper arrow) and 4.34 (lower arrow). PA: periamygdaloid cortex; PC; prepyriform cortex; V: ventricle. Nissl stain.

prepyriform cortex has a curved surface that extends 2 cm posteriorly from the posterior edge of the bulb. The olfactory receptors lie in the olfactory mucosa that lines the nasal cavity and extends over a centimeter anteriorly from the bony plate at the anterior edge of the bulb.

The in-depth structure of the two masses is shown in a low-power view (10 ×) of a horizontal section (Fig. 4.22) in which the nuclei in the cell bodies have been stained (methylene blue). Each neural mass has a laminar structure in which groups of cell bodies form layers of grey matter parallel to the surface. The input axons to each mass form a layer at the surface, and the output axons contribute heavily to the mass of myelinated axons (white matter) at the inner aspect or base of each mass. The layers in the bulb are folded around a fluid-filled cavity called the *ventricle*. Domains limited to the lateral or medial walls can be treated as planes. The whole surface can be treated as a segment of an ellipsoid or, in the case of the bulb in the rabbit, as an incomplete sphere (Rall & Shepherd, 1968). The anterior half of the prepyriform cortex can be represented by a segment of a hemicylinder (Horowitz & Freeman, 1966).

The depth of the bulb is 1.6–1.8 mm from the surface to the ventricle. Three typical sections stained by different techniques are shown in Fig. 4.23a. Each shows the prominent masses of synaptic complexes called *glomeruli* that form a layer (GL) between the input axons in the primary olfactory nerve (PON) and a mass of interwoven dendrites and axons forming the

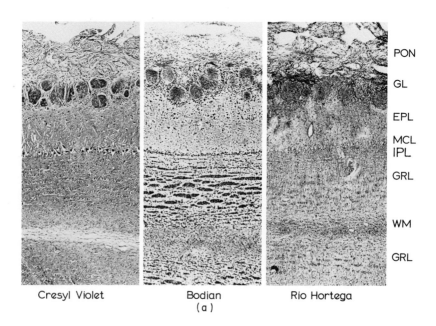

			PON
			GL
			EPL
			MCL
			IPL
			GRL
			WM
			GRL

Cresyl Violet	Bodian	Rio Hortega
	(a)	

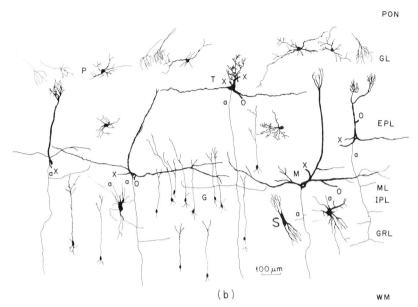

FIG. 4.23. (a) Vertical sections through the lateral wall of the olfactory bulb that are perpendicular to the PON and to the bulbar surface. (b) Camera lucida drawings of neuron types in the olfactory bulb in the indicated layers. GL: glomerular layer; EPL: external plexiform layer; MCL: mitral cell layer; IPL, internal plexiform layer; GRL: granule cell layer; WM: white matter; P: periglomerular cell; T: tufted cell; M: mitral cell, G: granule cell; S: stellate cell; a: axon; x, o: basal dendrites extending into or out of plane of section. Rapid Golgi preparations (Freeman, 1972d).

external plexiform layer (EPL). A thin layer of cell bodies, the mitral cell layer (MCL), separates the EPL and the internal plexiform layer (IPL) that consists mainly of small axons. Beneath the IPL there are multiple laminae of cell bodies comprising the granule cell layer (GRL). At the base there is a layer of white matter (WM) that contains efferent axons and centrifugal axons (from other parts of the brain to the bulb). The efferent axons form the lateral olfactory tract (LOT) on the surface of the prepyriform cortex. These seven layers are all parallel to the surface (cf. Fig. 4.22).

2. Local geometry. The principal four types of neurons in the bulb are shown in camera lucida drawings from Golgi preparations in Fig. 4.23b. The finely branched terminals of each PON axon are restricted to a part of one glomerulus. Small neurons known as periglomerular neurons (P) occupy the glomerular layer (GL) and have axons and dendrites radiating in directions parallel to the surface. From their radial symmetry they are expected to generate closed fields.

The spatial structure of the glomerular layer is shown in a low-power composite photomicrograph of a histological section cut parallel to the bulbar surface (Fig. 4.24a). The outside dimensions of the figure are 3.5 × 3.5 mm and are equal to the dimensions of the recording array shown by the larger rectangle on the bulb in Fig. 4.21. (The larger inset is 2 × 2 mm, the size of the smaller rectangle.) Each glomerulus is a mass of axonal and dendritic endings with small numbers of cell bodies. Large numbers of cell bodies are found between the glomeruli, which give the appearance in cross section of a mosaic of paving stones set in gravel. Each glomerulus is partially or wholly encapsulated in a layer of glial processes (larger inset, Rio Hortega stain). The cell bodies in the intervening spaces are mainly those of periglomerular cells. An example is shown from a Golgi preparation at the same size scale as the glomeruli (the marker is 100 μm). The dendrites

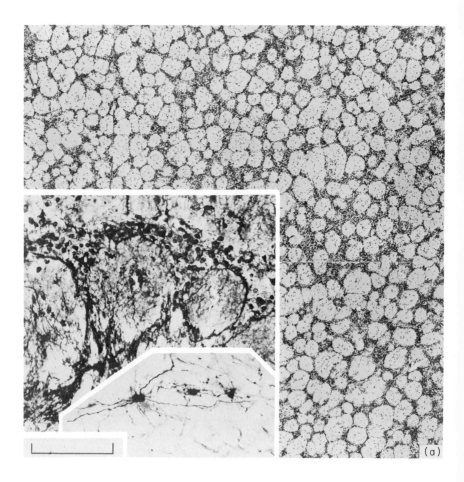

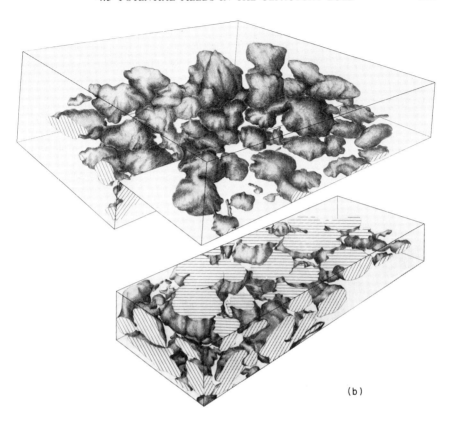

(b)

FIG. 4.24. (a) Composite photomicrograph of a section in the plane of the glomerular layer (GL in Fig. 4.23). Outer square is 3.5×3.5 mm; inner square is 2×2 mm (see squares in Fig. 4.21). The marker represents 100 μm for the scale of the two insets. Outer square: cresyl violet stain to show the nuclei of the periglomerular cells and the mosaic of the glomeruli. Inner square: Rio Hortego stain to show the partial glial encapsulation of the glomeruli. Small inset: Golgi stain to show the size and structure of representative periglomerular cells. (b) Reconstruction from serial sections of the outlines of glomeruli (cresyl violet stain) in a 1×1 mm section. View is from inside the bulb looking outwardly. The glomeruli are irregularly shaped globules, often confluent, with an average diameter of 135 μm.

extend between glomeruli for distances up to 4 or 5 glomerular diameters, but generally less far.

A perspective drawing made by reconstruction of serial sections through the layer (1×1 mm, Fig. 4.24b) shows the irregular globular form of the glomeruli. Each has very roughly the shape of a sphere, as suggested by the cross sections in Fig. 4.24a, but they are both irregular and confluent. From measurements of the maximal diameters of the clumps in the reconstruction (as well as others not shown), the mean glomerular diameter is 135 ± 30 μm. The density is 18.3/mm^2, and the total is about 3200 in each bulb.

The next layer, called the EPL, is organized very differently. There are large numbers of long dendrites extending in all directions parallel to the surface at all depths. These arise from large neurons with cell bodies in the EPL called *tufted cells* (T) and in the MCL called *mitral cells* (M). Each has an apical dendrite normal to the surface extending into a part of one glomerulus or occasionally two glomeruli, and each has three or four basal dendrites extending for long distances (up to 1 mm) in all directions parallel to the surface. Each has an axon with multiple collaterals (side branches), which branch off as it extends to the white matter. From the high degree of radial symmetry the mitral and tufted cells are predicted to generate closed fields on generalized activation, or dipole fields when the active membrane is restricted to the glomerular tufts of the apical dendrites.

The many small neurons with cell bodies packed together in the GRL are called *granule cells*. Each has a few short basal dendrites and a single sparsely branched ascending dendrite oriented normal to the surface, which is studded with gemmules. The axial symmetry implies that these neurons generate dipole fields, when input is restricted to either end. The neurons have no axons, which implies that they do not generate action potentials.

Scattered through the EPL and GRL are relatively large neurons with dendrites and axons radiating in all directions. They are called *stellate* cells (S) and are predicted to generate closed fields when the input is distributed over the dendrites. Unlike the other three types, they do not densely populate a single layer.

3. Topology. The topology of connections defining the neural sets in the olfactory bulb (and cortex) is shown in Fig. 4.25. Each receptor (R) has one axon that extends to the bulb in the PON and ends in one of the glomeruli. The ending is a densely branched tuft (Fig. 4.23b). The approximately 140 million receptors for each bulb have no interconnections and form the KO$_R$ set. Periglomerular neurons (P) receive axodendritic synapses from PON axons, are densely interconnected by axodendritic synapses in and between glomeruli, and form the KI$_P$ set. The mitral–tufted cells (M, T) receive axo- and dendrodendritic synapses from PON axons and periglomerular neurons. They form the KI$_M$ set by virtue of their axodendritic and axosomatic synaptic interconnections through axons in the EPL and IPL. The granule cells (G) interact and form the KI$_G$ set, though the channel of the interaction is not known. The mitral–tufted cells both deliver and receive synaptic input to and from granule cells, because most of the dendrodendritic synapses between mitral–tufted and granule cells are reciprocal (Shepherd, 1972). The interconnection between the mitral–tufted

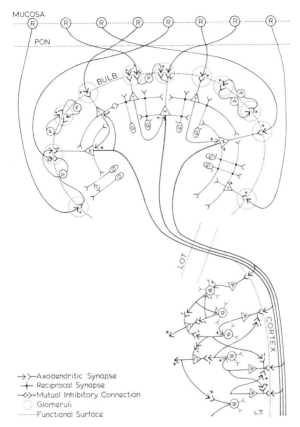

FIG. 4.25. Schematic diagram of principal types of neurons, pathways, and synaptic connections in the olfactory mucosa, bulb, and cortex (see Fig. 1.5) (Freeman, 1972f).

KI_M set and the granule cell KI_G set forms a KII_{MG} set in the neural mass of the olfactory bulb (see Fig. 1.5d).

4.3.2. ANALYSIS OF THE SPATIAL FUNCTION OF POTENTIAL

The coordinates of the lateral wall of the bulb are designated x (increasing in the main direction of orthodromic (forward) propagation of action potentials on the PON axons), y (in directions normal to the PON and parallel to the surface), and z (in directions normal to the surface and the PON). On single-shock stimulation of the PON at $x = y = 0$, the AEP, monopolarly recorded and averaged from a site on the activated bundle ($x = x_0, y = y_0$, and usually $y_0 = 0$) at the surface ($z = 0$) which is $\hat{v}_{x,y,z}(T)$, shows a triphasic action potential followed by a complex response consisting of a damped sine wave superimposed on a nonoscillatory baseline shift (Fig. 4.26). The successive negative peaks (upward) are labeled N1, N2, ... The successive positive peaks are labeled P1, P2, ..., even if they are greater than zero. The amplitude of the action potential attenuates rapidly to zero with increasing x (see Section 2.3.3).

The field of potential manifested by the AEP, $\hat{v}(T, x, y, z)$, is broadly distributed over and through the lateral wall of the bulb. The field recorded with 64 electrodes (Fig. 4.27a) on the bulbar surface $z = 0$ is $\hat{v}_{T,z}(x, y)$ and is shown for several representative values of T in Fig. 4.27b–g, including the rising phase, crest, and falling phase of N1, and the crests of N2, N3, and N4. The potential is unimodally distributed over a portion of the surface (the 8×8 rectangular array of electrodes is 3.5×3.5 mm), and the crest N1 moves across the surface in the direction of propagation of the PON axons. The crests of N2, N3, ... recur at increasing values for x.

The surface location, $x = x_0$, $y = y_0$ and $z = 0$, of the maximum for the potential of N1 over all values of T, x, and y, is called the *epicenter* of the bulbar response domain. The potential field in a plane transecting the bulb at $x = x_0$, $\hat{v}_{T,x}(y, z)$, is shown in Fig. 4.28 for three values of T corresponding to the crest of N1, the zero crossing between N1 and P1, and the crest of P1. During N1 there is a dipole field with a zero isopotential surface in the deep half of the EPL, a negative pole in the EPL, and a positive pole in the GRL. During the zero crossing at the surface there is a closed field with a negative pole centered in the lower half of the EPL. During P1 there is a dipole field with a zero isopotential at the MCL, a positive pole in the EPL, and two negative poles in the IPL (see AEPs in Fig. 4.38).

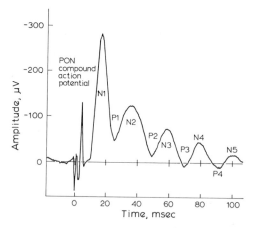

FIG. 4.26. Typical bulbar AEP, $\hat{v}_{x,y,z}(T)$, following electrical stimulation of the PON with $N = 335$ (Freeman, 1972a).

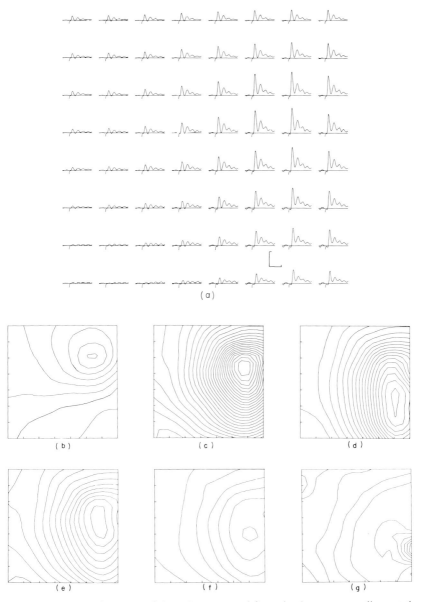

FIG. 4.27. (a) Set of 64 AEPs, $\hat{v}_z(T, x, y)$, constructed from simultaneous recordings at the surface $z = 0$. Array size: 3.5×3.5 mm (see Fig. 4.21). Top: anterior. Left: dorsal. Amplitude: 200 μV. Time: 25 msec. (b)–(g) Maps of fields of potentials $\hat{v}_{T,z}(x, y)$ at times of (b) onset, 11 msec, (c) crest, 16 msec, and (d) decline, 21 msec, of the first peak of the AEP, N1 (see Fig. 4.26), and at crests of (e) N2, 40 msec, (f) N3, 64 msec, and (g) N4, 86 msec (Freeman, 1974a).

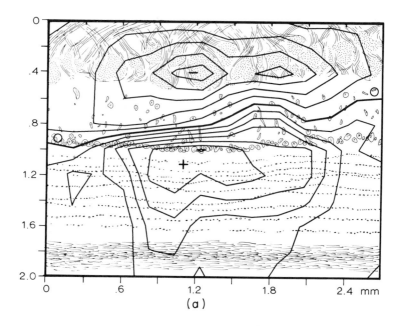

(a)

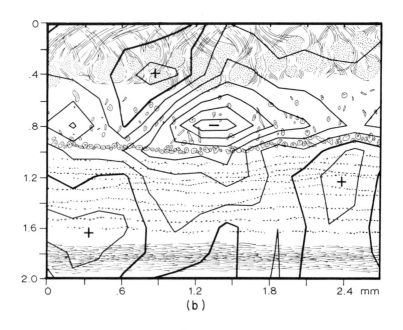

(b)

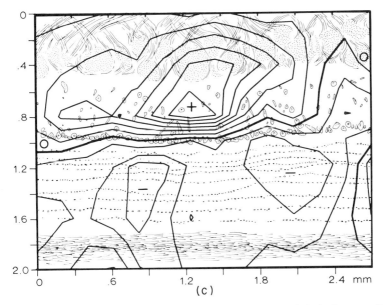

FIG. 4.28. Maps of fields of potential $\hat{v}_{T,x}(y,z)$ in a cross section of the bulb perpendicular to the PON and to the bulbar surface. Contour intervals are in microvolts. Poststimulus times refer to the crest of N1, the time midway between N1 and P1, and the crest of P1 (see Fig. 4.38) (Freeman, 1972d). (a) $T = 13.1$ msec at 60 μV; (b) $T = 22.5$ msec at 20 μV; (c) $T = 29.4$ msec at 20 μV.

The center of the response domain is at x_0, y_0, z_0, where z_0 is the depth of the zero isopotential surface at N2, N3, ... The potential as a function of time at selected points along an electrode track through the epicenter is designated $\hat{v}_{x_0, y_0}(T, z)$. The two examples in Fig. 4.29 are AEPs in response to PON stimulation (a) and LOT stimulation (b) for selected values of z. The AEPs have the same form but with different amplitudes, except near $z = z_0$. For $z < z_0$ and $\hat{v}_{x_0, y_0}(T, z)$ the amplitudes of N1 and of the baseline shift are negative; for $z > z_0$, the amplitudes of N1 and of the baseline shift are positive. At and near $z = z_0$, the amplitudes of N1 and the baseline shift are minimal, and the oscillation lags about 90° (1.57 rad) from the oscillation recorded at the surface $\hat{v}_{x_0, y_0, z=0}(T)$.

For analysis by stimulation the following assumptions are made: (1) $\rho(x, y, z) = \rho$ is constant. (2) The input velocity $\theta(x)$ is constant over x, and there is negligible delay in the y and z coordinates. (By this assumption we neglect events seen near $z = z_0$ during the rising phase and crest of N1, when the distribution of emf is being established in the EPL). (3) The number of sets is $\mu = 2$. [By this assumption we omit consideration of action potentials in the PON and mitral–tufted cells, which are more suitably

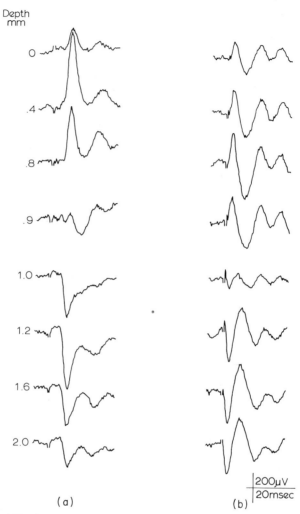

FIG. 4.29. AEPs $\hat{v}_{x_0,v_0}(T,z)$ from an electrode track through the epicenter of a response domain on (a) PON and (b) LOT stimulation and recorded in the olfactory bulb of a cat (Freeman, 1972d).

dealt with in the context of single axons and KO sets of neurons—see Section 3.1.6, 4.1.4, and 4.1.5, and reports by Rall (1962), Rall and Shepherd (1968), and Nicholson and Llinás (1971)]. (4) The representation of source–sink geometry for each local subset of neurons by equivalent point charge is the same for every local subset within the same set. (5) The representation of the time dependence of charge magnitude for each local subset is by the same time function within the set. (6) The potential fields of all subsets are superimposed in the mass.

There is inferred to be a dipole field $v_G(X)$ as in Fig. 4.11 which is generated by the KI set of granule cells. These are the only neurons having axial symmetry, which extend across the zero isopotential surface. There is inferred to be a closed field $v_M(X)$, as in Fig. 4.12, generated by the mitral–tufted cells, which lies in the EPL, MCL, and IPL layers. These are the predominant radially symmetric neurons in or near those layers. The time function for $f_G(T)$ is inferred to be represented by the AEP at the epicenter $\hat{v}_{x_0, y_0, z=0}(T)$. The time function for $f_M(T)$ is inferred to be represented by the AEP at the center $\hat{v}_{x_0, y_0, z_0}(T)$. The potential field of the response domain is inferred to be

$$\hat{v}(T, x, y, z) = v_M(X) f_M(T) + v_G(X) f_G(T) + \varepsilon(T, x, y, z). \qquad (65)$$

The parameters of the dipole field $v_G(X)$, are evaluated in the following way. The values for potential along an electrode track through the epicenter $v_{T, x_0, y_0}(z)$ are shown as means and standard errors for four sets of measurements in Fig. 4.30, for T at the crest of N1 on PON stimulation. At this time, $f_M(T) = 0$. A predicted potential function is calculated as follows. The subset of granule cells in each local domain $\Delta x \, \Delta y$ is treated as equivalent

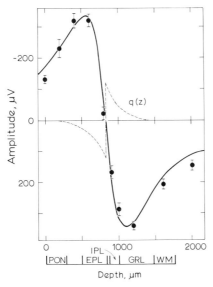

FIG. 4.30. Depth gradient of potential $\hat{v}_{T, x_0, y_0}(z)$ at crest of N1 on PON stimulation. Dots: means $\pm$ SE (N = 4); solid curves: from Eqs. (69); dashed curves: from Eqs. (66) (Freeman, 1972d).

to a core conductor, which is infinite in extent and uniformly depolarized over its superficial half $z < z_0$. From Example A in Section 4.1.3, the distributed source and sink are represented by an equivalent charge density distribution

$$q(x_i, y_j, z_k) = \begin{cases} -\xi(x_i, y_j)\exp[(z_k - z_0)/\lambda], & z_k > z_0, \\ \xi(x_i, y_j)\exp[-(z_k - z_0)/\lambda], & z_k < z_0, \end{cases} \tag{66}$$

where $k = 1, ..., 50$. The density of the active state of each subset and the current source–sink density is inferred to decrease monotonically in all directions of x and y from x_0 and y_0. The distribution is approximated by a bivariate normal density function that determines the values for the source density in each local subset over the whole set (Fig. 4.31a):

$$\xi(x_i, y_j) = \exp[-\tfrac{1}{2}(x_i/\sigma_x)^2 - \tfrac{1}{2}(y_j/\sigma_y)^2], \tag{67}$$

where σ_x and σ_y are standard deviations, and $i = 1, ..., 50$, $j = 1, ..., 50$. The charge at each point is

$$q_a = \xi(x_i, y_j)\, q(z_k). \tag{68}$$

For calculation of $v_{T, x_0, y_0}(z)$, the delay in activation T is fixed at one value T_a for all q_a because the contributions from q_a for all $x < x_0$, where

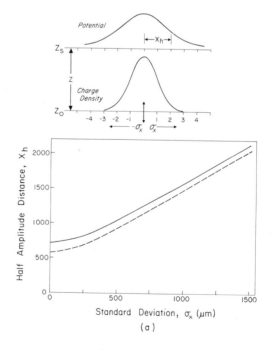

(a)

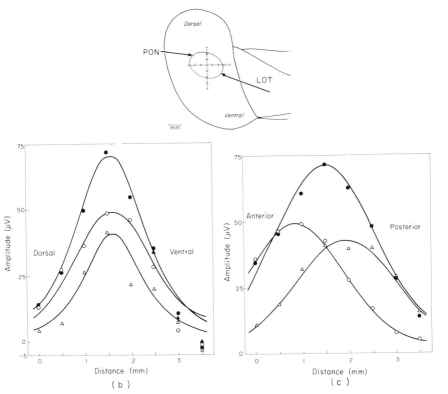

FIG. 4.31. (a) Calculated relation between the standard deviation σ_x of a normally distributed set of activated granule cells and the half-amplitude radius of the surface field potential $v_{T,z}(x, y)$ at $z = 0$ (Freeman, 1972d). Solid line: $z_0 = 1000$ μm; dashed line: $z_0 = 800$ μm. (b, c) Measurements of surface distributions of potential $\hat{v}_{T,x_0,z}(y)$ and $\hat{v}_{T,y_0,z}(x)$ from the bulb of a cat on PON stimulation at three times during N1. Fitted curves: from Eq. (69) with $\lambda = 170$ μm and $z_0 = 820$ μm. Inset shows locations of 1×8 recording arrays and the half-amplitude ellipse (Freeman, 1974a). (b) $N = 100$ at $1.5\times$ threshold for 3 pps. $\bigcirc$: $t = 14.4$ msec, $\sigma = 560$ μm; $\bullet$: $t = 17.6$ msec, $\sigma = 465$ μm; $\triangle$: $t = 20.8$ msec, $\sigma = 320$ μm. (c) $\bigcirc$: $t = 14.4$ msec, $\sigma = 770$ μm; $\bullet$: $t = 17.6$ msec, $\sigma = 880$ μm; $\triangle$: $t = 20.8$ msec, $\sigma = 880$ μm.

$T < T_a$, are added to those from q_a for $x > x_0$, where $T > T_a$. The potential along the z axis at $x_0 = y_0 = 0$ is

$$v_{T,x_0,y_0}(z_n) = \sum_{i=1}^{50} \sum_{j=1}^{50} \sum_{k=1}^{50} q_a/\eta, \qquad \eta = [x_i^2 + y_j^2 + (z_k - z_n)^2]^{.5}.$$

$$(69)$$

Curves for $v_{T,x_0,y_0}(z_n)$ are fitted to $\hat{v}_{T,x_0,y_0}(z)$ by trial and error selection of values for λ and z_0 (Fig. 4.30). The optimal values are $\lambda = 170$ μm, $z_0 = 820$ μm, and $\sigma_x = \sigma_y = 900$ μm.

The mean length of 82 granule cells in the cat is 320 μm (Freeman, 1972d), so the electrotonic length is 320/170 or 1.88. This is similar to the value 1.7 estimated for the mean electrotonic length of the granule cells in the rabbit (Rall & Shepherd, 1968). The summation in Eq. (69) is truncated at $z - z_0 = \pm 3\lambda$, or 510 μm. This corresponds approximately to the range of distribution of the dendrites of granule cells over the combined depth of the EPL, IPL, and GRL. The range is greater than the mean length, because the cell bodies are distributed through the GRL.

The potential computed at the surface $z = 0$ is sufficiently far from the dipole source–sink distribution that $q(z_k)$ can be replaced for each subset by a point source and sink $q(z_k) = 1$ at $z_k = z_0 + \lambda$ and $q(z_k) = -1$ at $z_k = z_0 - \lambda$. For fixed values of z_0, λ, σ_x, and σ_y, the potential at the surface along any line through the epicenter is given by

$$v_{T, z_0}(x, y) = \sum_{i=1}^{50} \sum_{j=1}^{50} \sum_{k=1}^{50} q_a/\eta, \qquad \eta = [(x_i - x)^2 + (y_j - y)^2 + z_k^2]^{.5},$$

(70)

and Eqs. (67) and (68). The predicted surface potential is a unimodal bivariate distribution in x and y (Fig. 4.31a).

The half-amplitude distance x_h or y_h of the response domain is the distance from the epicenter of activity to a location at which the surface amplitude is half the amplitude at the epicenter. The value for y_h increases with increasing σ_y at fixed values for λ and z_0. The relation is linear (Fig. 4.31a).

$$\sigma_y = y_h - (z_0/2).$$

(71)

Also,

$$\sigma_x = x_h - (z_0/2).$$

Equation (71) holds to a good approximation for $\sigma_y > 300$ μm. Below that value for σ_y, y_h approaches a minimal value of 600 to 700 μm, depending on z_0. The value for σ_y is insensitive to changes in σ_x or λ. Equation (71) suffices to predict the standard deviations of a bivariate random distribution of active granule cells, for which the mean is beneath the epicenter, from the half-amplitude widths of the surface field of potential (Fig. 4.31b and c).

4.3.3. TIME-DEPENDENT ACTIVITY

The bulbar response is established over a domain in the bulb by propagating action potentials in the PON at a mean velocity $\theta_x = .42$ m/sec. The questions are considered whether the delay in the PON can account for the apparent movement of the field of potential across the bulb, whether the effect of the delay persists as a phase gradient across the response domain, and whether a phase gradient exists radiating from the epicenter, similar to the phase gradient of waves radiating from the site of an object dropped in water. Answers are sought by measuring the frequency and phase of the oscillatory component of the AEPs at each of 64 points, and by predicting the phase gradient using the distributed dipole model.

The delay is introduced into the array of fixed modules representing source–sink density in the response domain as an ordered delay in onset of activity T_x, increasing in x by $T_x = x_i/\theta_x$ where $\theta_x = .42$ m/sec is PON mean conduction velocity (Section 2.3.3). Once activity is established in each local subset of granule cells, the activity is assumed to have the same time function, but with varying amplitude dependency on location. The function is estimated from the AAEP, an ensemble average, $v_x(T) = \mathscr{E}[\hat{v}_{x,y,z=0}(T)]$, of the set of 64 AEPs recorded at the surface.

The AAEP is measured by fitting it with the sum of basis functions (Section 2.5.3) specified by $v_x(T) = v_1(T) + v_2(T)$:

$$v_1(T) = V_1[\sin(\omega T + \varphi)e^{-\alpha T} - \sin\varphi\cos\omega T\,e^{-\beta T}],$$

$$v_2(T) = V_2\left[\frac{-ae^{-aT}}{(b-a)(c-a)} + \frac{-be^{-bT}}{(a-b)(c-b)} + \frac{-ce^{-cT}}{(a-c)(b-c)}\right], \tag{72}$$

where $v_1(T)$ represents the damped sine wave oscillation and $v_2(T)$ represents a baseline shift (Section 2.5.3). The frequency of the damped sine wave is ω in radians per second; the phase is φ in radians; the decay rate is α in reciprocal seconds; the rise time of N1 is β in reciprocal seconds. The rise time, decay rate, and rate of recovery from a positive overshoot of the baseline shift are, respectively, b, c, and a.

An example of the AAEP is shown in Fig. 4.32a by the plotting symbols; $v_x(T)$ is shown by the solid curve, and $v_1(T)$ and $v_2(T)$ are shown by the dashed curves. The relation is

$$\mathscr{E}[\hat{v}_{x,y,z=0}(T)] = v_1(T) + v_2(T) + \varepsilon(T), \tag{73}$$

where $\varepsilon(T)$ is the minimized least squares deviation.

Equation (72) is then fitted to each of the 64 AEPs from the surface electrode array. Parts (b) and (c) of Fig. 4.32 show the isopotentials based on the 64 values for V_1 and for V_2 (see Fig. 4.27c). The frequency ω varies insignificantly over x and y. The 64 values for decay rate α and phase φ are represented by contours in, respectively, parts (f) and (e) of Fig. 4.32. The arrow denotes the line $y = z = 0$. The observed values for $\varphi(x)$ at $y = 0$, $z = 0$ are plotted in the part (d) as the filled circles. The straight line segment indicates the nature of a uniform phase gradient.

The potential as a function of time for selected points along the line x_n

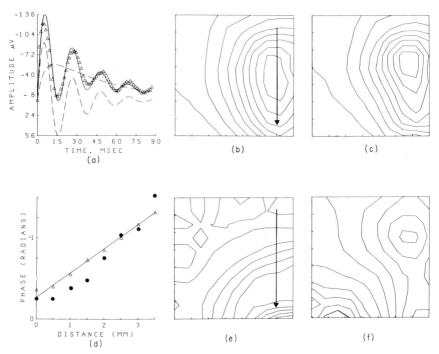

FIG. 4.32. (a) Average AEP ($\triangle$). Solid curve: fitted from Eq. (72); dashed curves: dominant and minor components (see Section 2.5.3). (b) Contour plot for amplitude V_1 in Eq. (72). (c) Contour plot for amplitude V_2. (d) Comparison between observed phase ($\bullet$) and predicted phase ($\triangle$) from Eq. (72) fitted to the wave forms constructed with Eq. (74) with $\theta = .42$ m/sec mean PON conduction velocity. (e) Contour plot for phase φ. (f) Contour plot for decay rate α.

for fixed $y = 0$ and $z = 0$ is

$$v_{y,z}(x_n, T) = \sum_{i=1}^{50} \sum_{j=1}^{25} \sum_{k=1}^{2} q_d v(T - T_x)/\eta,$$

$$q_d = q_y(x_i, y_j, z_k), \qquad \eta = [(x_i - x_n)^2 + y_j^2 + z_k^2]^{.5}, \tag{74}$$

where y_j is summed over half the field by virtue of symmetry. The function $v_{y,z}(x_n, T)$ is the predicted waveform for the AEP at each site x_n. Comparison with the observed AEPs is made most easily by fitting $v_{y,z}(x_n, T)$ with Eq. (72). The predicted frequency $\omega(x_n)$ for the damped sine wave is everywhere the same. The predicted amplitude distributions for V_1 and V_2 over x_n are very similar to the observed distributions for $\sigma_x = 900$ μm and $\sigma_y = 720$ μm. The predicted phase $\varphi(x_n, y, z)$ at $y = z = 0$ (triangles) is compared with the observed phase $\varphi(x, y = 0, z = 0)$ in Fig. 4.32d. The direction and amount of change in phase lag with increasing x_n, as predicted from the designated values of θ, z_0, λ, σ_x, and σ_y introduced into the model, are close to the observed change over $x_n = x_i$.

The predicted and observed AEPs differ in one important respect. Whereas the predicted value for $\alpha(x_i)$, the decay rate of the damped sine wave in Eq. (72), is everywhere the same, the observed values are distributed. High values are found at the epicenter and low values at the margin of the response domain. This is not compatible with the assumption of constancy of $v_G(T)$ over the response domain. This is an important property that is discussed in detail in Section 6.1.4.

Analysis of responses to low-level LOT stimulation shows that the same general properties hold, but the conduction velocity is much faster, and the direction of spread is reversed, as expected from the direction of antidromic propagation (in reverse of the normal direction of flow) of LOT input to the bulb (see arrows in inset in Fig. 4.31b, c).

Analysis has also been carried out for single–shock responses to supra-maximal stimulation of the LOT (Rall & Shepherd, 1968). In this case the delay in activation is assumed to be fixed, and the distribution of input is assumed to be to the entire set of mitral cells in the bulb. The gross geometry of the sets of mitral and granule cells in the rabbit is represented by a "punctured sphere." The predicted and observed absolute amplitudes $v_{t,x,y}(z)$ and $v'_{t,x,y}(z)$ are greater inside the bulb $z < z_0$ than at the surface $z = 0$ for every value of t.

The phase gradient in depth $\varphi_{x_0,y_0}(z)$ is also useful. A set of AEPs on low-level PON stimulation as a function of depth $\hat{v}_{x_0,y_0}(z, T)$ is fitted with the basis functions designated in Eq. (72). Additionally a set of AEPs on low-level LOT stimulation is fitted with another set of basis functions (Section 3.5.3)

$$v_n(t) = \sum_{m=1}^{2} v_m [\sin(\omega_m T + \varphi_m) e^{-\alpha_m T} - \sin(\varphi_m) \cos(\omega_m T) e^{-\beta T}]. \quad (75)$$

The values for φ and φ_m are plotted as functions of depth in Fig. 4.33. The phase is constant with increasing depth to within about 100 μm of a reversal point, and then, within an additional 200 μm of depth, reverses by an average of 3.13 rad (3.14 rad = 180°). The narrow range of phase reversal $z_0 \pm 100$ μm is evidence that the contribution of the closed field in the EPL, MCL, and IPL is much less in amplitude and spatial extent than the contribution of the dipole field.

There are two spatial components in both the orthodromic and antidromic fields of potential evoked by PON and LOT electrical stimulation. The dominant component $v_1(T, X)$ is a distributed dipole field $v_G(X)$ with its zero isopotential surface in or near the MCL, which is assigned to the granule cells. One pole is in the EPL and the other pole is in the GRL.

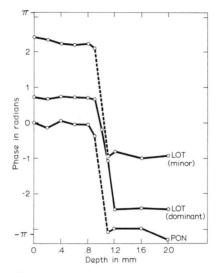

FIG. 4.33. Phase of oscillatory components of AEPs as a function of depth in bulb along a line passing through the epicenter of response domains (Freeman, 1972d).

The secondary component $v_{II}(T, X)$ is a closed field $v_M(X)$ with its main pole located in the EPL and the MCL, and which is attributed to the mitral–tufted cells. The time function of the dipole field $f_G(T)$ has an oscillatory transient superimposed on a baseline shift. The time function of the closed field $f_M(T)$ is oscillatory. The oscillation lags the oscillation in $f_G(T)$ by about one-quarter cycle. Explanation of the significance of the time functions is deferred to Section 5.4.4.

Next we consider the relation between $v_{x_0, y_0, z}(T)$ and the active state of the KI_G set. The activation of the set depends on input paths with constant conduction velocities. There is a delay in onset of activation of each local subset, which is a function of conduction distance. The oscillating impulse response manifested in the dipole field at the surface $\hat{v}_{x, y, z=0}(T)$ displays a phase gradient in the direction of propagation of the input. Because the delay is continuously increasing along x across the epicenter at $x = x_0$ and because the activity on both sides of the epicenter is in the form of a damped sine wave, the sum of waves from subsets for $x < x_0$ with phase lead and of waves from subsets for $x > x_0$ with phase lag is equal to the phase of activity of subsets for $x = x_0$, in the formation of an ensemble average over subsets near the epicenter. Then we need not consider the delay in further analysis of the active state in the neighborhood of the epicenter.

At and near the center of the dipole field the zero isopotential surface is plane and the isopotential surfaces are parallel to it. The lines of extracellular current of the field are normal to the isopotentials and parallel to the axes of the generating neurons oriented perpendicular to the surface. The set of conditions is formally identical to the condition of a nerve suspended in air in which the extracellular action current is constrained to flow parallel to the axons and in the reverse direction of intracellular current. The extracellular potential function at any time T with depth from the epicenter, $T, \hat{v}_{T,x_0,y_0}(z)$ is proportional to the intracellular potential function along the axes of the neurons, except that the scale and reference potential for the two fields may differ (see Section 4.1.3, Example D).

From this principle we infer that an extracellular AEP recorded on a line passing through the center and epicenter is proportional to the time-varying average transmembrane potential over an ensemble of subsets of neurons surrounding the center of the response domain, which contribute current to the line at the center. This geometric condition holds if the site of recording at z lies outside the domain of the closed field centered at $z = z_0$. The average deviation in transmembrane potential difference from resting potential $v_m(T) - v_0$ is defined as the active state in the wave mode for a subset of neurons (Section 1.3.2). Then the AEP from any point between the epicenter and the superficial pole of the dipole field is a measure of the active state of the subset of neurons at the center of the response domain.

$$\mathscr{E}_G[v_m(T) - v_0] = k\hat{v}_{x_0,y_0,z}(T), \qquad 0 \leqq z < z_0, \tag{76}$$

where $v_m - v_0$ is the average deviation from rest of the transmembrane potential of each KI_G subset near the site of transmembrane current reversal over z; k is an empirical proportionality constant; and $\mathscr{E}_G[\cdot]$ denotes the ensemble average over KI_G subsets in the vicinity of the center of the response domain of the olfactory bulb.

Equation (76) holds for other recording sites located on the line joining the epicenter to the superficial pole, because the phase gradient along that line segment is zero (Fig. 4.33). Because of the smoothing property of summation of potential, it holds to a good approximation within the half-amplitude width of a response domain. For a plane dipole field it holds for sites in and deep to the deep pole $z > z_0$, provided the sign of k is reversed. For curved dipole fields that are convex at the surface, it holds for both poles. The domain of the ensemble average $\mathscr{E}[v_m(T)]$, which is related to $\hat{v}_{x,y,z}(T)$ by Eq. (76), is asymmetric with respect to sites on the outer side $z < z_0$ and inner side $z > z_0$. The ensemble domain is smaller on the outer side and larger on the inner side. In summary, the proportionality expressed by Eq. (76) between the AEP and the KI_G active state depends on the local and global architecture of bulbar neurons and on their time and space activity distributions. Within the specified limitations, Eq. (76) provides the principal basis for testing the dynamic models described in Chapters 5 and 6.

4.4. Potential Fields in the Prepyriform Cortex

4.4.1. CORTICAL GEOMETRY AND TOPOLOGY

The primary olfactory cortex is coextensive with the area of termination of the LOT axons on the ventrolateral surface of the brain. It is divided into two main parts, frontal and temporal, where it is crossed by the middle cerebral artery (MCA, Fig. 4.34). Only the frontal part is shown. This part is further divided into the anterior olfactory nucleus (AON), which includes the areas in Fig. 4.34 marked A1 and A2, and prepyriform cortex

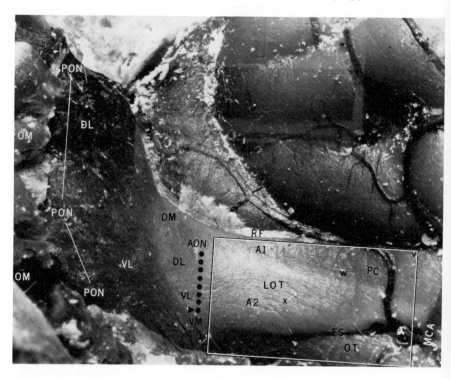

FIG. 4.34. Lateral view of forebrain of a cat at the angle shown by the lower arrow in Fig. 4.22. Rectangle is 4.0 × 7.2 mm (6 × 10 electrode recording array). ●: represent 1 × 8 electrode array for stimulation. DL: dorsolateral bulb; VL: ventrolateral bulb; DM, DL, VL, VM: locations of axons in the LOT from the designated quadrants of the bulb; A1, A2: parts of anterior olfactory nucleus AON; PC: prepyriform cortex; RF: rhinal fissure; ES: endorhinal sulcus; OT: olfactory tubercle; MCA: middle cerebral artery; V, W, X, Y: selected recording sites (see Fig. 4.38).

(PC). The LOT covers most of the lateral surface of the nucleus in its trajectory from the bulb to the other parts of the primary olfactory cortex. It converges to the medial edge of the prepyriform cortex. Its axons and axon collaterals turn laterally, diverge, and intersperse over the surface of the cortex. The distribution is diffuse over the entire cortex extending from the entorhinal sulcus (ES) medially to the deepest part of the rhinal fissure (RF) laterally.

The lateral aspect of the nucleus (AON) in the cat is sufficiently flat to be represented by a plane. The axons in the LOT in its trajectory over the nucleus are topographically arranged in such a way that the most dorsal axons come from the dorsomedial quadrant of the bulb (DM), and the most ventral come from the ventromedial quadrant (VM). Those between come from the dorsolateral (DL) and ventrolateral (VL) quadrants. The bulb projects into the LOT as if it were cut on its medial surface and spread flat (Shepherd and Haberly, 1970). Mitral–tufted axons from the medial bulb divide to pass above and below the ventricle in the bulb (Fig. 4.22). This arrangement implies that there is a degree of topographical order in the bulbar projection to the nucleus, such that neurons in each horizontal strip of the bulb project to a horizontal strip in the nucleus.

The cortex (PC) can be represented geometrically by a hemicylinder of radius r. The long axis of the cylinder is parallel to the LOT and is labeled x. The y axis is along the diameter of the cylinder, and the z axis is perpendicular to the midpoint of the cylinder (Fig. 4.35). The LOT axons converge to the ventromedial edge of the hemicylinder, and their branches turn 90° to diverge over the convexity of the hemicylinder. There is no detectable topographic order in the distribution. Axons from each part of the bulb end in all parts of the cortex.

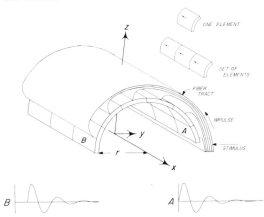

FIG. 4.35. Schematic diagram of the geometrical pattern of spread of activation over the hemicylindrical prepyriform cortex after single-shock stimulation of the LOT (from Horowitz & Freeman, 1966).

One effect of the curvature is that much of the nuclear and cortical surface is buried in the rhinal fissure (Fig. 4.34) forming the lateral border. Plane arrays of electrodes are placed only over the exposed part of the surface by applying sufficient light pressure to the surface (Fig. 4.34 in which the 4 × 7 mm rectangle represents a 6 × 10 electrode array).

The thickness of the cortex is 1.0–1.2 mm. There are three main layers (Fig. 4.36). Layer I is called the *molecular layer* and is divided into Ia, the LOT, and Ib, a layer of superficial dendrites and axon collaterals. The outer half of Ib contains LOT collaterals, and the inner half contains axon collaterals of cortical neurons. Layer II is formed by densely packed cell bodies of small neurons called *superficial pyramidal cells.* Layer III contains the cell bodies of deep pyramidal cells, short axon cells, and polymorphic cells. The cortex is bounded at its base by a mass of myelinated axons that is part of the white matter of the interior of the brain.

There are three main neuron types (O'Leary, 1937; Ramón y Cajal, 1955; Valverde, 1965; Heimer, 1968; Stevens, 1969; Price, 1973; for nomenclature, see the work of Pigache, 1970). The superficial pyramidal or polymorphic cells (Type A) have multiple short, branched, apical dendrites (Fig. 4.37a) extending from the cell bodies in Layer II mainly into Layer Ib. Their axons descend and radiate into Layers Ib, II, and III. They receive axo-dendritic synapses from LOT axon collaterals over the superficial half

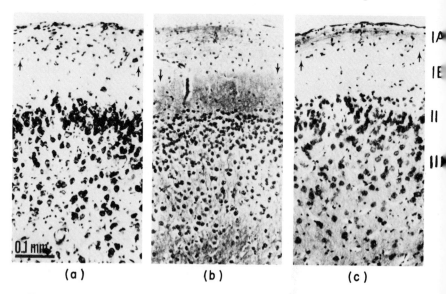

(a)   (b)   (c)

FIG. 4.36. Histological sections through the prepyriform cortex, showing the layers with three stains: (a) Nissl; (b) Bodian; and (c) Weil. The arrows mark the inner border of Layer IA containing the axons from the bulb (Price, 1973).

and axon collaterals from other cortical neurons in the deep half of their extent in Layer Ib. Because of the axial alignment of their dendrites and the location of synapses in Layer Ib, they are expected each to generate a dipole field. On activation only by LOT axons, the field is expected to be asymmetric with the greater source–sink density and absolute amplitude of potential in the superficial pole. This is because the active membrane areas are limited to the superficial terminals of the dendrites (see Fig. 4.2a and b). On activation, however, also by axons of intracortical origin, the dipole field is expected to be less asymmetric due to the extension of the active membrane to the area of the soma. In the second case, the zero isopotential surface should be located nearer the surface (see Fig. 4.42 in the next section) relative to the zero isopotential surface in the first case (see also Fig. 5.31).

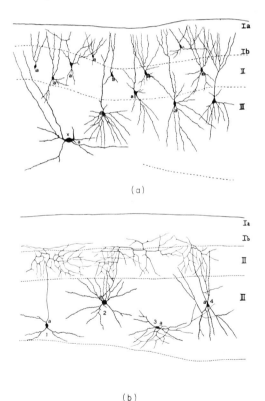

FIG. 4.37.   (a) Distribution and appearance of prepyriform superficial and deep pyramidal-type cells drawn from Golgi preparations of immature mice. (b) Distribution and appearance of four short-axis cylinder cells (prepyriform interneurons or granule cells) with axons extending principally into Layers Ib and II (from O'Leary, 1937, with omission of his distinction of layer III into two parts III and IV).

The second type of neuron is characterized by dendrites radiating in all directions for relatively short distances from a cell body in Layer III, but not into the outer third of Layer Ib (Fig. 4.37b). Its axon ascends and radiates into Layers Ib, II, and III. This type has been labeled as "deep neuron," "pyramidal cell," "granule cell," and "short-axis cylinder cell" by various authors. It is here called the "Type B cell." The star-shaped radial symmetry of its dendrites gives the expectation of a closed field of potential on uniform synaptic activation.

The third type of neuron, called *deep pyramidal cell*, has a pyramid-shaped or irregularly shaped cell body in Layer III and relatively extensive branched dendrites in Layers II and III (lowest cell, Fig. 4.37a). The axon of this cell is known to give off collaterals in Layer III and occasionally Layer II, and its main axon is known often to leave the cortex (Valverde, 1965). The cortex is known to have a well-developed efferent axon system (Heimer, 1969; Price, 1973), and in keeping with the cytoarchitecture of other areas of cortex, it is reasonable to believe that the larger neurons maintain the axons forming the efferent system. The efferent neurons of the cortex comprising the third type are grouped here under the label "Type C" neurons.

The proposed principal connections are shown schematically in Fig. 4.25. The Type A neurons receive input from the LOT and are densely interconnected with each other by axon collaterals in Layers Ib and II. They are known to be mutually excitatory (Section 1.3.1), so they form the KI_A set. The Type B neurons receive input from Type A neurons but not from the LOT, and they are densely interconnected with each other. They are mutually inhibitory and form the KI_B set (Section 5.4.4). Their axons have dense connections onto the dendrites of Type A neurons, which is the basis for the existence of a KII set in the cortex. The intracortical connections of the efferent neurons, here called Type C are inadequately known and they are provisionally designated as the KO_C set. By virtue of the laminar geometry, the KI_A set of Type A neurons is expected to generate an asymmetric distributed dipole field centered in Layer Ib, and the sets of Type B and C neurons are expected to generate closed or nearly closed fields centered in Layers II and III.

4.4.2. Observed Fields of Cortical Potential

Single-shock electrical stimulation of the LOT at the surface in the mid-regions of the cortex, $z = 0$, results in a compound action potential in the LOT. This propagates orthodromically over the cortex along the x axis at a velocity of 5 to 10 m/sec. The amplitude decreases rapidly with increasing x (Fig. 4.38b). The volley is carried over the convexity by collaterals

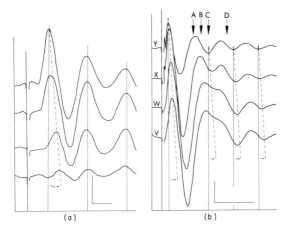

FIG. 4.38. Comparison of AEPs $\hat{v}_{x,y,z}(T)$ from (a) surface of bulb on orthodromic PON stimulation and from (b) surface of cortex on LOT stimulation. Recording sites on cortex are shown in Fig. 4.34. Dashed lines: preservation of a phase gradient along the cortex due to conduction delay in the LOT; amplitude: 200 μV; time: 20 msec.

at a lower velocity (1–2 m/sec). It is followed by an oscillatory evoked potential, which is shown after averaging as a selected set of AEPs, $\hat{v}_{x,y,z}(T)$ in Fig. 4.38b. The positions of the monopolar recording and stimulating electrodes are shown in Fig. 4.34 by the black rectangle and the letters, Y, X, W, and V, and by the 1 × 8 array of black dots.

The frequency of the oscillation differs for different locations on the cortical surface. In this respect the cortical AEPs are unlike the bulbar AEPs on PON stimulation which have a common frequency (Fig. 4.38a).

The potential at the surface $v_{T,z}(x, y)$, $z = 0$, is shown in Fig. 4.39 for selected instants during the first surface negative peak, N1. Each arrow has its tail at the location of the maximal potential in that frame and its head at the location of the maximum in the succeeding frame. There are two maxima of potential in the surface coordinates. The anterior maximum overlies the anterior olfactory nucleus (A2). It shows little tendency to move during N1 and recurs at approximately the same location during N2, N3, etc. The posterior maximum moves upwardly in the frame (dorsolaterally over the cortex, PC) in the direction of the LOT axon collaterals. By the conclusion of N1 in the anterior part of the cortex, the peak is moving into the inaccessible part of the lateral surface.

The distribution of potential over the surface during subsequent peaks, P1, N2, P2, ..., is rather complicated. Four representative distributions are shown in Fig. 4.40. The patterns suggest that the impulse input initiates

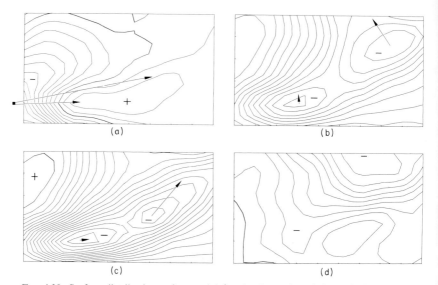

FIG. 4.39. Surface distributions of potential $\hat{v}_{T,z_0}(x, y)$ at selected times during N1 of the cortical AEP on LOT stimulation (see Fig. 4.34). Time: (a) 1.28 msec; (b) 384 msec; (c) 5.12 msec; (d) 6.40 msec.

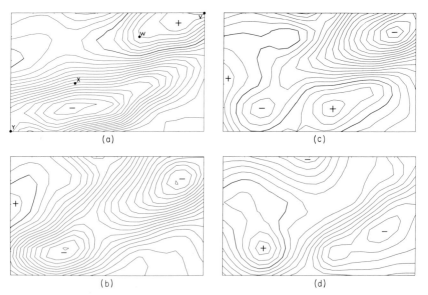

FIG. 4.40. Surface distributions of potential $\hat{v}_{T,z_0}(x, y)$ at selected times indicated by letters, A, B, C, D, in Fig. 4.38 and corresponding to parts (a), (b), (c), (d), respectively.

oscillatory events in two domains of the cortex underlying the electrode array. The potential fields of the domains partially overlap, so that the locations of the epicenters cannot be precisely determined by inspection. The successive maxima in potential over the nucleus (A1) occur in the same location, whereas the successive maxima of potential oscillation over the cortex move dorsolaterally.

The depth distribution of potential of single-shock response $v'_{T_m,x}(y, z)$, is shown for four coronal planes in Fig. 4.41. The planes of mapping at A18 and A16 shown by parts (d) and (c), respectively, pass through the frontal part, and those at A14 and A12, parts (b) and (a), respectively, pass through the temporal part of the cortex. The planes lie about 30° from the yz plane that is perpendicular to the LOT. The values at T_m are taken from the peak of N1 recorded at each site without regard to its

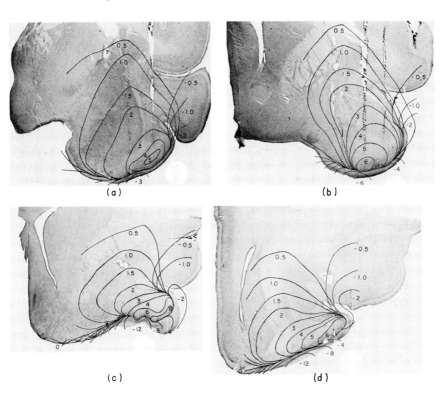

(a)   (b)

(c)   (d)

FIG. 4.41. Depth distribution of single-shock response $v'_{T_m,x}(y, z)$ at the time of the maximal amplitude of the first surface-negative, deep-positive peak. Use of this technique gives rise to overlapping isopotentials in the lateral aspects of the field due to conduction delay. (a) A12; (b) A14; (c) A16; (d) A18 in millimeters anterior to midaural plane.

latency, in order to represent the maximal amplitude distribution in one set of figures. As the result, the isopotentials for the peak positive and negative values cross each other over the lateral convexity, where the delay is greatest. The field is a curved distributed dipole field. During N1 the superficial pole is negative and is centered near the LOT. The deep pole is positive and is located within the concavity of the curvature. The zero isopotential surface is located near the base of Layer Ib, where the trunks of the dendrites approach the cell bodies of the superficial pyramidal cells.

The precise location of the zero isopotential surface for any point in depth is determined by making a small lesion or electrolytic deposit with a micro-electrode. When the location of selected points has been histologically verified, the change in location of the zero isopotential surface with time is determined with respect to the verified points. Partly because of the technical difficulties in making and reading a large number of small lesions, and partly because of spatial distortions in processing the histological sections of the brain in which the recordings are made, the maps of isopotentials based on selected sampling sites are subject to uncontrollable local distortions. The sections and the maps are only approximately superimposable.

An example of the movement of the zero isopotential surface $\hat{v}_x(T, y, z) = 0$, which implies the movement of all other isopotential surfaces, is shown in Fig. 4.42 at intervals of 1.25 msecs from the crest of N1. By the crest of N1 it is established as a curved surface AA, part (a) corresponding to the curvature of Layer II and known from use of electrolytic deposits to lie in the inner third of Layer Ib. During the next 3.75 msec (to DD) it rotates around the convexity of the cortex. By 5 msec from the crest (EE), part (b), the polarity of the dipole field is totally reversed. The zero isopotential surface is reestablished in Layer Ib, but during P1 it continues to rotate about the convexity, similarly to a rotating tangent to the base of Layer Ib.

The pattern of spread is shown in the schematic diagram in Fig. 4.43a of a cross section of the cortex through PC in Fig. 4.34 (see also Fig. 4.37). On the right is shown a selected set of recording sites [A–F, part (b)] and a representative set of AEPs from those sites [part (c)]. Each element represents a subset of cortical neurons that generates a dipole field. The start latency increases with distance from the medial edge of the cortex. One effect of the delay is seen at the start of the AEP labeled F, where the initial deflection is downward (positive). This is due to recording the deep positivity of the dipole field established at A and B before the activating volley has reached E and F. The same phenomenon can be visualized in maps of the contours of potential superimposed on photo-micrographs of the plane of mapping. In this case the isopotentials move with poststimulus time.

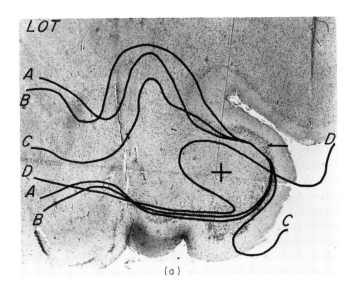

(a)

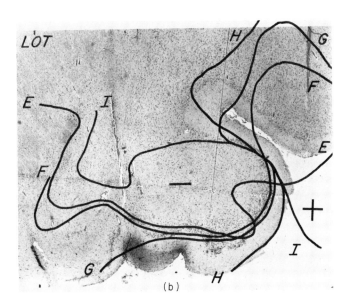

(b)

FIG. 4.42. Location of the zero isopotential surface of the field of potential $\hat{v}_{T,x}(y, z)$ in the plane perpendicular to the LOT and to the cortical surface. (a) Locations during N1; (b) locations during P1.

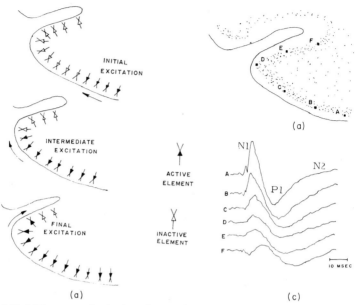

FIG. 4.43. (a) Sequence of activation of prepyriform cortical dipole generators (see PC in Fig. 4.34) following LOT stimulation. (b) Location of elements deep to surface recording sites. (c) AEPs at designated sites in the plane A17 (with permission of J. M. Horowitz).

The dipole field is attributed mainly to the KI_A set of Type A neurons, because these neurons have the appropriate local and global geometry and the required location of synaptic input to account for the position of the zero isopotential surface and the locations of both poles. This conclusion holds for both surface-negative and surface-positive polarities of the dipole field. It is supported by intracellular recordings from Type A cells, which show EPSPs followed by IPSPs (LOT stimulation, Biedenbach & Stevens, 1969b); by the effects of small lesions in the cortex, which reduce both N1 and P1 if made in Layer Ib and have no effect if made in Layers III and IV (Fig. 5.32); and by source–sink analysis based on differencing (Haberly & Shepherd, 1973; see footnote in Section 4.1.2).

In summary, both the anterior olfactory nucleus and the prepyriform cortex generate dipole fields of potential. Both oscillate at some characteristic frequency on impulse driving, and both oscillations are initially surface-negative. Both dipole fields reflect an oscillatory active state in the KI_A sets in the respective parts of the primary olfactory cortex. The location of the oscillatory active state in the nucleus bears some topographic relation to the part of the LOT which activates it, and the location of the event is fixed. The oscillatory active state in the prepyriform cortex shows a systematic lag in the direction of delay in initial activation. That is, there is a phase lag or phase gradient in the direction of LOT conduction delay. It is the phase gradient that gives the appearance of a rotating dipole field. There is no present evidence for the existence of a topographic relation between the bulb and the prepyriform cortex.

4.4.3. RELATION OF POTENTIAL FIELDS TO ACTIVE STATES

The chief desideratum in extracellular recording in multineuronal fields of potential is a measure of potential $\hat{v}$ that is proportional to the ensemble means of the active states of the generating neurons $\mathscr{E}(v_m)$. We have seen (Section 4.3.3) from the analysis of a plane dipole field that if a coherent domain can be identified, the potential at the epicenter is a function [Eq. (76)] of the active state of the neural subset comprising the domain. This principle also holds for epicenters on the convexity of curved surfaces. It cannot, however, hold if the surface potential is determined by dipole fields of two or more KI sets forming a neural mass. Types B and C neurons are expected to generate closed fields on the basis of their local dendritic and synaptic geometry, but the possibility exists that incomplete radial symmetry may lead to the formation of a dipole component of the fields of subsets of Types B and C neurons that could degrade the relation between the surface potential and the active states of the set of Type A neurons.

The problem is analyzed in the following way. The cortical mass consists of three sets of neurons. The KI_A and KI_B sets are more densely populated than the KO_C (or possibly KI_C) set, so only these two are considered. The KI_A set generates a dipole field $v_A(X)$ with its zero isopotential surface at the base of Layer I. The active state for impulse input can be assigned the time function of a damped sine wave $f_A(T) = V_A \sin(\omega T + \varphi_A) e^{-\alpha T}$. The KI_B set generates a field of potential $v_B(X)$, which is inferred to be a closed field centered in Layer II. The active state also has the time function of a damped sine wave $f_B(T) = V_B \sin(\omega T + \varphi_B) e^{-\alpha T}$. The frequency and decay rate in $f_A(T)$ and $f_B(T)$ are identical, but the active state of KI_B must lag by one-quarter cycle the active state of KI_A. (This will be proven in Chapter 5.) Therefore, $\varphi_B - \varphi_A = -90°$.

The field potential at the surface $v_{x,y,z}(T)$, $z = 0$, reflects only the closed field $v_B(X)$ and the time function $f_B(T)$. The field potential in Layer II, $v_{x,y,z}(T)$, $z > z_0$, is the sum of the deep pole of the dipole field and the monopole field $v_A(X) + v_B(X)$. The time function is the vector sum of $f_A(T)$ and $f_B(T)$, which is $v_{AB} \sin(\omega T + \varphi_{AB}) e^{-\alpha T}$, where φ_{AB} depends on the phases and relative amplitudes of the two damped cosines.

These phase relations are shown in Fig. 4.44. In parts (a)–(c) there are, respectively, two AEPs from the deep pole that are initially positive (downward) in potential and a third AEP (the lowest) that is from the surface pole and is initially negative (upward). The active state of the KI_A set is shown by the lower PSTH, which oscillates in phase with the surface AEP. The active state of the KI_B set is shown by the upper PSTH, which oscillates with a quarter cycle phase lag from the surface AEP. (These phase relations also hold between the pulse probability waves of Types A and B units and the cortical EEG as shown in Sections 3.3.3, 3.3.5, and 5.4.4). This implies that the surface AEP has the same phase, frequency and decay rate as the active state of the KI_A set in this stimulus-recording arrangement.

In part (b) the lower AEP is from the surface recording and conforms to a damped cosine wave, $\cos(\omega T)e^{-\alpha T}$. The phase $\varphi_A = 90°$, and relative amplitude v_A are shown by the vector at **A** in part (e) at 90°. The middle AEP is from the base of Layer I at the minimum for the amplitude of peak N1. The amplitude v_{AB} is relatively low, and the phase φ_{AB} is 180°. The AEP in fact conforms to an initially positive damped sine wave. The KI_B set is maximally excited at the first downward crest of the sine wave. The Type B neurons in the set have dense current sources in their cell

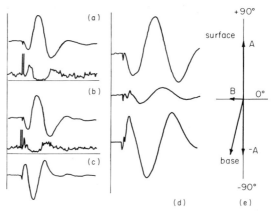

FIG. 4.44. Evidence that a prepyriform field of evoked potential consists in the superposition of a dipole field generated by the Type A neurons $v_A(X)$ and a monopole field generated by the Type B neurons $v_B(X)$. The time function $f_A(T)$ is obtained in the AEP recorded at the cortical surface [(d), lower AEP], and the time function $f_B(T)$ is obtained in the AEP recorded at the zero isopotential surface of $v_A(X)$, where $v_B(X)$ is near maximal [(d), middle AEP]. Elsewhere the AEP reflects the weighted sum of $f_A(T)$ and $f_B(T)$ [(d), upper trace], as shown in (e) the vector diagram. The forms for $f_A(T)$ and $f_B(T)$ are predicted from PSTHs as in (a)–(c) (see also Section 5.4.4) (Freeman, 1968b). (a) $N = 450$ for 450 μm at 125 msec; (b) 270 μm; (c) -300 μm; (d) $N = 92$ for the three curves at 370, 0, and -180 μm, respectively, at 62.5 msec. Distances are heights above zero isopotential in μm.

bodies and broader but less dense current sinks in their radial dendrites that are concentric with their cell bodies. As shown in Figs. 4.10 and 4.12, the high density of the source gives the closed field its polarity. The initially positive (downward) sine wave, therefore, represents a field of potential $v'_B \sin(\omega T + 180°)e^{-\alpha T}$, which is 180° out of phase with the active state $f_B(T) = v_B \sin(\omega T + 0°)e^{-\alpha T}$. That is, the active state $f_B(T)$ lags the active state $f_A(T)$ by 90°, but the field potential v'_B leads the active state $f_A(T)$ by 90°. This is shown by the vector **B** in part (e). The upper AEP in part (d) is taken from Layer II. The potential predicted for the deep pole of the dipole field is $v'_A \sin(\omega T - 90°)e^{-\alpha T}$, because it is 180° out of phase with the surface recording. This is shown by the vector $-$**A**. The vector sum of $-$**A** and **B** predicts the phase and amplitude of the AEP from the deep pole, which typically has about 30° of phase lag from the inverted surface AEP. It is concluded that the cortical field consists of a KI_A dipole field and a KI_B closed field, and that surface recordings reflect the active state of the KI_A set.

Another determinant of the phase of AEPs in the cortex is the combination of curvature and delay in activation (see also Section 4.3.3). This combination, however, gives a different pattern of phase relations than that attributable to the KI_A and KI_B sets. This is shown by setting up a hemi-cylindrical array of dipole charge elements (Fig. 4.35), and assigning to each element a delay in impulse input, and an impulse response consisting of a damped sine wave. The potential is calculated for selected points representing specified recording sites. The order and amount of delay for each element, the size and curvature of the cylinder, the frequency and decay rate of the impulse response, and the distances of the recording sites from the zero charge surface at z_0 are adapted to correspond to the dimensions of the cortex and its response.

Predicted responses at three points on the surface are shown in Fig. 4.45a. They show the predicted phase lag of the oscillation in the direction of LOT impulse propagation. The predicted functions of potential with depth are

$$v_1(T) = v_{x,y}(T, z), \quad z = 0; \qquad v_2(T) = v_{x,y}(T, z), \quad z = z_0;$$

$$v_3(T) = x_{x,y}(T, z), \quad z > 0$$

(Fig. 4.45a). There is a disparity between the absolute amplitudes at the inner and outer recording sites. For the designated parameters of frequency and delay, the outer absolute amplitude exceeds the inner absolute amplitude $|v_1(T)| > |v_2(T)|$. The relation is the reverse of the intuitively predicted relation (Example B in Section 4.2.2 and Section 4.3.3). It occurs because the potential at site 2 inside the cylinder is the sum of contributions that

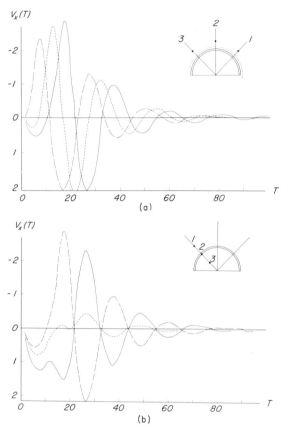

FIG. 4.45. (a) Predicted phase lag of calculated AEPs that is designed to conform to experimental observations (Fig. 4.43). Dashed line: V_1; dotted line: V_2; solid line: V_3. (b) Calculation of the predicted AEPs at the cortical surface (1), midpoint (2), and depth (3) shows that the absolute amplitude outside the cylinder V_1 exceeds the absolute amplitude inside the cylinder V_3. This conforms to observation (Fig. 4.41) in reverse of the expectation for a curved dipole surface without afferent delay. However, the predicted AEP at the center of the dipole sheet V_2 does not conform to observation (middle AEP, Fig. 4.44d). Therefore, the cortical field of potential is not accounted for by a curved dipole sheet generator with activation delay; a monopole generator must be included (from Horowitz & Freeman, 1966).

are weighted more heavily toward those from the limits of the cylinder than is the case for the site 1 outside the cylinder. This results in amplitude reduction inside the cylinder owing to phase dispersion. It occurs in the prepyriform dipole field (Fig. 4.41), as shown by the greater absolute amplitude of the surface pole over the deep pole.

Although the weighted summation across the response domain is sufficient to reverse the ratio of absolute amplitudes, it is not sufficient to change the phase relation between $\hat{v}_1(T)$ and $\hat{v}_2(T)$ by the amount required. Moreover, there is no significant phase shift in the predicted function $\hat{v}_3(T)$ with respect to the mirror image of the function $\hat{v}_1(T)$.

It is concluded that the surface potential $\hat{v}_x(T)$, $x = x_0$, $y = y_0$, $z = 0$, is proportional to the ensemble average of the active states of the subset of neurons in the KI_A set $\mathscr{E}[v_m(T)]$ which forms a coherent domain centered under the recording site. Therefore Eq. (76) derived for the KI_G set in the olfactory bulb holds also (within the specified limitations) for the KI_A set. The same conclusion cannot be drawn for surface recording sites at the margins of coherent domains or for sites beneath the cortical surface or the zero isopotential surface.

4.5. Divergence and Convergence in Neural Masses

4.5.1. THE OPERATION OF DIVERGENCE

The active state o_μ of each set μ in a neural mass can be described by the functions of time, amplitude, and distance $o_\mu(t, x, y, u)$, where t is real time, X is x, y, and z, and u is a variable representing amplitude in either pulse mode p or wave mode v. Under the assumptions given previously, each function and mode can be separated into three parts:

$$o_{\mu v}(t, x, y, u) = g_{\mu v}(u) h_{\mu v}(x, y) f_{\mu v}(t), \qquad \text{wave mode,} \qquad (77)$$

$$o_{\mu p}(t, x, y, u) = g_{\mu p}(u) h_{\mu p}(x, y) f_{\mu p}(t), \qquad \text{pulse mode.} \qquad (78)$$

The global potential field generated by the mass and manifesting its active states in the wave mode $v'(t, X)$ is the sum of the fields of potential of a number of sets M that make detectable extracellular contributions in the wave mode. The procedure has been described for postulating on anatomical grounds the existence of a number of sets in a mass, determining the probable location and spread of active states by locating afferent tracts and synaptic sites, predicting source–sink distributions from local and global neural geometry, and calculating a potential function $v_\mu(X)$ for each set. This function is weighted by a characteristic time function $v_\mu(X) f_\mu(T)$ for each set, and the sum over M is evaluated from $\hat{v}(T, X)$.

Each function $f_\mu(T)$ is dependent on the active state in the wave mode $o_{\mu v}(t, x, y, u)$. Each function $v_\mu(X)$ is determined by $q_\mu(X)$, representing the source–sink distribution. The time dependency of the active state $f_\mu(T)$ for a local subset of neurons is given by the ensemble average of transmembrane potential for the neurons in the subset $\mathscr{E}(v_m(T))$. Certain conditions have been described in which this is proportional to $\hat{v}_X(T)$. We now ask how the equivalent charge function $q_\mu(X)$ depends on the active state $h_{\mu v}(x, y)$. Two transformations are needed:

$$q_\mu(X) = H_{1v}[h_v(x, y), z], \tag{79}$$

$$v_\mu(X) = H_{2v}[q_\mu(X)]. \tag{80}$$

The first transformation H_{1v} is the step of converting a proposed activity density function $o_{\mu m}(t, x, y)$ to the accompanying source–sink distribution and then to a distribution of equivalent charge. An example has been given in Section 4.4.3 for the KI_B set. The neurons are radially symmetric and are concentrated in Layer II of the cortex. When they are excited, they generate concentric source–sink distributions with central high-density sources. In large numbers the fields of individual neurons add without vector components, so the expected field of the excited KI_B set is a closed centrally positive field. This is represented by a concentric charge distribution $q_B(X)$ with its outer limits in the deeper part of Layer I. The second transformation H_{2v} is the step of summing the potential contributed by all the charge to determine the potential field $v_B(X)$.

The observable electrical activity of a neural mass manifests distributions of activity in the pulse mode $o_{\mu p}(t, x, y, u)$. The pulse trains recorded and averaged in a mass, $p'(t, X)$ and $\hat{p}(T, X)$, are generated by a number of sets M. The averaged pulse density function of each set $p_\mu(T, X)$ is separated into time- and distance-dependent parts $p_X(T)$ and $p_T(X)$, where $p_{\mu X}(T)$ may be determined by PSTHs, and $p_T(X)$ is found by recording pulse trains at multiple sites in an active domain. Again, two transformations are defined and evaluated:

$$\psi_\mu(X) = H_{1p}[h_{\mu p}(x, y), z], \tag{81}$$

$$p_\mu(X) = H_{2p}[\psi_\mu(X)], \tag{82}$$

where $\psi_\mu(X)$ is the spatial (three-dimensional) distribution of impulses determined by the active state $q_{\mu p}(x, y)$ and is homologous with $h_\mu(X)$, and where $p_\mu(X)$ is the distribution of action potentials determined by electrical recording.[†] Again, the first transformation H_{1p} is the prediction of the relation between an active state and a pulse density function. The predicted pulses may occur in the dendrites, in axonal initial segments, or for some neurons

[†] An assumption that has not been thoroughly tested but can and should be with the multiple microelectrode technique described in Example A in Section 7.2.2 is that the pulse density function $p_{\mu T}(X)$ is constant over z through the depth of the KI_μ set as well as over small distances x and y. This assumption is needed in order to establish an equivalence between $\psi_\mu(X)$ and $h_{\mu p}(x, y)$ by the operation H_{1p} in Eq. (81). Some evidence for its validity is found in the fact that the neurons in each column in somatosensory and primary visual neocortex have very similar receptor field properties (Hubel & Wiesel, 1962; Mountcastle, 1966).

not at all. The second transformation H_{2p} is required to establish the spatial relation between the spatial distribution of pulses and a spatial field of potential. The field may be quite different from the distribution of pulses, as for example the compound action potential is not the same as any single action potential (Fig. 2.11) and in fact may be everywhere zero in the presence of a large volley of action potentials (Fig. 2.14). In general, $\psi_\mu(X)$ is not identical to $p_\mu(X)$ because the field of the action potential extends beyond the neuron generating the impulse.

For any set that contributes both to $\hat{v}(T, X)$ and $\hat{p}(T, X)$, if the active states of the set are defined with respect to transmembrane potential and pulse probability at or near the trigger zone of each neuron, then

$$h_{\mu v}(x, y) = h_{\mu p}(x, y). \tag{83}$$

More generally, the conversions from waves to pulses and from pulses to waves that are the bases for defining $G(v)$ and $G(p)$ in neural masses (Section 3.3.6) can be conceived as taking place at points, so that it is feasible to define a single function $h_\mu(x, y)$ for each neural set in a mass, which is independent of mode and may be estimated from observed activity in either mode.

Evaluation of the transformation implied by H_{2v} has been undertaken in the preceding sections. Analysis and evaluation of H_{1v}, H_{1p}, and H_{2p} is given in the following sections. Transmission of activity from one set μ to another $\mu + 1$ involves two complementary processes. The projection of many neurons in set μ onto each neuron in set $\mu + 1$ is convergence. The projection of each neuron in set μ onto many neurons in set $\mu + 1$ is divergence. If either occurs, both must occur, and the choice of label is determined by whether the input or the output is identified on a single neuron. If divergence occurs, then the spatial functions of the active states for the sets are related but not equal. Let $h_\mu(x, y)$ denote $h_{\mu v}$ or $h_{\mu p}$ depending on the mode for the μth transmitting subset. Then the relation

$$h_{\mu+1} = H(h_\mu, z) \tag{84}$$

defines the operation H of divergence of neural activity on transmission from the active state of set μ to the active state of set $\mu + 1$.

The spatial distribution of an active state is defined over the xy plane of a neural set. Divergence takes place in the xy plane in directions orthogonal to the topological trajectory of transmission. The description and measurement of divergence is based on measuring two appropriate functions, $\hat{h}_\mu(x, y)$ and $\hat{h}_{\mu+1}(x, y)$ in the x and y dimensions with appropriate sets of basis functions in x, and on comparing the parameters of the sets of basis functions. The most useful basis function is the normal density function. The measure of the active state on this basis in the x and y coordinates is the variance σ_μ^2 (the square of the standard deviation σ_μ) and $\sigma_{\mu+1}^2$ of the normal curves fitted to them. The operation of divergence is expressed as the ratio $\sigma_{\mu+1}^2/\sigma_\mu^2$, or the difference $\sigma_{\mu+1}^2 - \sigma_\mu^2$ of the output and input variances.

Divergence takes place during transmission at synapses and over compound nerves and tracts. The mechanisms differ, so we will distinguish between two basic classes of divergence-convergence and call them, respectively, *synaptic divergence* and *tractile divergence*.

Tractile divergence has three mechanisms. Each tract or nerve has a set of cross-sectional areas over its trajectory. The tract is coextensive with the areas of the transmitting and receiving neural sets at the start and end of each tract, but many tracts are funneled through small areas in transit, by dense packing of the axons. If a volley is induced in a small area of high density by an electrical stimulus, the set of action potentials spreads out over the target neural set. The dilation of the volley from onset to termination is in proportion to the ratio of output to input cross-sectional areas. The number of pulses is not changed. This is *dilative divergence*. If the axons of neurons in each local subset of a transmitting set become interspersed among the axons of other local subsets on arrival at the receiving set, the representation of the transmitting subset (after any correction for dilation) is larger at reception than on transmission. If there is no branching, neither the total number of pulses nor the pulse density is affected. This we call *interspersive divergence*. If each axon gives off collaterals that are interspersed with the collaterals of other axons, both the total number of pulses and the pulse density are increased. This we call *collateral divergence*. Dilative divergence is described by the ratio of variances. The other forms of synaptic and tractile divergence are described by the difference between variances.

The complementary facet of divergence $H(X)$ is convergence $H^{-1}(X)$, in which each point on the receiving surface receives from a distribution of points on the transmitting surface. In this point of view the various types and mechanisms of divergence do not appear explicitly. The operation is most familiar in the form of the *receptor field* of a single sensory neuron (e.g., Barlow, 1953; Hubel & Wiesel, 1962; Mountcastle, 1966) from which input converges to that neuron. That is, the input to the neural system is a spatial distribution of excitation and/or inhibition, and the output is the pulse rate of a single neuron or a unit cluster. The convergence operation $H^{-1}(X)$ can also be described by means of Gaussian basis functions (Rodieck & Stone, 1965), and where both $H(X)$ and $H^{-1}(X)$ have been measured in the same preparation (see Fig. 4.46) the two facets of the operation are found to be congruent. Typically, only one of the two facets of operation is accessible to measurement, but there is no definite reason at present to question the complementarity, so that either type of measurement should suffice.

4.5.2. EVALUATION OF SPATIAL DISTRIBUTIONS OF ACTIVE STATES

The spatial distribution of an active state $h_\mu(x, y)$ is defined by an activity density function (see Section 1.3.2) at any time T over the surface normal to the direction of transmission z. The current source–sink distribution of the active state is represented by an array of fixed charge $q(X)$ that has been tested by comparing its potential field $v(X)$ with an observed field $\hat{v}_T(X)$. In order to determine the activity density function, an operation must be performed on the array of charge to determine its extent in the x and y dimensions. The nature of the required operation depends on the system under study and its mode of operation.

Some appropriate examples are taken from the olfactory system of the cat. The main sequence of events following monopolar single-shock electrical stimulation of the PON is listed in Table 4.2 (Fig. 4.25). The stimulus current

TABLE 4.2

DEFINITION OF SYMBOLS FOR NEURAL ACTIVITY DISTRIBUTIONS[a]

Distribution	Symbol	Operation	Symbol
Source of stimulus current[b]	σ_s	Current spread	$\sigma_{s \cdot a}$
PON axons[b]	σ_a	Dilation	$d_{a \cdot b}$
Glomerular PON endings[c]	σ_b	Interspersion	$\sigma_{a \cdot b}$
Periglomerular neurons[b]	σ_p	Excitation of periglomerular neurons by PON axons	$\sigma_{b \cdot p}$
Excited mitral-tufted neurons[b]	σ_e	Excitation of mitral-tufted neurons by PON axons	$\sigma_{b \cdot e}$
Excited granule cells[b]	σ_g	Excitation of granule cells by mitral-tufted neurons	$\sigma_{e \cdot g}$
Inhibited mitral-tufted neurons[b]	σ_i	Inhibition of mitral-tufted neurons by granule cells	$\sigma_{g \cdot i}$

[a] Sequence in list shows order of transmission through olfactory bulb.
[b] Observable experimentally.
[c] dorsal: σ_{gd}, $\sigma_{a \cdot gd}$, etc.; ventral: σ_{gv}, $\sigma_{a \cdot gv}$, etc.

excites a certain distribution of axons in the PON that conducts action potentials to the glomeruli in the bulb. There is dilative and interspersive divergence between the stimulus site and the glomeruli. The PON input excites distributions of periglomerular neurons in the glomerular layer and mitral–tufted cells in the EPL and MCL. The mitral–tufted cells excite a distribution of granule cells that then inhibits another distribution of mitral–tufted cells. The widths of distributions have been measured for PON axons, periglomerular neurons, excited mitral–tufted cells, excited granule cells, and inhibited mitral–tufted cells.

Example A. The compound action potential of the PON is shown in Fig. 2.13. The set of traces on the left is from monopolar recording at surface sites along the z axis of transmission, $x_0 = 0$, $y_0 = 0$, $\hat{v}_{x_0, y_0}(T, z)$. The set of traces on the right is from surface sites, $x_0 = 0$, along a line y normal to the transmission axis $\hat{v}_{x_0, z_0}(T, y)$ at a value for z_0 of 1.0 mm from the stimulating electrode at $z = 0$. The x axis is normal to the surface of the PON.[†]

A time T_0 is selected at which the value $\hat{v}_{T_0, x_0, y_0}(z) = v_0(0)$, maximally negative, corresponding to the negative-upward crest of the compound action potential. The functions, $\hat{v}_{T_0, x_0, y_0}(z)$ and $\hat{v}_{T_0, x_0, z_0}(y)$, are digitized. The values are normalized by dividing each by the maximum $v_0(0)$. On the basis of the analysis given in Section 4.1.3, the function $\hat{v}_{n, T_0, x_0, y_0}(z)$ is treated as proportional to the source–sink density along z and is used to specify a source–sink distribution along the z axis:

$$q(x, y, z_k) = \begin{cases} \xi(z_k) \Delta z, & x = 0, \quad y = 0, & (85) \\ 0, & x \neq 0, \quad y \neq 0, & (86) \end{cases}$$

$$\xi(z_k) \Delta z = \hat{v}_{T_0, x_0, y_0}(z_k), \qquad k = 1, \dots, 50. \qquad (87)$$

The potential as a function of distance from the transmission axis along y is calculated at n points

$$v_n(y) = \rho \sum_{k=1}^{50} q_k(x, y, z_k) / \eta, \qquad (88)$$

$$\eta = [y_n^2 + (z_k - z_0)^2]^{.5}, \qquad \eta \geq \Delta z / 2.$$

The values are normalized by division by $v_0(0)$. The half-amplitude width of the potential function is less than that observed, so Eq. (86) is not valid.

[†]The convention being followed here is that the z axis conforms to the main direction of transmission in a neural set, and the xy plane is the set of directions in which divergence takes place. When divergence is evaluated in the PON, the z axis lies parallel to the PON axons. When divergence is evaluated in the bulb, the z axis lies perpendicular to the PON on the bulbar surface, and the x axis is aligned with the PON. We use a convention based on local functional topologies rather than on anatomical or stereotaxic coordinates for the whole brain, because the tracts and layers in the brain are usually curved and are not readily described in Cartesian coordinates. Hence, each computation of divergence must be preceded by specification of the coordinates.

Next, the active axons are postulated to lie in a bivariate random distribution $h(x, y)$ around the z axis with the mean at $x_0 = y_0 = 0$ and with standard deviation σ_a. The distribution of charge in x and y is

$$q(x_i, y_j, z_k) = \xi(z_k)\,\Delta z \exp[-(x_i^2 + y_j^2)/2\sigma_a^2], \qquad (89)$$

where $h(x, y)$ is represented by a bivariate normal density function. The potential along y is

$$v(y) = \rho \sum_{i=1}^{40} \sum_{j=1}^{20} \sum_{k=1}^{50} q(x_i, y_j, z_k)/\eta, \qquad (90)$$

$$\eta = [x_i^2 + (y_j - y_n)^2 + (z_k - z_0)^2]^{.5}, \qquad \eta \geq \Delta x/2.$$

The values of $v(y)$ are normalized by division by $v_0(0)$. The value of σ_a is varied, until the observed and computed half-amplitude widths x_a of the fields of potential coincide. The empirical relation of x_a to σ_a is approximately a straight line for $\sigma_a > 50\ \mu m$:

$$\sigma_a = 1.5(x_a - 92) \qquad (91)$$

in microns. An example of the observed potential (points), calculated potential (curve), and equivalent charge distribution in y (dashed curve) is shown in Fig. 4.46. The average of 31 measurements is $\sigma_a = 190 \pm 49\ \mu m$

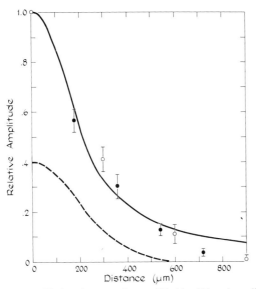

FIG. 4.46. Experimental (filled and open points, $\pm SE$, $N = 12$) and predicted distributions of potential [solid curve; Eqs. (85)–(90)] as a function of the perpendicular distance (y) from the axis (x) of a set of activated axons, which are distributed about the x axis in accordance with the normal density (dashed curve, $\sigma_a = 300\ \mu m$). See Fig. 2.13b (Freeman, 1974c).

(SD). This is the desired mean value and range for the activity density function of the PON on monopolar stimulation $h(x, y)$ when measured with the normal density curve as the basis function.

The PON axons are parallel to each other over their main trajectory so that the same results are obtained whether the stimulating electrode [to determine $H^{-1}(x)$] or recording electrode [to determine $H(x)$] is moved in steps over y (Fig. 4.46, respectively, filled and open points).   □

Example B.   The evaluation of the activity density function for periglomerular neurons on monopolar PON stimulation is based on measurements of pulse rates of single neurons in PST histograms (Section 1.3.3), $\hat{p}_{x_0, y_0, z_0}(T)$, where T is poststimulus time. The x axis is parallel to the direction of PON transmission and passes through the epicenter of the response domain at $x = x_0$, as determined from AEPs (Section 4.3.2); y is the line normal to x at the surface through the epicenter at $y = y_0$; z_p is the depth of the glomerular layer. The mean pulse rate is found for a time interval ΔT starting at the onset of an evoked response of the neuron and ending 10 msec later (Fig. 5.10).

The monopolar stimulus site is changed to successive sites along y_n as the basis for determining $H^{-1}(x)$, and the PSTH from a pulse train at a fixed recording site is obtained on stimulation at each stimulus site. The distribution of the mean induced firing rate for 17 neurons is shown in Fig. 4.47 over the range of variation in stimulus site. The epicenters have been superimposed. The values are fitted with the normal density function with $\hat{\sigma}_p = 410$ μm. On the basis of results shown in Fig. 4.46, it is inferred that the function relating mean response rate at one site on variation of input site is congruent with the variation in mean response rate over a set of recording sites for a fixed input site.

The field of the action potential around each neuron may be detected as far as 100 μm from the maximal potential at or near the neuron. If 100 μm is adopted as an outside value for the standard deviation σ_{vp} of the distribution of the field of the action potential, the observed variance $\hat{\sigma}_p^2$ is the sum of variance due to the distribution of the active state σ_p^2 and the variance σ_{vp}^2 due to the field of each neuron. For $\hat{\sigma}_p = 410$ and $\sigma_{vp} = 100$, $\sigma_p = 397$. The difference between $\hat{\sigma}_p$ and σ_p is less than the error of measurement, so the inclusion of the effect of the field of the action potential is unnecessary, and $\sigma_p = \hat{\sigma}_p$. That is, $p_p(X) \approx \psi_p(X)$ in Eq. (82) and $h_p(x, y)$ is evaluated by $\hat{\sigma}_p$.   □

Example C.   The distribution of potential at the surface as measured during N1 of the AEPs is inferred (Section 4.3.2) to be generated by a random distribution of active granule cells at a depth $z_0 = 820$ μm with the

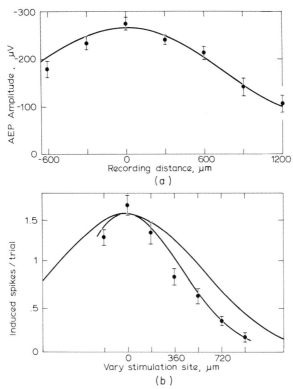

FIG. 4.47. (a) Experimental (points ±SE, $N = 17$) and theoretical distribution (curve) of AEP amplitude during N1 at surface of bulb (see Fig. 4.31); $x_h = 975$ μm. (b) Experimental distribution (points, ±SE, $N = 17$) of periglomerular KI_P activity ($\sigma_P = 410$ μm) as a function of distance from the epicenter of response domains, compared with estimated distribution (wider curve) of KI_G activity ($\sigma_g = 560$ μm). Spontaneous rate is .07 spikes per trial lasting 10 msec (equivalent to 7 pulses/sec) (Freeman, 1974d).

mean at the epicenter and standard deviations σ_x and σ_y in microns. The potential functions $v_{T_{N1}, y_0, z_0}(x)$ and $\hat{v}_{T_{N1}, x_0, z_0}(y)$ are fitted with curves from Eq. (70) to evaluate σ_x and σ_y. For the example in Fig. 4.47, $y_h = 970$ μm and $\sigma_y = 560$ μm. It is inferred that the source–sink distribution in x and y is identical to the activity density function, so that $\sigma_g = \sigma_y$.

Mean values for x_h, y_h, σ_x, and σ_y that are derived from measurement of response domains at multiple sites to determine $h_G(x, y)$ on stimulation at fixed sites on the dorsal and ventral PON are listed in Table 4.3. The widths of the domains in the ventral quadrant (VL in Fig. 4.34) are greater than the widths in the dorsal quadrant (DL), because interspersive divergence is greater in the ventral PON than in the dorsal PON (LeGros Clark, 1957; Freeman, 1972a). The grand mean for σ_g is the geometric mean. □

TABLE 4.3

WIDTH OF ACTIVE FOCUS ON PON STIMULATION

Recording location	Recording axis[a]	N	x_h, y_h (μm)	SD	σ_{gv}, σ_{gd} (μm)
Ventral	dv $= y$	13	1420	277	1010
	ap $= x$	13	1540	216	1130
Mean:					1063
Dorsal	dv $= y$	11	911	158	501
	ap $= x$	11	1465	202	1055
Mean:					818
Grand mean		48	1335	215	925

[a] dv is dorsoventral and ap is anteroposterior (Freeman, 1974a).

Example D. A monopolar stimulating electrode is placed on the PON, and the location of a response domain is established by surface recording (see Fig. 4.27). A microelectrode is inserted to the base of the EPL or the MCL, and PST histograms are constructed from pulse trains of mitral–tufted cells recorded at that level $z = z_0$ for different values of x and y (Fig. 4.48a). Three classes of PSTH are found. Those mitral–tufted cells, which undergo excitation at time T_e followed by inhibition at time T_i, form a central domain (Fig. 4.48b), for which the diameters are D_e in the x (anteroposterior, ap) and y (dorsoventral, dv) directions. Those cells which undergo inhibition without preceding excitation are found to occupy an area surrounding the excitatory zone with diameters $D_i > D_e$. Inhibition

TABLE 4.4

DIAMETERS OF EXCITATORY AND INHIBITORY FOCI[a]

Set	Axis[b]	D_e	D_i	$D_e - D_i$	x_h, y_h
1	dv	1900	3100	1200	1000
2	ap	1600	2700	1100	925
3	dv	1850	3000	1150	1130
4	ap	2650	3600	950	1260
5	dv	1500	3000	1500	970
6	dv	1900	3200	1300	930
7	dv	2000	3000	1000	1020
8	dv	2200	3100	900	1100
Mean:		1950	3087	1138	1042
SE:		118	84	70	41

[a] Values are given in microns (Freeman, 1974b).
[b] dv is dorso ventral and ap is anteroposterior.

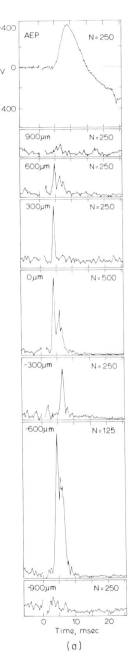

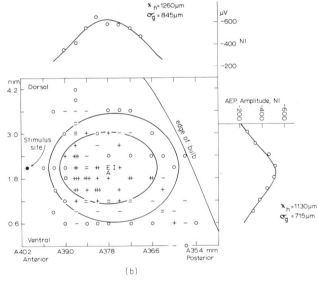

FIG. 4.48. (a) Mitral–tufted cell PSTHs as a function of distance from the epicenter of a response domain (Freeman, 1972c). (b) Distribution of unit clusters showing initial excitation followed by inhibition ($+$), inhibition without initial excitation ($-$), and no effect (0) in relation to AEP amplitude during N1 (Freeman, 1974b). Computed values for dv × ap: $D_e = 1850 \times 2650 \, \mu m$; $\sigma_e = 412 \times 590 \, \mu m$; $D_i = 3000 \times 3600 \, \mu m$; $\sigma_i = 667 \times 800 \, \mu m$.

occurs everywhere at the same latency T_i so that the boundary at D_i encloses a region of an inhibitory event. Outside D_i there is no response to the stimulus.

The configuration consists of a relatively small excitatory focus $\hat{p}_{T_e,z_0}(x, y)$, followed by a relatively larger inhibitory focus $\hat{p}_{T_i,z_0}(x, y)$, where T_e and T_i refer to the poststimulus times at which maximal excitation and inhibition are observed. The surface distributions of potential $\hat{v}_{T_{N1},z_0}(x, y)$, at the time of the crest of N1, are recorded for the same response domain. Estimates for x_h and y_h are obtained as in Example C. Values for the parameters from several experiments are listed in Table 4.4 The values in Table 4.4 are used to estimate values for standard deviations, σ_e and σ_i, of excitatory and inhibitory activity density functions for mitral–tufted cells, represented as normal distributions, which are manifested by the excitatory and inhibitory foci at T_e and T_i. The method is given in the next section. □

4.5.3. EVALUATION OF SYNAPTIC DIVERGENCE

Calculation of the extent of divergence of activity among the bulbar neurons is based on three general assumptions.

(a) Each neural activity distribution evoked directly or indirectly by electrical stimulation is random about its mean located at the epicenter and can be fitted with a bivariate normal density function $h_\mu(x, y)$. The size of the distribution is given by its standard deviation in microns σ_μ or its variance σ_μ^2.

(b) From each small region within an activity distribution, the divergence of neural transmission from subset μ to subset $\mu+1$ is random over x and y. The impulse response of the divergence operation $h_{\mu,\mu+1}(x, y)_T$ is a normal density function. The width of the transmission divergence is given by the standard deviation $\sigma_{\mu,\mu+1}$ or variance $\sigma_{\mu,\mu+1}^2$ of the distribution of the transmission. Departures from radial symmetry (in the form of elliptical or irregular distributions) are neglected.

(c) Except for the difference of interspersive divergence between the dorsal and ventral PON layer, the bulbar connections are spatially homogeneous. The transmission divergence $h_{\mu,\mu+1}(x, y)$ from neurons in each local subset of a response domain is independent of the location of the region, both with respect to the bulb, x, y, and the epicenter, x_0, y_0, of the distribution.

From assumption (a) it is inferred that the distributions of initially excited mitral–tufted cells, excited granule cells, and inhibited mitral–tufted cells are all random. From inspection of the results it is inferred that they have a common mean or epicenter within any given focus, within the limits of experimental error. From assumptions (b) and (c), it is inferred that when an activity distribution is transmitted, the variance σ^2 of the new activity distribution is the sum of the variance of the input activity distribution and the transmission variance. In terms of the symbols in Table 4.2 the variance of the distribution of initially excited mitral–tufted cells σ_e^2 is added to the transmission variance from mitral–tufted cells to granule cells $\sigma_{e \cdot g}^2$ to give the predicted variance of the distribution of excited granule cells σ_g^2:

$$\sigma_g^2 = \sigma_e^2 + \sigma_{e \cdot g}^2. \tag{92}$$

The same relation holds for transmission from the distribution of excited granule cells σ_g^2 to the distribution of inhibited mitral–tufted cells σ_i^2 with transmission variance $\sigma_{g \cdot i}^2$.

$$\sigma_i^2 = \sigma_g^2 + \sigma_{g \cdot i}^2. \tag{93}$$

The distance of transmission from mitral–tufted to granule cells depends on the combined lengths of the dendrites of both cell types, in directions parallel to the bulbar surface, and not on either alone. The same holds for subsequent transmission from granule cells to mitral–tufted cells. That is, transmission from any one mitral–tufted cell to any one granule cell depends on the serial lengths and functional states of the two dendritic trees connecting them, and transmission in the reverse direction depends on the serial lengths and states of the same two dendritic trees. Reciprocal transmission for any large number of such neurons is inferred to be symmetric in the surface coordinates. This is a corollary of assumption (c), from which it is inferred that

$$\sigma_{e \cdot g} = \sigma_{g \cdot i}. \tag{94}$$

Equations (92)–(94) are combined and solved for $\sigma_{e \cdot g}$.

$$\sigma_{e \cdot g} = (\tfrac{1}{2}\sigma_i^2 - \tfrac{1}{2}\sigma_e^2)^{.5}. \tag{95}$$

The experimental measurements on the distributions of initially excited and inhibited mitral–tufted cells are in terms of diameters, D_e and D_i (Table 4.4). These are converted to estimates of σ_e and σ_i in the following way. The curves drawn as boundaries of the excitatory and inhibitory foci are conceived in probabilistic terms as enclosing most (between 95 and 99%) of the designated response types, but probably not all of them. From a table of the cumulative normal density function, the radius of a focus in units of the standard deviation σ can be specified for a given percentage of responding units included within that radius. Furthermore, the diameter of the focus can be expressed in units of standard deviation, or alternatively, the standard deviation can be obtained by dividing the diameter by a dimensionless factor η_x

$$\sigma_e = D_e / \eta_x, \qquad \sigma_i = D_i / \eta_x. \tag{96}$$

The value of the conversion factor η_x is determined by the relationships between D_e, D_i, and the standard deviation of the distribution of activated granule cells σ_g from the same response focus as follows. The half-amplitude radius x_h of the surface field of evoked potential at N1 is measured along the same surface lines as D_e and D_i. The values for x_h in Table 4.5 are used to estimate the standard deviation of the distribution of excited granule cells σ_g by Equation (71) previously derived.

$$\sigma_g = x_h - (z_0/2), \tag{97}$$

where $z_0 = 820 \ \mu m$ is the depth of the zero isopotential surface of the dipole field at N1 (Section 4.3.2). The mean and standard error (Table 4.5) $\sigma_g = 632 \pm 41 \ \mu m$.

TABLE 4.5

DERIVATION OF MITRAL–TUFTED TO GRANULE CELL TRANSMISSION DISTANCE[a]

Set	x_h, y_h	σ_g	η_x	σ_e	σ_i	$\sigma_{e \cdot i}$
1	1000	590	4.36	436	711	397
2	925	515	4.31	371	626	357
3	1130	720	3.46	534	867	482
4	1260	850	3.72	713	968	468
5	970	560	4.24	354	708	434
6	930	520	5.06	375	632	360
7	1020	610	4.18	479	718	378
8	1100	690	3.90	565	796	396
Mean:	1042	632	4.15	478	753	409
SE:	41	41	.17	43	41	17

[a] Values are given in microns.

Equations (92)–(94) are combined to give

$$\sigma_i^2 - \sigma_g^2 = \sigma_g^2 - \sigma_e^2, \tag{98}$$

which is solved for σ_g:

$$\sigma_g = (\tfrac{1}{2}\sigma_e^2 + \tfrac{1}{2}\sigma_i^2)^{.5}. \tag{99}$$

Equations (96) are substituted into Eq. (99), and it is solved for η_x:

$$\eta_x = (\tfrac{1}{2}D_i^2 + \tfrac{1}{2}D_e^2)^{.5}/\sigma_g. \tag{100}$$

A value for η_x is computed for each case in Table 4.5. The mean for η_x is 4.15. From a table of the cumulative normal density function, the mean diameter of 4.15 standard deviations includes 96% of a normal distribution.

The locations of recording sites at which initial excitation are found is reviewed in relation to the designated boundaries. Of 105 such points in 6 foci, 100 are found to be on or within the boundaries, or 95%. This shows that the estimated values of η_x are consistent with the experimental data. A similar check on η_x cannot be made for the inhibitory foci, because the observed distributions are too irregular.

Equations (96) are substituted into Eq. (95),

$$\sigma_{e \cdot g} = (\tfrac{1}{2}D_i^2 - \tfrac{1}{2}D_e^2)^{.5}/\eta_x. \tag{101}$$

Equation (101) is combined with Eq. (100),

$$\sigma_{e \cdot g} = [(D_i^2 - D_e^2)/(D_i^2 + D_e^2)]^{.5}\sigma_g. \tag{102}$$

Values for $\sigma_{e \cdot g}$ are computed for each case in Table 4.5. The mean and standard error for $\sigma_{e \cdot g}$ for 8 cases is $\sigma_{e \cdot g} = 409 \pm 17$ μm. The 95% confidence interval is ± 39 μm (370–448 μm, $t_{.05} = 2.36$, df $= 7$).

The mean value designated for $\sigma_{e \cdot g}$ is compatible with anatomical observations on the lengths of mitral–tufted basal dendrites. It is commonly stated that the lengths from the soma are about 1 mm. A set of 50 measurements of selected long dendrites in Golgi preparations (see Fig. 4.24) in cats showed that the longest was 903 μm. If 900 μm were treated as the 97.5% inclusion radius of the distribution of basal dendrites from any point in the external plexiform layer in directions parallel to the surface, the standard deviation would be 900/2.25, or 400 μm. The branching of granule cell dendrites would add to the anatomical basis for spread, which implies that the structural basis required for the observed magnitude of transmission variance exists.

The measurements used to evaluate $\sigma_{e \cdot g}$ are based on responses to PON stimuli at moderately high-stimulus intensity. The estimate is inferred to hold at lower intensity, because the standard deviations of the distributions of excited PON axons σ_a and of excited granule cells σ_g do not vary with stimulus intensity up to $4 \times$ threshold. The results cannot be extrapolated to observations at higher intensity. However, the lower range includes the range of normal EEG activity (Section 3.3.1) so the results should hold for analysis of activity induced by odors.

The same assumptions are applied to the analysis of excitation of periglomerular cells by PON axon terminals (Section 4.5.2, Example B). An afferent volley is inferred to evoke a distribution of input to the glomeruli σ_b, which induces a distribution of periglomerular activity σ_p by synaptic transmission with divergence, $\sigma_{b \cdot p}$. The expected relation from assumptions (b) and (c) as for Eq. (92) is

$$\sigma_p^2 = \sigma_b^2 + \sigma_{b \cdot p}^2. \tag{103}$$

The precision of measurement is such that distributions differing by less than

$\pm 10\%$ in width are difficult to distinguish, so that reliably detectable differences would occur only for the cases where $\sigma_p > 1.11\sigma_b$. Equation (103) can be reformulated as

$$\sigma_b^2 + \sigma_{b\cdot p}^2 > 1.24\sigma_b^2. \tag{104}$$

On solving for σ_b, the result is

$$\sigma_b < 2\sigma_{b\cdot p}. \tag{105}$$

This relation implies that the size of the test input distribution cannot exceed twice the size of the expected transmission distribution, unless the precision of measurement is better than $\pm 10\%$.

Periglomerular neurons are considerably smaller than mitral–tufted cells, and it is reasonable to suppose that their mean transmission divergence is less than half the input divergence on PON electrical stimulation, which averages more than 630 μm. This implies that divergence from PON terminals to periglomerular neurons is negligible on electrical stimulation, so that $\sigma_{b\cdot p} \approx 0$, and

$$\sigma_p = \sigma_b, \qquad \sigma_b \gg \sigma_{b\cdot p}. \tag{106}$$

The apical dendrites of mitral–tufted cells lie parallel to each other in their trajectory from the glomeruli to the cell bodies. They are inferred to contribute negligible divergence in so far as mitral–tufted unit responses to PON stimulation are concerned, so that $\sigma_{b\cdot e} \approx 0$, and

$$\sigma_e = \sigma_b, \qquad \sigma_b \gg \sigma_{b\cdot e}. \tag{107}$$

These inferences are tested as follows. The distribution of evoked periglomerular unit activity has been measured across a focus in response to PON stimulation (Freeman, 1974a). The intensity of response varies with distance from the epicenter in accordance with a normal density function with $\sigma_p = 410$ μm. The concomitantly measured distribution of N1 has a value of $\sigma_g = 560$ μm. From Eqs. (92), (106), and (107),

$$\sigma_{e\cdot g} = (\sigma_g^2 - \sigma_p^2)^{.5} \tag{108}$$

and $\sigma_{e\cdot g} = 382$ μm. This value lies within the 95% confidence intervals established for $\sigma_{e\cdot g}$, by recording mitral–tufted unit responses. It is concluded that Eqs. (106) and (107) hold for bulbar responses to electrical stimulation.

4.5.4. EVALUATION OF TRACTILE DIVERGENCE

From Section 4.5.2, Example A, the size of the distribution of excited axons around a stimulating electrode in the PON is $\sigma_a = 190 \pm 49$ μm, and also the dilation of the set of action potentials due to gross geometrical factors is by $d_{a \cdot b} = (11)^{1/2}$, yielding an expected size of the volley averaging $d_{a \cdot b} \sigma_a = 630\ \mu m$. The estimated geometric mean size of the distribution of activated granule cells in the dorsal bulb is $\sigma_{gd} = 818\ \mu m$, and in the ventral bulb $\sigma_{gv} = 1063\ \mu m$ (Table 4.3). From Eqs. (92) and (107), and assumption (c) in Section 4.5.3,

$$\sigma_{bd} = (\sigma_{gd}^2 - \sigma_{e \cdot g}^2)^{.5}, \qquad \sigma_{bv} = (\sigma_{gv}^2 - \sigma_{e \cdot g}^2)^{.5}. \tag{109}$$

From $\sigma_{e \cdot g} = 409\ \mu m$, $\sigma_{bd} = 710\ \mu m$ and $\sigma_{bv} = 982\ \mu m$. The values in excess of $630\ \mu m$ are inferred to result from interspersion of axons in the PON layer. From assumption (b) the interspersion is treated as random from each point in the PON layer, with a standard deviation in microns of $\sigma_{a \cdot b}$. The variance introduced by interspersion $\sigma_{a \cdot b}^2$, is added to the variance of activity in the PON volley $11\sigma_a^2$ to give the expected variance of activity in the glomeruli at the PON terminals σ_b^2:

$$\sigma_b^2 = 11\sigma_a^2 + \sigma_{a \cdot b}^2. \tag{110}$$

Therefore,

$$\sigma_{a \cdot bd} = (\sigma_{bd}^2 - 11\sigma_a^2)^{.5}, \qquad \sigma_{a \cdot bv} = (\sigma_{bv}^2 - 11\sigma_a^2)^{.5}. \tag{111}$$

The above values for σ_a, σ_{bd}, and σ_{bv} give us $\sigma_{a \cdot bd} = 332\ \mu m$ and $\sigma_{a \cdot bv} = 756\ \mu m$. These figures imply that the 95% inclusion diameter ($\pm 2\sigma_{a \cdot b}$) for the distribution of PON axons arriving at the bulb form each stimulated subset in the PON layer is 1.3 mm in the dorsal bulb and 3.0 mm in the ventral bulb. This is up to half the anteroposterior extent of the bulb in the cat (5.7 mm) and one-quarter the dorsoventral extent (11.6 mm). The fractions are still larger for the rabbit in which the bulb is smaller than in the cat.

The analysis given here is based on measurements on excitatory foci in the dorsal bulb averaging $1950\ \mu m$ in diameter and inhibitory foci averaging $3087\ \mu m$. The width of the fringe zone in which cells are inhibited without preceding excitation is $569\ \mu m$ or 30% diameter of the excitatory focus. The typical excitatory focus in the ventral bulb is larger and has a narrower predicted fringe of inhibition without preceding excitation, for the following reasons.

The variance of the PON volley σ_a in the ventral bulb is occasionally $(275\ \mu m)^2$ or larger. With dilation by $d_{a \cdot b}$ the input variance is $d_{a \cdot b}^2 \sigma_a^2 = (920\ \mu m)^2$. The addition of interspersive variance $\sigma_{a \cdot bv}^2 = (756\ \mu m)^2$ yields distributions of glomerular and of mitral–tufted excitation with $\sigma_b = \sigma_e = 1190\ \mu m$ by Eq. (107) and Eq. (110). The transmission from mitral–tufted cells with $\sigma_{e \cdot g} = 409\ \mu m$ activates granule cells in a distribution with $\sigma_g = 1260\ \mu m$ by Eq. (92) and $x_h = 1670\ \mu m$ by Eq. (97). The expected distribution of inhibited mitral–tufted cells has $\sigma_i = 1320\ \mu m$ by Eq. (93) and (94). From the factor $\eta_x = 4.15$ the predicted diameter of the excitatory focus is 5000 μm, and the predicted width of the inhibitory fringe is about 250 μm, or 5% of the diameter of the excitatory focus by Eqs. (96). Thus the ventral response foci are not only larger, but the inhibitory fringe is narrower and correspondingly more difficult to locate and measure.

The general principle emerges that when the input variance is increased in the face of a fixed level of transmission variance, the difference between the input variance and the output variance decreases to the vanishing point. A special case has been described in Eqs. (103)–(105). Because electrical stimulation of the PON excites a distribution of axons having a variance σ_a^2 that cannot be reduced below a certain minimum, and because dilation and interspersion impose additional variance, the variance of the distribution of excitatory input to the glomeruli σ_b^2 always exceeds the variance of the following stages of synaptic transmission, $\sigma_{b \cdot p}^2$, $\sigma_{b \cdot e}^2$, and $\sigma_{e \cdot g}^2$. Only the variance $\sigma_{e \cdot g}^2$ is sufficiently large to be measured on PON stimulation. It is not detectable in the bulb on LOT stimulation, because the dilation of antidromic LOT input to the bulb is twice the dilation of orthodromic PON input to the bulb. This does not mean that divergence does not occur within the distribution of activity established by the input. It means that the divergence cannot be measured as a detectable outward spread of activity evoked by electrical stimuli in the PON or LOT unless the variance of the test input is sufficiently small. Moreover, it seems reasonable to believe that the variance of PON input to the glomeruli evoked by odors is much larger than $\sigma_{b \cdot p}$ or $\sigma_{e \cdot g}$, although as yet no evidence has been found to demonstrate this in controlled conditions. Then the response domain in the bulb is predicted to be fixed by the input, and travelling waves analogous to those resulting from throwing a handful of gravel into still water are predicted not to occur.

The high transmission variance of the PON is compatible with a high degree of topographic organization of the PON, which is revealed in a close dependence of the location of the epicenter of a response domain on the position of a stimulating electrode. An example is shown in Fig. 4.49a–c in which the monopolar surface stimulus site is moved in steps of 180 μm in the y direction. The corresponding shift in the epicenter of the response domain is shown by the isopotentials.

This fact holds also for the LOT. There is a clear topographic organization of the mitral–tufted axons in the LOT as it emerges from the bulb onto the brain surface (Fig. 4.34). The most dorsal part (DM) contains axons from the dorsomedial quadrant of the bulb. The upper and lower middle sectors of the LOT contain axons from the dorsolateral (DL) and ventrolateral (VL) quadrants of the bulb. The ventromedial (VM) quadrant sends axons into the most ventral part of the LOT (Shepherd & Haberly, 1970).

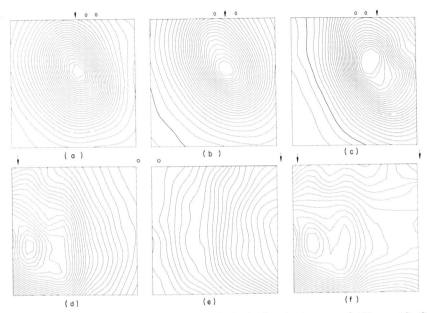

FIG. 4.49. (a)–(c) Effect of changing the PON stimulus site in steps of 180 μm. (d)–(f) Results of stimulating separately [(d) and (e)] at two sites and then simultaneously (f). Time of each frame is at crest of N1. Contour interval is 15 μV with 2 × 2 mm array of 64 recording electrodes (Freeman, 1974a).

However, in the further trajectory of the LOT to the cortex there is a high degree of collateral divergence, such that each local region of the bulb projects to a large but indeterminate fraction of the cortical area. This high transmission variance is reflected in the fact that stimulation almost anywhere on the LOT can evoke unit activity in neurons in different parts of the cortex. Conversely, stimulation at any point on the cortical surface off of the visible LOT (PC in Figure 4.34) evokes a distributed dipole field covering the DL, VL, and VM quadrants of the bulb. (Stimulation at A1 over the dorsal part of the anterior olfactory nucleus evokes a dipole field covering the DM quadrant of the bulb.)

The contour maps of the fields of AEPs at the brain surface show that the spread of activity evoked by LOT stimulation in the nucleus (AON, A1 and A2) is different from the spread in the prepyriform cortex (PC in Fig. 4.34). For each stimulus site on the LOT just posterior to the bulb, there are two domains of maximal evoked activity, of which one overlies the AON and the other the PC (Figs. 4.39 and 4.50). The location of the epicenter over the nucleus depends on the location of the LOT stimulus site, and as the stimulus site is moved in small steps from the dorsal to the

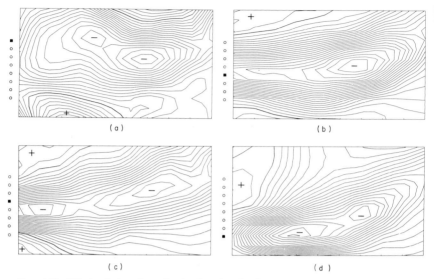

FIG. 4.50. Effects of changing stimulus location in the LOT in steps of 300 μm on the AEP field of the prepyriform cortex during N1 with $T = 2.56$ msec. Each response field has two components. (b, d) Anteriorly over the AON (see Fig. 4.34) the crest of the field changes location with change in stimulus site, and the response domain is standing. (a, c) Posteriorly over PC the field rotates over the surface (see Fig. 4.42), and there is no evidence of topographic order between the LOT and PC.

ventral LOT, the epicenter shifts in the same direction (Fig. 4.50). The epicenter does not move significantly in the dorsoventral direction with time during N1 and it recurs in the same location during N2, N3, etc. In contrast, the location of the epicenter over the prepyriform cortex is independent of the LOT stimulus site, and it moves with time during N1 from anteroventral to posterodorsal over the cortex (Figs. 4.39 and 4.40). This movement gives rise to the appearance of a rotating dipole field as shown in Fig. 4.42.

These observations imply that the AON receives input from the bulb with a degree of topographic specificity, which is similar to the projection of the PON onto the bulb. That is, each small region in the LOT projects in a spatial distribution over the nucleus, and the location of the spatial mean of the distribution depends on the location of the small region. This occurs during the passage of the LOT over the AON to the PC. The LOT axons converge to the anteroventral edge of the PC, intersperse, and then diverge over the PC in the posterodorsal direction. The conduction velocity over the PC (<2 m/sec) is slower than over the AON branches (5 m/sec) because the axons divide, and the branches have smaller diameter. The delay from one side of the PC to the other is apparently about the same as the duration of a half-cycle of the AEP, which accentuates the appearance of the rotating dipole field.

The quantitative assessment and interpretation of these patterns of projections are still to be made. At present, we can say that measurements made of the surface potential functions $\hat{v}_{T,z}(x, y)$, $z = 0$, for AEPs (Figs. 4.38, 4.39, and 4.50) and for EEG waves have shown that coherent domains commonly exist with half-amplitude radii exceeding 1 mm and not un-commonly an entire electrode array of 4×7 mm. Irrespective of whether the extent of coherence is due to externally imposed covariance or to intracortical interactions, the extent is sufficiently great to establish the condition in the cortex, as in the bulb, that a recording at the epicenter of a domain $\hat{v}_{x_0,y_0,z}(T)$, $z = 0$, is a mirror image time function of the ensemble average of the mean transmembrane potential $\mathscr{E}[\hat{v}_m(T)]$ of the subsets of neurons comprising the coherent domain. That is, in circumscribed conditions the surface recording of potential can be treated as a measure of a state variable of the cortical neural mass.

This is particularly useful in the analysis of the dynamics of the cortical KII set as a lumped circuit in Section 5.4. The reduction to a lumped circuit is assumed to be valid in the analysis of averaged cortical responses to single-shock stimulation of the LOT, because the collateral divergence in the LOT is extensive, and the size of a coherent domain established by the input is sufficiently large to define an epicenter and establish proportionality between the surface record and the active state of the superficial pyramidal KI_A set. The function $H(X)$ is then replaced by a linear function. The functions, $V_\mu(s, X, U)$ and $P_\mu(s, X, U)$, for the KI_A set, as given by the Laplace transform of Eqs. (77) and (78) become lumped approximations.

$$V_\mu(s, X, U) \propto h_{\mu v} G_{\mu v}(U) F_{\mu v}(s), \tag{112}$$

$$P_\mu(s, X, U) \propto h_{\mu p} G_{\mu p}(U) F_{\mu p}(s). \tag{113}$$

For a fixed input range of amplitudes U in both modes, P and V, Eqs. (112) and (113) can be reduced to lumped linear forms

$$V_\mu(s, X, U) \propto g_{\mu v} h_{\mu v} F_{\mu v}(s), \tag{114}$$

$$P_\mu(s, X, U) \propto g_{\mu p} h_{\mu p} F_{\mu p}(s), \tag{115}$$

comparable to those derived in Section 3.3.4. On this basis we are now prepared to undertake analysis of feedback properties in lumped circuit approximations in Chapter 5.

CHAPTER 5

Interaction:
Single Feedback Loops with Fixed Gain

5.1. General Properties of Single Feedback Loops

We have reviewed the basic properties of neurons and neural masses and described them in terms of their topologies and their dynamics with respect to time, amplitude, and distance. We are ready to consider explicitly the properties resulting from interactions within masses. As described in Section 1.3.1 a neural mass is any identifiable collection of neurons for which mass analysis is proposed, such as the visual cortex, primary visual cortex, neocortex, superior olivary nucleus, superior colliculus, thalamus, any nucleus of thalamus, etc. Each mass consists of KO and KI sets, and there are functional interconnections within sets and between sets. Each mass has multiple channels for interaction.

It is unreasonable for either explanatory or heuristic purposes to attempt to analyze quantitatively all of the major interactions in a mass at the outset. The preferred procedure is to identify one channel of interaction as the primary determinant of the dynamics of a neural mass in an appropriate experimental condition. The topology of the mass is then abstracted or reduced to a simpler form in which the primary channel of interaction is described by a lumped feedback loop, and the other channels of interaction are described by lumped input channels. By this approach we gain a nucleus of understanding that can be expanded by introducing further complexities as the opportunities and needs for description arise.

The process of abstraction is intuitive and highly particularized for each neural mass. There is no escaping the need for detailed understanding of the neuroanatomical and neurophysiological properties of a mass if the result is to be a description of the dynamics of the mass and not an untestable hypothesis. This chapter begins with a description of the general properties of single feedback loops and concludes with detailed examples of the analysis of the mammalian olfactory system at three levels. Additional examples of the style of analysis have been published for the hippocampus (Horowitz, 1972; Horowitz, Freeman & Stoll, (1973) and the cerebellum (Bantli, 1974a, b), in addition to analytic studies of the compound eye of the horseshoe crab, *Limulus* (e.g., Knight, Toyoda & Dodge, 1970). There are numerous sensory and motor systems (e.g., Spekreijse, 1969; Lopes da Silva, van Rotterdam, Storm van Leeuwen & Thielen, 1970; Elul, 1972; Wilson & Cowan, 1973) for which analysis en masse is being undertaken, but for which mass-action transfer functions have not yet been derived, evaluated and tested. There are no easy generalizations from these examples and perhaps cannot be, because each mass has its peculiarities, but the method does yield testable predictions and appears to be widely applicable.

5.1.1. TYPES OF NEURAL FEEDBACK

The concept of feedback was familiar to biologists over a century ago, and to engineers yet a century before that. Feedback occurs whenever the output of an element in a dynamic system in part determines the input of that element (Sections 1.3.4) as shown by a topological flow diagram (Fig. 5.1a), where $o_1, ..., o_4$ are functions of any variables, including time, and where the output of an element having the operator B_1 in part determines its own input through the operator B_2. This is a general description that holds for any system with a single feedback loop. The element B_1 comprises the forward channel and B_2 the feedback channel of the loop.

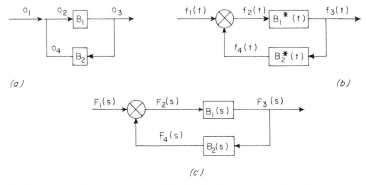

FIG. 5.1. Conventional representations of feedback, where the asterisk indicates convolution.

If the operators B_1 and B_2 are time-invariant linear functions for domains of input and ranges of output, o_1, o_2, o_3, o_4, such that $o_j(t)$ are approximated by functions only of time $f_j(t)$ and if the combination of $o_1(t)$ and $o_4(t)$ to give $o_2(t)$ is additive, the system is linear and time invariant. By convention, if $f_4(t)$ is added to $f_1(t)$, there is a $+$ at the summation point to denote a positive feedback loop as shown in Fig. 5.1b. If $f_4(t)$ were subtracted, there would be a $-$ to denote negative feedback. The operators are denoted by capital letters and the state variables in time are denoted by lower case letters. Following the Laplace transformation, the state variables are shown by capital letters (Fig. 5.1c). The output as a function of input is derived by means of the convolution theorem (Section 2.3.2). For negative feedback,

$$F_3(s) = [F_1(s) - F_3(s)B_2(s)]B_1(s). \tag{1}$$

Because the functions are linear, the order of operations can be changed. Equation (1) is solved for the ratio of output to input to give the transfer function of the closed loop system:

$$F_3(s)/F_1(s) = B_1(s)/[1 + B_1(s)B_2(s)]. \tag{2}$$

If there is a positive feedback loop, the sign in the denominator is minus. If the input is a unit impulse (Sections 2.1.4 and 2.3.3), then $F_1(s) = 1$. For the transfer function of the impulse response, $V(s) = F_3(s)$,

$$V(s) = B_1(s)/[1 - B_1(s)B_2(s)]. \tag{3}$$

Feedback occurs in almost every part of the nervous systems of every animal, and it is so well known and recognized that a list of examples is not needed. In virtually all known instances of single-loop feedback, however, both the operators B_1 and B_2 are nonlinear, so that the state variables, $o_1, \ldots, o_4$, are not functions only of s. Moreover, the operators are distributed in space. The construction of partial differential equations with multiple non-linearities is not easy, and the solutions are very difficult to obtain and require a high order of mathematical talent and training. Most solutions take the form of general statements concerning the existence of classes of output for classes of input, which are difficult or impossible to test against experimental data. When analytic or computer simulated solutions are formed for particular systems, they cannot be generalized to related but differing systems.

An alternative to nonlinear analysis is piecewise linear approximation. The advantages are simplicity and precision. The construction and solution of linear differential equations with fixed coefficients is relatively straight-forward and according to well-known rules. The solutions take the form of predicted space–time functions of potential which can be tested by fitting them to the data. The difficulties are chiefly experimental. The necessary simplifying assumptions must be justified by data analysis which is usually indirect and qualitative. The conditions of stimulation and observation must be adapted to correspond to the specifications of the assumptions. These conditions must be shown to include the conditions holding during normal physiological activity, when the neural masses under study are performing their normal functions, so that the models and inferences made from them can be generalized to predict function during behavior.

There are two circumstances that make piecewise linear approximation feasible. First, the input–output function for the KO set (Section 3.3.6) is sigmoid, which reflects the presence of bilateral saturation in the two nonlinear conversion mechanisms for each set. Second, most neurons function most of the time in the middle region of the sigmoid curve during background activity and low-level evoked activity. These facts suggest that for a given domain of input the range of output can be predicted by a straight-line approximation to the segment of the sigmoid curve subtended by the input domain. The slope of the approximating line is the forward gain of the set. The slope decreases with each increase in the domain of input, corresponding to a decrease in forward gain by saturation. The gain is amplitude-dependent (Section 3.3.6). Given the input domain or output range, the gain is fixed, and the system function is treated as linear for that domain and range.

5.1.2. DERIVATION OF THE LUMPED PIECEWISE LINEAR APPROXIMATION

The KI set is defined (Section 1.3.1) as a collection of neurons having a common source of input, a common sign of output, and a nonzero level of interaction. We propose to derive a measure for the level of interaction that is a definitive property of the set. The topological aspect of interaction is expressed by dividing the set into two subsets, the transmitting and receiving subsets (Section 1.3.4). Each neuron is at all times a member of either subset but never both, because of the refractory period. The dynamic aspects of interaction are expressed by the transfer function of subsets at the KO level (without interaction) $O(s, X, U)$, in the dimensions of time (or frequency) s, amplitude U, and space X. The transfer function O includes a set of fixed parameters that are listed below and a set of variable parameters that represent interaction strengths and are evaluated as feedback gains.

The first step is separation of the transfer function into parts representing the three sets of independent variables. This separation is based on a set of assumptions regarding the parameters. The assumptions can be grouped in two general classes: (i) The parameters of neurons and subsets are uniform and time-invariant both with respect to the set and to active states of the set. (ii) The ranges for the amplitudes and rates of change of relevant active states are small relative to the ranges for possible active states. The substance of these assumptions is as follows.

(1)   The properties of each neuron and each subset are independent of location X within the set. In particular the passive membrane rate

coefficient a (Section 2.4.3) is the same for every cell and is constant with respect to X.

(2) The passive membrane rate coefficient is constant with respect to time and thus s (Section 5.3.3).

(3) The spatial distribution of each input channel over each neural dendritic tree is invariant with respect to the neuron, so that the lumped delay owing to terminal axonal dispersion and to dendritic cable delays (Sections 2.3.3–2.3.5) and designated by the rate coefficient b is constant with respect to X and s.

(4) The conduction delays T_c within the set are sufficiently small that T_c is constant with respect to X (Section 4.2.2).

(5) The density of the active states of the set and its input channel are sufficiently low that the passive membrane rate coefficient a is not affected by synaptic conductance changes (Section 3.2.4) or by the occurrence of action potentials and is constant with respect to U.

(6) The dispersive and cable delay is independent of the active states. (An exception is described in Section 5.2.1.)

(7) The conduction and synaptic delays are sufficiently small to be lumped into a single rate constant.

(8) The rates of change in active states are sufficiently low that threshold for each neuron is not dependent on the rate constants of g_{Na^+} (Section 3.1.5). The mean rates of firing of single neurons are sufficiently low that time-varying phenomena such as facilitation and adaption (Section 3.2.4) are not significant. The distribution of thresholds and the rate constants of refractory periods are time invariant. These several factors are the determinants of the empirical rate constants, γ_e and γ_i, which are constant with respect to s (Section 3.3.4).

(9) The amplitudes and rates of change of active states are low enough so that the levels of excitatory and inhibitory synaptic equilibrium potentials $\tilde{v}_i$ and $\tilde{v}_e$ and the chemical kinetics represented by the empirical rate constants ζ_i and ζ_e are time invariant (Section 3.3.5).

(10) The functions of the pulse to wave and wave to pulse conversion mechanisms are independent of location in the set [by assumption (1)] and of location with respect to any activity density function.

(11) The parameters (Section 4.5.1) of divergence $\sigma_{\mu \cdot \mu + 1}$ and the length constants of neurons λ_k are dependent on the passive electrical and geometric properties of neurons in the set and are time invariant.

(12) The parameters $\sigma_{\mu \cdot \mu + 1}$ and λ_k are independent (Section 4.5.2) of the amplitudes of active states and (with some exceptions) of location X.

These assumptions are inferred to hold over the ranges of amplitudes and rates of change displayed by background activity in the wave mode (Section 3.3.1) and pulse mode (Section 3.3.2), and for evoked activity within those ranges. The time periods over which time invariance can be said to hold are seconds to minutes in anesthetized animals, and in waking animals for durations depending on the imposition of behavioral controls. For this reason the observation, measurement, and comparison of background and evoked activity from a neural set in relation to behavior is essential to establish the appropriate range for analysis by piecewise linear approximation (see Freeman, 1963). By the above assumptions, O is replaced by an expression of the form

$$O(s, X, U) \propto G(U)H(X)F(s). \tag{4}$$

The description of the topological property of feedback for a KI set under these assumptions is shown in Fig. 5.2. Part (a) shows the topology of the linear and nonlinear elements. The input $I(s, X, P)$, on the afferent tract undergoes dispersion $F_f(s)$ (Section 2.3.3), divergence $H_f(X)$ and pulse to wave conversion (Section 3.3.5) $G_i(P)$. Tractile and synaptic divergence (Section 4.5.1) are both included in $H_f(X)$. The transformed input is weighted, summed, and smoothed by the low-pass characteristic of the passive post-synaptic membrane $F_{1v}(s)$ and establishes an extracellular field of potential $V_1(s, X, U)$ through the operator $H_{v1}(X)$ which is one form of output of the set. The activity is also converged and transmitted $H_{1v}(X)$ to the wave to pulse conversion mechanism $G_1(V)$. A transmitting subset is established within the receiving subset which, through the operator $H_{p1}(X)$, forms a spatial distribution of observable action potentials in the pulse mode $P_1(s, X, U)$.

The pulses undergo the sequence of frequency-dependent $F_{2p}(s)$, space-dependent $H_{2p}(X)$, and amplitude-dependent $G_2(P)$ transformations and sign specification ($\pm$) described for the input, as they are transmitted to the receiving subset. The activity in the form of dendritic current is smoothed $F_{2v}(s)$, establishes an output $V_2(s, V, U)$ through $H_{v2}(X)$, and is transmitted $H_{2v}(X)$ to the wave to pulse mechanism $G_2(V)$. A new transmitting subset is formed. The pulses in the feedback path are detectable through the operator $H_{p2}(X)$ as a distribution of action potentials $P_2(s, X, U)$. Following the standard sequence of transformations, $F_{1p}(s)$, $H_{1p}(X)$, and $\pm G_1(P)$, the activity in the feedback path is delivered to a receiving subset that includes neurons that contributed to the input. The loop is closed at the summation point of those neurons in the KI set.

The system representing the set is linearized by means of a third general assumption: (iii) For a given domain of pulse input to the set in a specified time interval $\Delta T, I_{p, \Delta T}(s, X)$, the functions $G(V)$ and $G(P)$ can be approximated by a straight line (Section 3.3.6), provided the output of each set is determined over ΔT. The slope of the straight line is dependent on the domain of input for each nonlinear element, and it is constant over ΔT. The forward gains of the elements in the vth KO subset are fixed at positive real numbers

$$G_v(P) \propto g_{vp} P, \qquad G_v(V) \propto g_{vv} V. \tag{5}$$

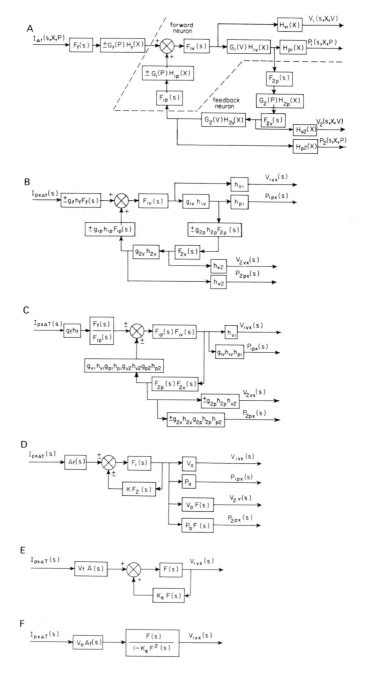

FIG. 5.2. Topological reduction of a KI set to a lumped, piecewise linear approximation.

In part (b) under assumptions (i)–(iii) the domain of input is fixed at $I_{p,X,\Delta T}(s)$ for both amplitude and spatial distribution. The range and spatial distribution of the active states for each subset v in the set are fixed and the operators become fixed real numbers. For pulse to wave conversion,

$$G_f(P)H_f(X) \propto g_f h_f P, \qquad G_1(P)H_{1p}(X) \propto g_{1p}h_{1p}P,$$
$$G_2(P)H_{2p}(X) \propto g_{2p}h_{2p}P. \tag{6}$$

For wave to pulse conversion,

$$G_1(V)H_{1v}(X) \propto g_{1v}h_{1v}V, \qquad G_2(V)H_{2v}(X) \propto g_{2v}h_{2v}V. \tag{7}$$

For AEP output,

$$H_{v1}(X) \propto h_{v1}, \qquad H_{v2}(X) \propto h_{v2}. \tag{8}$$

For PSTH output,

$$H_{p1}(X) \propto h_{p1}, \qquad H_{p2}(X) \propto h_{p2}. \tag{9}$$

The model is transformed to a lumped linear feedback system with fixed gain coefficients depending on the fixed range of input.

In part (c) the linearized elements are rearranged by block substitution to consolidate the frequency-dependent functions and the fixed gain coefficients. In part (d), the transfer functions for the input channel, the forward channel, and the feedback channel are redefined:

$$A_f(s) \triangleq F_f(s)/F_{1p}(s), \qquad F_1(s) \triangleq F_{1p}(s)F_{1v}(s), \qquad F_2(s) \triangleq F_{2p}(s)F_{2v}(s). \tag{10}$$

The forward gain coefficients are

$$V_a \triangleq g_f h_f h_{v1}, \qquad P_a \triangleq g_f h_f g_{1v}h_{1v}h_{p1},$$
$$V_b \triangleq g_f h_f g_{2p}h_{2p}h_{p2}, \qquad P_b \triangleq g_f h_f g_{2v}h_{2v}g_{2p}h_{2p}h_{v2}. \tag{11}$$

The feedback gain coefficient is

$$K \triangleq g_{v1}h_{v1}g_{p1}h_{p1}g_{v2}h_{v2}g_{p2}h_{p2}. \tag{12}$$

In part (e) the loop is specified as a positive feedback loop, and the output is taken only in the wave mode from the forward channel. By assumption (1),

$$F_1(s) = F_2(s) = F(s). \tag{13}$$

In part (f) the transfer function for the loop is represented by the feedback equation. The input to the loop is $V_a A(s) I_{p,X,\Delta T}(s)$ and the transfer function is

$$C(s) = F(s)/[1 - K_e F^2(s)]. \tag{14}$$

where $K_e = K$ is excitatory positive feedback gain. This is the form desired [see Eq. (3)] for analysis by piecewise linear approximation in which for each function $I_{p,x,\Delta T}(s)$ there is a positive real number K_e. The problem for analysis is to evaluate K_e by comparing solutions to Eq. (14) with the output of KI sets in neural masses. The value for K_e represents the magnitude of interaction in the set for the designated conditions. This is important because the interaction is the defining characteristic of the KI set and a principal determinant of its properties. It is essential that we be able to measure it.

5.1.3. ROOT LOCUS AS A FUNCTION OF FEEDBACK GAIN

The expanded form of the feedback Eq. (14) in $F(s)$ is the ratio of two polynomials in s (Section 2.2.3)

$$C(s) = \frac{a_m s^m + a_{m-1} s^{m-1} + \cdots + a_1 s + a_0}{b_n s^n + b_{n-1} s^{n-1} + \cdots + b_1 s + b_0}, \qquad n \geq m. \qquad (15)$$

When the numerator and denominator are factored,

$$C(s) = a_m \prod_{j=1}^{m} (s + z_j) / b_n \prod_{j=1}^{n} (s + d_j), \qquad n \geq m, \qquad (16)$$

where z_j and d_j are real or complex numbers. The roots of the polynomial in the numerator are called *zeros* for as s takes the value of any $-z_j$, $C(s) = 0$. The roots of the polynomial in the denominator are called *poles* for when s equals $-d_j$, $C(s) = \infty$ (see Section 2.2.3).

The values for $s = -z_j$ and $s = -d_j$ are represented as points in the complex plane for $s = \alpha + j\omega$, and each point represents a damped sine wave or exponential (Fig. 5.3). The values for the coefficients in Eq. (15) depend on the rate coefficients in $F(s)$ which are a, b, ... (see list at beginning of Section 5.1.2), and on the value for K_e. Whereas the rate coefficients $F(s)$ are assumed to be fixed for all input and time, the value for K_e is dependent on the input domain and response range over time intervals ΔT. For a range of values for K_e, there is a range of values for each of the roots, $-z_j$ and $-d_j$. The range of values takes the form of a curve or line segment in the s plane, which is known as the *root locus* for $-z_j$ or $-d_j$. For each transfer function $C(s)$ there are m root loci for the zeros and n root loci for the poles.

For $K_e = 0$, $C(s) = F(s)$. This is called the *open loop state*, and the roots are the open loop poles and zeros. Open loop poles are shown as crosses $\times$ (double poles as $*$) and open loop zeros are shown as circles $\bigcirc$. For $K_e \neq 0$, the roots are closed loop poles (triangles $\triangle$) and closed loop zeros (squares $\square$). Whereas the open loop poles and zeros are constant, the closed loop roots are fixed at points on the root loci determined by K_e.

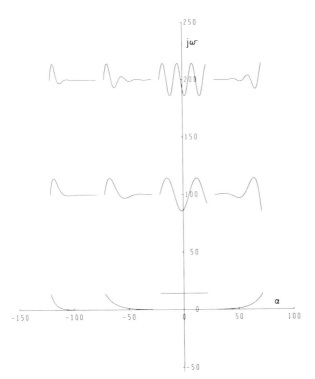

FIG. 5.3. Relation between location of a real pole or complex pole pair in the s plane and the form of the impulse response: frequency ω and decay rate α.

Example A. Let the time-dependent property of the KO subset be approximated by first-order differential equation with a single rate constant a so that the open loop transfer function is

$$C(s) = F(s) = a/(s+a). \tag{17}$$

From Eq. (14) the closed loop transfer function for positive feedback is

$$
\begin{aligned}
C(s) &= F(s)/[1 - K_e F^2(s)] \\[4pt]
&= \frac{a/(s+a)}{1 - [K_e a^2/(s+a)^2]} \\[4pt]
&= \frac{as + a^2}{s^2 + 2as + (1 - K_e)a^2}.
\end{aligned} \tag{18}
$$

On factoring, we obtain

$$C(s) = a(s + z_1)/(s + d_1)(s + d_2), \qquad z_1 = a, \qquad d_1, d_2 = a(1 \pm K_e^{.5}). \tag{19}$$

There is a closed loop zero at $s = -a$ and there are two real poles at $s = -a(1 \pm K_e^{.5})$. For $K_e = 1$, $s = -2a$ and $s = 0$. The two open loop poles for the forward and feedback channels are shown as a double pole (∗) at $s = -a$ in Fig. 5.4. The two root loci coincide with the real axis $s = \alpha$, one running to the left of $s = -a$ and the other to the right of $s = -a$, with K_e increasing above zero at $s = -a$. The inverse Laplace transform of Eq. (19) is in the form

$$c(t) = A_1 e^{-d_1 t} + A_2 e^{-d_2 t}, \tag{20}$$

where A_1 and A_2 are determined by partial fraction expansion (Section 2.2.3).   □

Example B.   The KII_{ei} set consists of a KI_e set interacting with a KI_i set. For a set of conditions to be described in Section 5.3.1, the KII_{ei} set can be reduced to the interaction of a KO_e set with a KO_i set. If $F_e(s) = F_i(s) = F(s)$, then

$$C(s) = F(s)/[1 + K_n F^2(s)], \tag{21}$$

where K_n is a positive real number evaluating the interaction strength as negative feedback gain. As in Example A let $F(s) = a/(s + a)$, so that

$$C(s) = a(s + z_1)/(s + d_1)(s + d_2), \qquad z_1 = a, \quad d_1, d_2 = a(1 \pm jK_n^{.5}). \tag{22}$$

The open loop double pole and closed loop zero appear as before. The root loci are vertical lines at $s = -a \pm j\omega$, starting from $s = -a$ at $K_n = 0$ (Fig. 5.5). The position of the closed loop poles is shown for $K_n = 1$. Poles having complex values always occur in conjugate pairs. The inverse Laplace

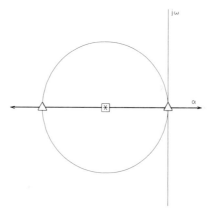

FIG. 5.4. Root locus plot for positive feedback between two first-order delay elements.

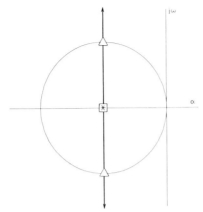

FIG. 5.5. Root locus plot for negative feedback between two first-order delay elements.

transform gives the predicted impulse response in the form

$$c(t) = A_0 \cos(\omega t + \varphi) e^{-\alpha t} \tag{23}$$

where A_0 and φ are determined by partial fraction expansion and Euler's theorem (Section 2.1.4). □

These simple examples illustrate certain features that also hold for second- and third-order approximations for $F(s)$. In the case of positive feedback there is one real-valued root that moves to the right of $s = -a$ with increasing K_e. For $0 < K_e < 1$, the root at $s = -a(1 - K_e^{.5})$ predicts that the impulse response [Eq. (20)] contains a term $A_1 e^{-d_1 t}$ that has a monotonic decay slower than the passive decay rate a of the open loop KO set. In this range of K_e, $d_1 \to 0$ as $K_e \to 1$. For $K_e = 1$, the predicted impulse response contains a step function. In the case of negative feedback for $K_n \neq 0$ there is a complex pole pair, which implies that the impulse response contains a damped sine wave. The frequency ω increases with increasing K_n.

Example C.   Let the dynamics of the KO subset be approximated by a second-order differential equation for which the transfer function is

$$F(s) = ab/(s+a)(s+b). \tag{24}$$

The closed loop transfer function is

$$C(s) = ab(s+a)(s+b)/[(s+a)^2(s+b)^2 - K_e a^2 b^2]. \tag{25}$$

On factoring,

$$C(s) = ab(s+a)(s+b)/\prod_{j=1}^{4}(s+d_j), \tag{26}$$

where the values for the four poles at $s = -d_j$ are determined by a, b, and K_e. The four root loci are shown as functions of K_e in Fig. 5.6. There are two open loop double poles and closed loop zeros at $s = -a$ and $s = -b$. Four closed loop poles are shown for $K_e = 1$. The inverse transform is

$$c(t) = \sum_{j=1}^{4} A_j e^{-d_j t}. \tag{27}$$

There are two real poles and one complex pole pair, so that

$$c(t) = A_1 e^{-d_1 t} + A_2 e^{-d_2 t} + A_3 \cos(\omega t + \varphi) e^{-\alpha t}. \tag{28}$$

For $K_e = 1, d_1 = 0$, and the predicted impulse response contains a step function and a highly damped sine wave (Fig. 5.3).   □

Example D.   Let the second-order approximation hold for the case of negative feedback, so that

$$C(s) = ab(s+a)(s+b)/[(s+a)^2(s+b)^2 + K_n a^2 b^2]. \tag{29}$$

On factoring,

$$C(s) = ab(s+a)(s+b)/\prod_{j=1}^{2} (s+\alpha_j+j\omega_j)(s+\alpha_j-j\omega_j). \tag{30}$$

There are two pairs of complex poles (Fig. 5.7) for which the values are determined by a, b, and K_n. The four root loci are curves, two of which move to the left and away from the $j\omega$ axis, and two of which move to the right toward and across the $j\omega$ axis. The inverse transform gives

$$c(t) = \sum_{j=1}^{2} A_j \cos(\omega_j t + \varphi_j) e^{-\alpha_j t}. \tag{31}$$

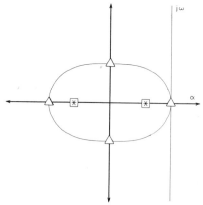

FIG. 5.6. Root locus plot for positive feedback between two second-order delay elements.

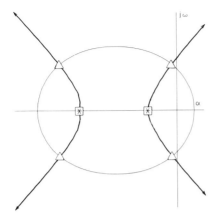

FIG. 5.7. Root locus plot for negative feedback between two second-order delay elements.

In this example, $\omega_1 = \omega_2$ and $\alpha_1 < \alpha_2$. The predicted impulse response consists of the sum of two damped sine waves, one of which is poorly damped α_1 and the other of which is highly damped, α_2. □

The root loci in these examples have been found by factoring the polynomials in the denominator for a set of values of K_e or K_n and interpolating smooth curves between the derived values for the closed loop poles. Especially for third-order or yet higher-order approximations for $F(s)$, this approach is easiest if a computer is available. If not, the root loci can be constructed by a trial and error graphic technique (DiStefano, et al., 1967). For each value of $s = -d_j$, the denominator of the polynomial is zero. That is,

$$1 - K_e F^2(s) = 0, \qquad 1 + K_n F^2(s) = 0. \tag{32}$$

For $s = -d_j$, $F^2(s) = C$, which is a complex number having an argument $|C|$ and a phase $e^{j\varphi}$. For positive feedback, $K_e = 1/C$ and

$$K_e = (1/|C|)e^{j\varphi}, \qquad \varphi = 0, 2\pi, 4\pi, \ldots. \tag{33}$$

For negative feedback, $K_n = -1/C$ and

$$K_n = (1/|C|)e^{j\varphi}, \qquad \varphi = \pi, 3\pi, 5\pi, \ldots.$$

For each value of $1/|C|$ there is a locus in the s plane called a *gain contour*. For positive feedback each root locus corresponds to a contour for phase φ of 0 rad ($0°$) or an even multiple of $n\pi$ rad (Fig. 5.6). For negative feedback each root locus corresponds to a phase contour of π rad ($180°$) or an odd multiple of $n\pi$ rad (Fig. 5.7). For a given value of K_e or K_n, the closed loop roots occur at the intersections of the gain and phase contours. These conventions are followed for labeling purposes in the following sections, but most of the root locus plots have been constructed by factoring, so that $|C|$ and φ are not explicitly evaluated.

5.1.4. AMPLITUDE-DEPENDENT GAIN AND STABILITY

The root locus plot is a valuable aid in the analysis of neural sets because it presents in a single visual display virtually all of the dynamic properties of each set. With practice it is relatively easy to estimate quickly from the pole–zero configuration how many terms the impulse response has, whether they are monotonic or oscillatory, and what their approximate amplitudes, decay rates, and frequencies are. Conversely, given the frequency ω and decay rate α of a component in an AEP, the location is specified for a real pole or pair of complex conjugate poles at $s = -\alpha \pm j\omega$ in the s plane (Fig. 5.3). The root loci show how each component in a predicted impulse response is expected to change in frequency and decay rate when the feedback gain is changed.

In general, the feedback gain can be expected to change whenever either of two conditions is changed. One condition is the mean level of activity without transient input when the KI set or reduced KII set is at equilibrium (Section 1.3.5). The other condition is the range of activity induced by input that drives the set away from equilibrium (Section 3.3.6).

The predominant nonlinearity in KI and KII sets is provided by the mechanism of wave to pulse conversion (Section 3.3.4). The input–output curve $G(v)$ is sigmoid (Section 3.36) and has the equation,

$$p = \begin{cases} p_o(3 - 2e^{-v}), & v \geq 0, \\ p_o e^{2v}, & v \leq 0, \end{cases} \tag{34}$$

where v is wave amplitude in dimensionless units of the empirical rate constant γ, and p_o is the mean pulse rate of the set. A set of input–output curves is shown in Fig. 3.20. We assume that pulse to wave conversion is linear and can be expressed by the fixed coefficient $\zeta \tilde{v}_i$ (Section 3.3.5).

Intuitively it is obvious in nonnormalized coordinates (Fig. 3.20) that the sigmoid curve can be approximated by a straight line for any given effective range of v. The slope of the straight line depends on p_o, which is a constant over any time period of linearization ΔT (Section 5.1.2), and also on the effective range (Fig. 3.20d). It is maximal for $v = 0$ at $p = p_o$, and steadily decreases for increasing v in either direction. The effective range is constant over ΔT. Further, there is a straight line which is parallel to the linear approximation to the sigmoid curve and tangent to the curve at a point with the value v_e^* or v_i^*. That value of v can be treated as representing the effective operating range (Section 3.3.6).

It is not possible to determine v_e^* or v_i^* directly from AEPs, but it is possible to determine the linearized loop gain and thereby the effective linearized forward gain and v_e^* and v_i^* from AEPs. This is described in Chapter 6. For the present it is sufficient to note that when the input amplitude is changed, the response amplitude then changes, and the altered range of v is accompanied by change in the slope of the linear approximation to the sigmoid curve. Hence the forward gains and the loop gains are changed, and the closed loop roots of the AEP are changed. When the KI or reduced KII set has been properly modeled, each AEP or PSTH should specify a set of points in the s plane that lie on root loci, and the closed loop gain is determined from the root loci.

The locations in the s plane at which root loci cross the $j\omega$ axis (Figs. 5.6 and 5.7) also convey some idea about the stability properties of a neural set (Section 1.3.5). For a linear system, the left half of the s plane, $s = -\alpha \pm j\omega$, is the domain of stable solutions, because all the terms e^{st} in the inverse transform have negative real parts. The exponentials and damped sine waves in the impulse response decay to zero. The right half of the s plane is the domain of instability, because all the solutions yield exponential terms having positive real parts. The exponentials and damped sine waves increase over time without limit (Fig. 5.3). At $s = \pm j\omega$ the decay rates are zero, and stability is to be defined. In this chapter consideration is restricted to solutions in the linear stable domain. Problems involving root loci that cross to the right half of the s plane are discussed first in Section 6.2.1.

5.2. Reduction from the KI Level

5.2.1. TOPOLOGICAL ANALYSIS OF THE GLOMERULAR LAYER

The impulse response at a point in a neural mass in the wave mode $o_v(t, x, y, u)$ or in the pulse mode $o_p(t, x, y, u)$ is manifested in the form of an AEP, $\hat{v}(T)$, or a PSTH, $\hat{p}(T)$, when the input is single-shock afferent electrical stimulation. The observed impulse response is fitted with a set of basis functions, $v(T)$ or $p(T)$. The Laplace transform gives $V(s)$ or $P(s)$, which represents the operation performed on the input by the mass and its afferent channel to give the response. The hypothesis may be put forward that the transfer function for the operation can be separated into a set of transfer functions in series or in parallel that represent separable operations of the mass and afferent channel. The inference can be made that one of the transfer functions is the operation $C_1(s)$ performed by a single feedback loop formed by a KI set in the mass, which is in series with a lumped transfer function for the afferent path $A_m(s)$ and an output transfer function in one of the forms described in Section 5.1.2, which are denoted generically by $N_u(s)$.

$$V_1(s) = A_m(s) C_1(s) N_v(s), \qquad P_1(s) = A_m(s) C_1(s) N_p(s), \qquad (35)$$

where $C_1(s)$ depends on the open loop transfer function of the KI set $A(s)$ and a feedback gain coefficient K_e or K_i (Section 5.1.3). Both give positive feedback:

$$C_1(s) = A(s)/[1 - KA^2(s)]. \qquad (36)$$

The immediate aim of analysis is to determine from the impulse response $\hat{v}(t)$ or $\hat{p}(t)$ the value for K which is the definitive property of the interactive mass. To this end it is necessary to describe and evaluate the open loop transfer functions $A(s)$ and the input and output transfer functions, $A_m(s)$ and $N_u(s)$. In practice the most difficult part of the analysis is the description and measurement of $A_m(s)$. A variety of methods can be used to do this. Common to all of them is topological analysis based on anatomical description and qualitative examination of input–output relationships.

An example of a KI set is the set of periglomerular neurons (Section 4.3.1). They receive external input from PON axons, and their output is in the form of pulse trains of single neurons. Intracellular recording in single periglomerular neurons has shown that their synaptic currents have properties that are generically the same as those of other neurons (Minor, 1969), and the KI$_p$ set can be predicted to generate a closed field centered in the glomerular layer (Section 4.3.2). However, this field is almost totally obscured by the powerful dipole field of the granule cells in the bulb. There is no directly observable output of the set in the wave mode.

The PSTH of single neurons in the set on single-shock PON stimulation consists (Fig. 5.8a) of a sustained increase in firing probability for 50 msec or more. There is a latency in onset of several milliseconds which varies between neurons and decreases with increasing stimulus intensity. No neurons are observed to undergo inhibition either at the start of the response or at any subsequent time. It is inferred that the neurons are excited by PON axons, and it is hypothesized that the long duration of the increase in poststimulus pulse probability is due to mutual excitation within the set.

From anatomical studies (Pinching & Powell, 1971a–d) PON axons form axodendritic synapses with periglomerular (P) dendrites and mitral–tufted (M) apical dendrites in the glomeruli (Fig. 5.9a). The periglomerular cells have observable output in the form of pulse trains $p_P(t)$. They have synaptic output by axodendritic synapses to each other, to other short axon cells (SA) in the glomerular layer, and to mitral–tufted apical dendrites (a) just external to the glomeruli. They also have synaptic connections to mitral–tufted cells by dendrodendritic synapses in the glomeruli (d), which are inferred to be excitatory (see Section 6.1.4). The periglomerular neurons receive secondary input from each other, by axodendritic synapses from

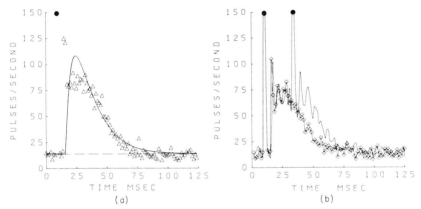

FIG. 5.8. PSTHs from a periglomerular unit on PON electrical stimulation (Freeman, 1974d). (a) Single-shock; (b) Paired shock.

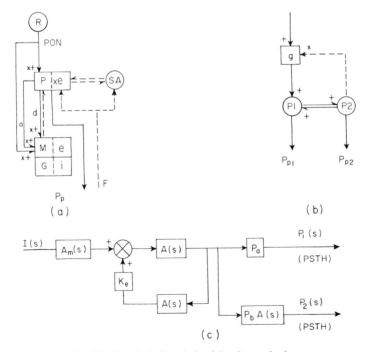

FIG. 5.9. Topological analysis of the glomerular layer.

short axon cells (SA), and from centrifugal axons (F) entering the bulb from the forebrain (Pinching & Powell, 1972a, b) but not in the lateral olfactory tract. There is anatomical evidence for input from mitral–tufted apical dendrites by dendrodendritic synapses. However, excitation of mitral–tufted axons by antidromic stimulation of the LOT, which leads to widespread excitation of both mitral–tufted and granule cells (G), does not change $p_P(t)$. It is inferred that there are not significant functional connections from the KII_{MG} set to the KI_P set.[†]

In topological reduction (Fig. 5.9b) the input is restricted to electrical stimulation of the PON, and the receptors (R) are omitted. The output is restricted $p_P(t)$, and there is assumed to be no feedback from the KII_{MG} set, so that set is omitted. The performance of the KI_P set is not significantly altered by cutting the bulbar stalk, and there is no deliberate input through F, so the centrifugal input channel is omitted. There is as yet no observable physiological output distinguished for short axon cells, and their possible role is unknown, so they are omitted. The interaction of the KI_e set is represented by mutual excitation between two KO_e sets (Section 1.3.4). Output is distinguished for the subset which is directly excited by a given PON volley, $p_{P1}(t)$, and for the subset which is indirectly excited through the initially excited subset $p_{P2}(t)$.

Nonlinearity in the operation of the system is revealed in two ways. First, with increasing input pulse intensity, the amplitude of output increases, but the decay rate from the crest of pulse probability increases (Fig. 5.10). This is the failure of proportionality. Second, when two stimuli are given in succession, the response to the second (test) stimulus is reduced in comparison with the response to the first (conditioning) stimulus (Fig. 5.8b). This is failure of both additivity and time invariance.

The reduction of response amplitude by preceding induced activity is called *glomerular transmission attenuation*. It is cumulative over a train of input pulses, and it also occurs in responses of mitral–tufted and granule

---

[†] The failure of strong LOT input to influence the PSTHs of periglomerular neurons is a bit puzzling because of the numerous reciprocal dendrodendritic synapses between peri-glomerular and mitral–tufted cells in the glomeruli. Gusel'nikova et al. (1970) have evidence that the distal dendrites of the mitral cells generate impulses in the same manner as do the apical dendrites of hippocampal pyramidal cells (Kandel & Spencer, 1961) and the dendrites of Purkinje cells (Llinas & Nicholson, 1971). We may suppose that the juxtaglomerular shaft of mitral-tufted apical dendrites contains a local region of spike-generating membrane which is triggered by PON and periglomerular excitatory input to the intraglomerular apical dendritic tuft, and by periglomerular axodendritic synapses on the apical dendritic shaft (Pinching & Powell, 1971c, d), whereas antidromic excitation of the mitral–tufted cell bodies is insufficient to trigger an apical dendritic spike and does not lead to an effective intra-glomerular dendritic depolarizing current loop. Confirmation will require intracellular recording in mitral–tufted cells.

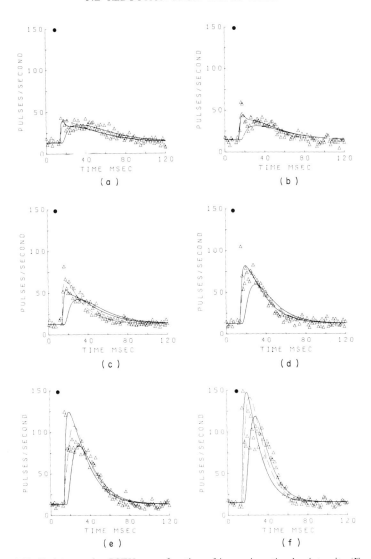

FIG. 5.10. Periglomerular PSTHs as a function of increasing stimulus intensity (Freeman, 1974e).

cells. This is shown by the reduction in AEP amplitude on PON stimulation, following a change in the stimulus rate from 1/sec to 6/sec (Fig. 5.11a and b). It occurs only when a nonoscillatory minor component is present in the AEP, in addition to the dominant oscillatory component (Fig. 5.11a and b compared with c and d). This minor component is principally due to KI_P output set through the KI_M set to the KI_G set (Section 6.1.4) and is absent

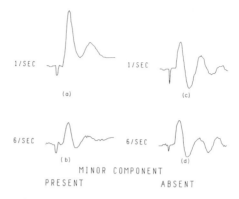

1/SEC

(a)

1/SEC

(c)

6/SEC

(b)

6/SEC

(d)

MINOR COMPONENT

PRESENT   ABSENT

FIG. 5.11. Demonstration that sensitivity of AEP amplitude to rate of PON stimulation depends on the existence of a prominent baseline shift in the AEP [(a) and (b)] (Freeman, 1974c).

on LOT stimulation. The attenuation effect is not induced by LOT input and it does not affect bulbar responses to LOT input.

On single-shock PON stimulation the attenuation effect increases in amplitude to a maximum around 50 msec after the stimulus and decays at a rate between 2/sec and 20/sec (Fig. 5.12c). The amplitude, rate of rise, and decay rate all increase with increasing input intensity. The spatial distribution of the attenuation effect is the same as the distribution of evoked periglomerular activity (Section 4.5.2, Example B). Its rise time and amplitude are closely related to the decay time and amplitude of evoked periglomerular activity (Fig. 5.12b). The effect is attributed (Freeman, 1974d) to a side affect of intense synaptic activity within the glomeruli, leading to the local accumulation of an unknown substance in the glomerular extracellular space, possibly potassium ions, which may depolarize all synaptic terminals in the glomeruli nonspecifically. This is inferred to decrease the output of each terminal for any given input (Sections 3.2.4 and 3.3.5; see also Example I in Section 1.3.1).

The nonlinear property of glomerular transmission is designated by the $x+$ symbol in Fig. 5.9a. Its specific role in determining PON input to periglomerular neurons is shown as a channel g in Fig. 5.9b, with an implied dependence $\times$ of the parameters of g on the output of KI_p.

Part (c) in Fig. 5.9 comprises a lumped circuit approximation and a piecewise linear approximation for the reduced system in part (b). For a given intensity of impulse input $I(s)$ the amplitude dependent gain is fixed at K_e, and the open loop transfer function for the KI_p set is designated $A(s)$. The output transfer function is $P_a = P_{P1}(s)$ for the forward channel and $P_b A(s) = P_{P2}(s)$ for the feedback channel. The nonlinearity in the input is

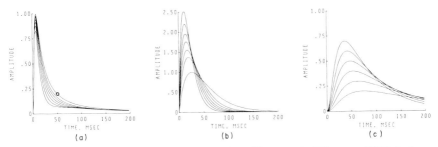

FIG. 5.12. (a) Experimentally estimated distribution of input to the KI_P set on PON single-shock stimulation. Amplitude is normalized to unity at peak. Curve marked O is without glomerular transmission attenuation; the underlying curves show the effect of increasing attenuation. (b) Time course of KI_P activity as experimentally determined for input of increasing intensity. The rise time is determined by the activity curves in (b). The integral of the curves in (b) determines the rise time of attenuation curves in (c) (from Freeman, 1974c–f).

incorporated into the transfer function $A_m(s)$. This completes the topological transformation preliminary to the construction of differential equations for $A(s)$ and $A_m(s)$.

5.2.2. DIFFERENTIAL EQUATIONS FOR THE KI_e SET

From Fig. 5.9c, the transfer functions for PON single-shock input and PSTH output are

$$P_{P1}(s) = \frac{P_a A_m(s) A(s)}{1 - K_e A^2(s)}, \tag{37}$$

$$P_{P2}(s) = \frac{P_b A_m(s) A^2(s)}{1 - K_e A^2(s)}. \tag{38}$$

In some other neural sets the open loop transfer function equivalent to $P_{P1}(s) = P_a A_m(s) A(s)$ can be obtained by administration of a large dose of general anesthetic that opens the loop by suppressing wave to pulse conversion without affecting pulse to wave conversion. Because there is no wave output for the KI_P set in the open loop state, $A(s)$ cannot be evaluated directly. It is done indirectly by measuring a set of closed loop impulse responses over a set of input intensities. With increasing input intensity K_e is decreased, and the values for the closed loop roots are changed. The roots for a set of input intensities are plotted in the s plane as an empirical root locus. The values for the open loop roots at $K_e = 0$ are determined by extrapolation (Fig. 5.13).

As a first approximation let

$$A_m(s) = 1, \qquad A(s) = ab/(s+a)(s+b), \tag{39}$$

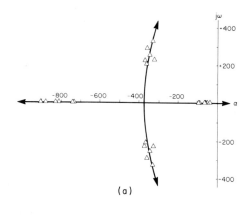

(a)

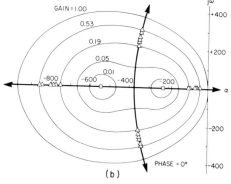

(b)

FIG. 5.13. Root locus plot for KI$_P$ set (Freeman 1974e). (a) Closed loop roots from Table 5.1. (b) Root loci and gain contours from Eq. (53).

where a represents the average passive membrane rate constant and b represents lumped synaptic and cable delay. Then

$$P_{P2}(s) = \frac{P_a a^2 b^2}{(s+a)^2(s+b)^2 - K_e a^2 b^2},$$

$$P_{P2}(s) = \frac{P_a a^2 b^2}{(s+\beta)(s+\gamma)(s+\alpha+j\omega)(s+\alpha-j\omega)}.$$

(40)

The inverse transform is

$$p_{P2}(t) = P_1 e^{-\beta t} + P_2 e^{-\gamma t} + P_3[\sin(\omega t + \varphi)e^{-\alpha t}].$$

(41)

There are two real poles. When curves from Eq. (41) are fitted to PSTHs of periglomerular units, the rate constant β is between 40/sec and 100/sec, representing the decay of the impulse response. The rate constant γ exceeds

700/sec. This term and the damped sine wave specified by the complex
roots represent the rising phase of the PSTHs.

The experimental complex root loci are found to be not compatible with
the root loci predicted for a positive feedback loop with $A(s)$ specified by
Eq. (39). The predicted complex root loci are parallel to the $j\omega$ axis (Fig. 5.4).
Moreover, the predicted impulse response for the operation specified by
Eq. (39) should show decreased rate of rise with decreasing values for
K_e, whereas the PSTH show increased rate of rise for high input intensities
and low values of K_e.

The model is improved by setting

$$A_m(s) = 1 + K' \exp[-(sT_b)^{1/2}].$$ (42)

This transfer function specifies the input to the periglomerular neurons as an
impulse accompanied by a transient having the form of a one-dimensional
diffusion process (Section 2.3.5). There is a rapid increase in PON input to
the glomeruli to a crest followed by a decay with a long tail (Fig. 5.12a,
uppermost curve marked by a zero). A rational approximation for the
exponential term (Section 2.2.5, Fig. 2.17c) is

$$A_m(s) \approx 1 + \frac{K'(s-z_0)^2}{(s+d_1)(s+d_2)},$$ (43)

where $d_1 = (\pi/2)^2/T_b$ and $d_2 = (3\pi/2)^2/T_b$. The values for z_0 are sufficiently
large that they can be replaced by a constant $d_1 d_2 \approx (s-z_0)^2$. On clearing
of fractions $A_m(s)$ is taken to be

$$A_m(s) = (s+z_1)(s+z_2)/(s+d_1)(s+d_2),$$ (44)

where

$$w = [(d_1+d_2)^2 - 4d_1 d_2(K'+1)]^{.5}, \qquad z_1 = (d_1+d_2-w)/2,$$
$$z_2 = (d_1+d_2+w)/2.$$ (45)

The input delivered to the KI_p set (Fig. 5.12) induces an increase in activity
of the set (Fig. 5.12b), which causes an increase in the attenuation effect
(Fig. 5.12c). The attenuation has little effect on the input prior to the crest
of the distributed volley, and it reduces the effectiveness of the declining
phase of the volley (Fig. 5.12a). The lower curves under the curve marked
zero are the result of attenuating the values for the curve marked zero.
This is done by multiplying the value at each time on the ordinate by the
attenuation amplitude at the same time in one of the curves in Fig. 5.12c.
The attenuation has little effect on the amplitude of input, but it decreases
the apparent dispersion of the input volley. The decrease of input dispersion
is represented in the model by a decrease in the value for T_b. The

negligible effect on pulse input amplitude is incorporated into the forward gain coefficients, P_a and P_b.

Equations (39) and (44) are substituted into Eq. (38). After clearing of fractions,

$$P_{P2}(s) = \frac{P_b\, a^2 b^2 (s + z_1)(s + z_2)}{(s + d_1)(s + d_2)(s + \gamma)(s + \beta)(s + \alpha + j\omega)(s + \alpha - j\omega)}. \tag{46}$$

The inverse Laplace transform gives

$$p_{P2}(T) = P_a\, e^{-\beta T} + P_b\, e^{-\gamma T} + P_c[\sin(\omega T + \varphi)\, e^{-\alpha T}] + P_{d1}\, e^{-d_1 T} + P_{d2}\, e^{-d_2 T}. \tag{47}$$

Equation (47) with 11 independent parameters is simplified for curve-fitting purposes by setting

$$P_b = -P_a + P_c \sin \varphi, \qquad P_1 \triangleq P_a, \qquad P_2 \triangleq P_c, \qquad P_3 \triangleq P_{d1} \triangleq -P_{d2},$$

$$p_{P2}(T) = P_1(e^{-\beta T} - e^{-\gamma T}) + P_2[\sin(\omega T + \varphi)e^{-\alpha T}$$
$$- \sin(\varphi)e^{-\gamma T}] + P_3(e^{-d_1 T} - e^{-d_2 T}). \tag{48}$$

Equation (48) has 9 independent parameters. Component P_1 represents the decay phase and components P_2 and P_3 represent together the rising phase of the PSTH.

Curves (dashed) from Eq. (48) fitted to PSTHs are shown in Figs. 5.10 and 5.14. A root locus plot for the four poles in $A(s)$ is shown in Fig. 5.13a. The poles at $s = -d_1$ and $s = -d_2$ are not shown. A set of values of the coefficients is given in Table 5.1. The values for T_b for two sets of PSTHs are also given in Table 5.2. The values decrease with increasing stimulus intensity.

The slight curvature of the empirical complex root loci implies that a second-order approximation for $A(s)$ is inadequate. The transfer function $A(s)$ is modified to include the effects of axonal transmission delay within the set by a rational approximation (see Section 2.3.3),

$$A(s) = ab(c - s)/(s + a)(s + b)(s + c), \tag{49}$$

where a and b are the same as in Eq. (39), and the axonal delay $T_c = 2/c$ is approximated by a zero at $s = c$ and a pole at $s = -c$. By trial and error approximation in the s plane, $a = 230/\text{sec}$, $b = 550/\text{sec}$, and $c = 2300/\text{sec}$:

$$P(s) = \frac{1.26 \times 10^5 (2300 - s)}{(s + 230)^2 (s + 550)^2 (s + 2300)^2 - 1.6 \times 10^{10} K_e}. \tag{50}$$

A set of root loci and gain contours is shown for Eq. (50) in Fig. 5.13b. The loci and contours near $s = \pm 2300/\text{sec}$ are not included. The observed

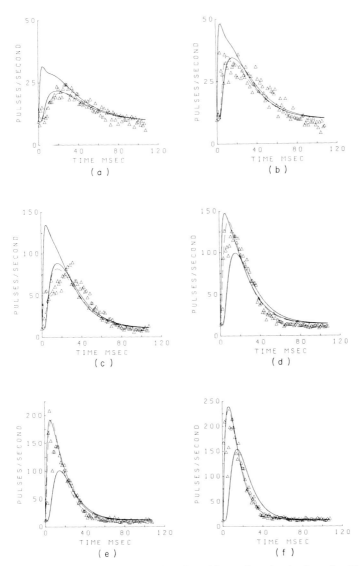

FIG. 5.14. Periglomerular PSTHs as a function of increasing stimulus intensity (Freeman, 1974e). See Table 5.2.

roots at $s = -\beta$ are plotted on the real axis near the origin. From the intersection of the gain contours over this range of values of β, the value for K_e empirically is given by

$$K_e = e^{-.017\beta} \tag{51}$$

for β in units of 1/sec. The relation is shown graphically in Fig. 5.15. Sets of values calculated from β are listed in Table 5.2. This completes the evaluation of the loop. In essence, the loop gain is determined from the decay rate of the PSTH as determined by Eq. (48).

The transfer function of the input channel is evaluated as follows. Estimates for T_b derived from AEPs on PON stimulation (Section 5.3.2) range from 39 to 28 msec with a mean of 32 msec. The same mean values hold for both open and closed loop conditions, as shown in Sections 5.3.2 and 5.3.3 from measurements on the AEPs taken at stimulus intensities near

TABLE 5.1

GLOMERULAR PST HISTOGRAMS[a]

Fig. 5.10	I (μA)	N	P_1 (pulses/ sec)	β (1/sec)	γ (1/sec)	P_2 (pulses/ sec)	ω (rad/ sec)	α (1/sec)	φ (rad)	P_3 (pulses/ sec)	T_b (msec)
(a)	25	200	84	40	927	27	318	337	−2.47	−64	46
(b)	27	200	159	49	807	65	328	371	−2.74	−117	45
(c)	29	200	205	57	845	85	245	381	−2.82	−130	41
(d)	31	200	276	67	908	146	208	401	−2.78	−209	26
(e)	33	200	944	79	899	265	218	402	−3.11	−844	25
(f)	35	200	919	95	1110	186	201	412	−3.17	−889	17

[a] Values are for coefficients in Eq. (48) and dashed curves in Fig. 5.14 with $N = 200$.

TABLE 5.2

CLOSED LOOP COEFFICIENTS FOR PST HISTOGRAMS FOR EQS. (49)–(51)[a]

Figure	K_a or (pulses/sec) forward limb	K_b (pulses/sec) feedback limb	K_e feedback gain	T_b (msec) PON delay
5.14a	.24	.23	.47	37
5.14b	.47	.63	.35	36
5.14c	1.49	1.97	.34	32
5.14d	1.57	2.22	.30	26
5.14e	2.05	3.32	.21	23
5.14f	4.99	3.96	.19	18
5.10a	.20	.32	.50	46
5.10b	.35	.38	.43	45
5.10c	.51	.75	.37	41
5.10d	.80	1.15	.31	26
5.10e	1.39	2.12	.26	25
5.10f	1.67	3.72	.19	18

[a] Fixed coefficients: $a = 230$/sec, $b = 550$/sec, $c = 2300$/sec, and $K' = 1.8$.

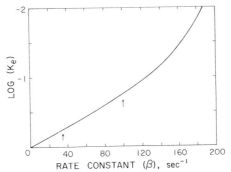

FIG. 5.15. Relation between KI_P feedback gain, K_e, and the rate constant of the predicted PSTH impulse response, derived from Fig. 5.13. Arrows show experimental range of observation (Freeman, 1974f).

the middle of the range of stimulus intensities. The respective means for T_b from two sets (including Table 5.1) are 29 and 33 msec with an overall range of 46 to 17 msec. Because the two means estimated from PST histograms conform to each other and to a result by a different technique, they are inferred to be correct as given.

The value for K' for glomerular PSTHs is estimated from the locations of the two zeros, $s = -z_1$ and $s = -z_2$, in Eq. (44). The root loci for the zeros lie on the real axis between the two poles, $s = -d_1$ and $s = -d_2$, and along a vertical line in the s plane midway between them. The negative values in Table 5.1 for P_3 in comparison to the positive values for P_1 imply that the zeros do not lie between the real roots at $s = -\beta$ and $s = -d_1$ or between $s = -\gamma$ and $s = -d_2$. The relatively small values for P_2 (on the average $P_1/P_2 = 3.6$) in comparison to both P_1 and P_3 (on the average $P_1/P_3 = -1.3$) in Table 5.1 imply that $s = -z_1$ and $s = -z_2$ lie closer to the complex roots at $s = -\alpha \pm j\omega$ than to the two real roots. The negative values for phase φ in Table 5.1 imply that z_1 and z_2 are complex, and that the positive imaginary part is less than ω. These conditions require that K' for glomerular cells lie between 1.5 and 1.8.

The axonal transfer function, Eq. (72), is evaluated by setting $K' = 1.8$ and taking the value of T_b for each case from Eq. (48)

$$A_m(s) = 1 + 1.8\exp[-(sT_b)^{1/2}]. \tag{52}$$

The overall transfer function $P_{P2}(s)$ is given by the product of $P(s)$ and $A_m(s)$. From Eqs. (44) and (49)–(52),

$$P_{P2}(s) = \frac{P_b 1.6 \times 10^{10}(s+g)(s+h)(2300-s)^2}{(s+\alpha+j\omega)(s+\alpha-j\omega)(s+\beta)(s+\gamma)(s+\delta)(s+\varepsilon)(s+d_1)(s+d_2)}. \tag{53}$$

The inverse transform of Eq. (53) is obtained by partial fraction expansion. The forward gain $K_b = P_b/K_e$ in Table 5.2 includes the effect of changing $I(s)$ and the effect of attenuation on input amplitude:

$$p_{P2}(T) = K_b[P_1 e^{-\beta T} + P_2 e^{-\gamma T} + P_3 e^{-\delta T} + P_4 e^{-\varepsilon T} + P_5 e^{-d_1 T} + P_6 e^{-d_2 T}$$
$$+ P_7 \sin(\omega t + \varphi)e^{-\alpha T}]. \tag{54}$$

There are three degrees of freedom in Eq. (54). The coefficients P_1–P_7 and φ are fixed by a, b, c, and K', and by the two variables K_e and T_b, derived from Eq. (48). Then K_b is evaluated by fitting curves from Eq. (54) to the PSTHs. Examples are shown as the solid curves in Figs. 5.10 and 5.14 which have the slower rise time.

The transfer function for the forward subset directly receiving PON input from Eqs. (37) and (38) is

$$P_{P1}(s) = (P_a/P_b) P_{P2}(s) A^{-1}(s). \tag{55}$$

In expanded form and using Eq. (49) for $A(s)$,

$$P_{P1}(s) = [P_a 1.6 \times 10^{10}(s+g)(s+h)(s+230)(s+550)(s+2300)(2300-s)^2]$$
$$\div [(s+\alpha+j\omega)(s+\alpha-j\omega)(s+\beta)(s+\gamma)(s+2200)(s+2400)$$
$$\times (s+d_1)(s+d_2)]. \tag{56}$$

The inverse transform is identical to that given by Eq. (54), but the values for P_1–P_7 and φ are different, and the forward gain coefficient $K_a = P_a/K_e^5$, is determined independently (Table 5.2).

The wave forms for $p_{P1}(t)$ are shown in Fig. 5.10 for six PSTHs as solid curves. They have the faster rise time and sharper crest. An additional example is shown in Fig. 5.14. At low stimulus intensity some glomerular units have short-latency increases in pulse probability (Fig. 5.10) and others have longer latency (Fig. 5.14). Either is compatible with the model, the short-latency units being members of the feed-forward subset and the longer-latency units being members of the feedback subset. At higher stimulus intensities almost all become members of the feed-forward subset, owing to the increased probability that any given neuron will receive PON input at high intensity.

The conformance of the solid curves from Eq. (54) to the data is taken as evidence that the positions of the closed loop zeros at $s = -z_1$ and $s = -z_2$ are substantially correct. Therefore the values for the open loop poles at $s = -d_1$, $s = -d_2$ and the value for dispersion gain K' are considered to be valid. The conformance of PST histograms to the inverse transforms of either Eqs. (53) or (56) is evidence that the open loop transfer function for $A(s)$ in Eq. (44) is correctly evaluated. This completes the model for PON afferent dispersion cascaded in series with KI_p excitatory interaction.

5.2.3. SELF-STABILIZATION OF THE KI_e SET

The neurons in the periglomerular layer generate background activity having the general properties described in Section 3.3.2. The particular characteristics are described elsewhere (Shepherd, 1972; Section 4.3.1) and need not be considered here. The background activity persists relatively unchanged after cutting the PON (thus completely deafferenting the bulb) and after cutting the bulbar stalk to remove all centrifugal input and most of the anterior olfactory nucleus (Section 5.4.1). The results of Section 5.2.2 lay the groundwork for explaining how the background activity is maintained.

By intuitive reasoning (Section 5.1.4) a feedback loop in which both channels have bilateral saturation of the kind described in Sections 3.3.4 and 3.3.5 must be stable for all input. For sufficient gain in the absence of saturation i.e., $K_e = K_0$ in an excitatory feedback loop, there must be steady state output for zero input at a steady state value $K_e = 1$. If there is nonzero steady state input, then $K_e \neq 1$.

In Fig. 5.1b the following conditions hold for a linear approximation in the steady state:

$$df_1(t)/dt = df_2(t)/dt = df_3(t)/dt = df_4(t)/dt = 0. \tag{57}$$

For the steady state let

$$\bar{F}_j = f_j(t), \qquad j = 1, \ldots, 4, \quad \bar{F}_2 \neq 0. \tag{58}$$

The excitatory feedback gain in the steady state (see Section 1.3.5) is

$$K_o = \bar{F}_4/\bar{F}_2. \tag{59}$$

From Eq. (57),

$$\bar{F}_2 = \bar{F}_1 + \bar{F}_4, \qquad K_o = 1 - \bar{F}_1/\bar{F}_2. \tag{60}$$

If $\bar{F}_1 > 0$ (steady state input is excitatory, as is expected for the background PON input), then $K_o < 1$. If $\bar{F}_1 < 0$ (steady state input is inhibitory), then $K_0 > 1$. Then $K_0 = 1$ only if the steady state input to periglomerular neurons is mixed excitatory and inhibitory with zero average, or if it is negligibly small in comparison to steady state input from other neurons in the KI_P set, $\bar{F}_1 \ll \bar{F}_2$.

One method for determining the steady state value for K_o is to extrapolate the values for β over the range of stimulus intensity of $\beta = 0$, where by Eq. (51), at threshold $K_e = K_o = 1$, and to determine whether the value of stimulus intensity at the intercept corresponds to the threshold stimulus intensity for the periglomerular response.

An example is shown in Fig. 5.16a for a set of values for β in Table 5.2.

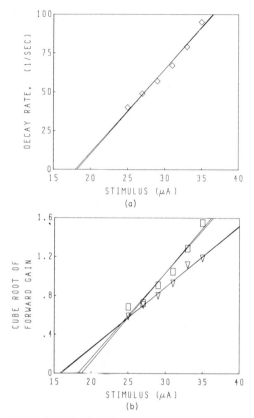

FIG. 5.16. (a) Extrapolation of values for β with decreasing stimulus intensity to zero. (b) Extrapolation of values for amplitudes in Table 5.2 of PSTHs to zero, following cube root transformation for $K_a(\triangledown)$ and $K_b(\square)$. By inference the decay rate is zero for zero input (Freeman, 1974f).

The intercept implies that if threshold input is $18\,\mu A$, then $K_o = 1$. However, the threshold cannot be determined directly, because the detection of near-threshold responses takes such prolonged averaging that time invariance probably no longer holds, and because the extrapolation required is probably not linear. Moreover, extrapolation cannot be based on measurements of crest amplitude of PST histograms, because the rates of rise and decay of periglomerular impulse responses change with input intensity.

PST histograms from the KI_P set are measured with Eqs. (48) and (54). The real-valued constants, P_a and P_b, are determined from response amplitude, which depends on stimulus intensity, glomerular transmission attenuation, and the forward gain through each channel of the feedback loop. The loop gain is K_e, and the forward gain is approximated by

$K_e^{.5}$. The attenuation has negligible effect on input amplitude (Fig. 5.12b) for impulse input and affects predominantly the apparent input dispersion. Therefore, the ratios, $K_a = P_a/K_e^{.5}$ and $K_b = P_b/K_e$, are determined by the stimulus intensity $I\delta(T)$, where I is in microamperes for an input current pulse of fixed duration.

The problem is to determine the relation between I and K_a or K_b, in order to find the value of I at which K_a and K_b extrapolate to zero. A tentative solution is based on the observation of the dependence of peak amplitude of the PON compound action potential (Sections 2.3.3 and 4.3.3) on stimulus intensity. Over the range used for stimulation of the KI_P set the amplitude increases as the cube of stimulus current (Fig. 5.17). The shape and latency of the compound action potential do not vary significantly with increasing stimulus intensity, provided the recording site is quite near the stimulus site and on the main axis of conduction (Section 4.5.2), which implies that the amplitude is proportional to the number of excited axons. It is assumed that the input of the PON to the KI_P set is proportional to that number, so

$$K_a = k_1(I-I_0)^3, \qquad K_b = k_2(I-I_0)^3, \quad I \geqq I_0,$$

where k_1 and k_2 are proportionality constants. The cube roots of K_a and K_b are plotted against stimulus current in Fig. 5.16b, together with pairs of regression lines computed from the correlation coefficients. The extrapolation to $K_a = K_b = 0$ gives intercepts on the ordinate that specify a range in which I is at threshold. The values of stimulus intensity between the intercepts include the extrapolated value of I_0 for $\beta = 0$.

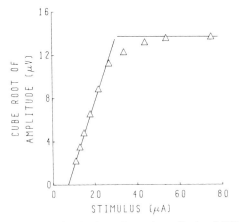

FIG. 5.17. Relation between stimulus intensity and amplitude of PON compound action potential, following cube root transformation. (Freeman, 1974f).

This conclusion derives from data taken in anesthetized animals with the PON intact. It has not been tested by repeating the measurements following transection of the PON, and it has not been examined in data from waking animals. However, the uncertainty concerns the precise value taken by K_o in the steady state, and whether background PON input affects that value. The data support the inference from Section 5.1.4 that the KI_P set is stabilized by saturation, at a nonzero steady state level of output. There is no requirement for inhibitory input to impose stability. When the set is perturbed by brief changes of input, the set returns to the same steady state, and the rate of return to the steady state increases with amplitude of perturbation.

An alternative method to Eq. (60) for evaluating K_o is derived from Eqs. (85) to (87) in Chapter 3 for nonlinear gain. In the absence of inhibitory input, $v \geq 0$, and

$$g(v) = g_o e^{-\gamma v}, \qquad v > 0, \tag{61}$$

$$g(p) = g_o [1 - v/(r\tilde{v}_i)], \qquad v > 0, \tag{62}$$

$$g_o = -2\gamma p_o \zeta \tilde{v}_i. \tag{63}$$

For a fixed level of activity, $g(v)$ and $g(p)$ are to be replaced by constants, g_v and g_p. The forward gain of each KO_P subset is $g_v g_p$, and in the steady state the forward gains of the two subsets are equal. Let

$$\tilde{K}_e \triangleq g_v^2 g_p^2. \tag{64}$$

Over the observed range of output it is assumed that $v/r\tilde{v}_i \ll 1$ in Eqs. (62). From Eqs. (61), (62), and (64),

$$\tilde{K}_e = g_o^2 e^{-2\gamma v}. \tag{65}$$

Under the same assumption and from Eq. (74) in Chapter 3,

$$dv/dp_d = -\zeta \tilde{v}_i. \tag{66}$$

On integration from p_o at $v = 0$ to p_d at v,

$$v = -\zeta \tilde{v}_i (p_d - p_o). \tag{67}$$

From Eqs. (63), 65, and (67),

$$\tilde{K}_e = g_o^2 \exp[-g_o(p_d - p_o)/p_o], \qquad v \geq 0. \tag{68}$$

That is, the negative logarithm of gain during an impulse response is given by the product of normalized induced pulse density input to the pulse to wave conversion mechanism, $(p_d - p_o)/p_o$, which is identical to the output of the preceding wave to pulse conversion mechanism $(p_d - p_o)/p_o$ times the gain at the preceding and following steady state levels of activity g_o plus a constant given by $-\ln(g_o^2)$.

As defined, $\tilde{K}_e$ is the instantaneous gain which according to assumption (3) in Section 1.1.3 cannot exist. The value for K_e is fixed at a level representing an appropriate average value over the duration impulse ΔT of the impulse response (Section 5.1.2). To obtain an average value for $\tilde{K}_e$ comparable to K_e, the value for p_d in Eq. (68) is set to the average pulse rate over the PSTH, $\bar{p}$. From the results in Fig. 5.16, $g_o = 1$. The time average of $\tilde{K}_e$ is designated K_e^*

$$K_e^* = \exp[-(\bar{p} - p_o)/p_o]. \qquad (69)$$

Sets of values for p_o, $\bar{p}$, and K_e^* are given in Table 5.3, and K_e^* is compared graphically with K_e in Fig. 5.18. The straight line at $45°$ is the expected relation. The scatter of points is too great to determine whether the premise that $K_o = 1$ is valid. However, the correlation of K_e and K_e^* is more interesting from another point of view. Equation (51), which determines K_e from the decay rate of PSTHs, has been derived from feedback analysis of periglomerular neurons.[†] Equation (69) which determines K_e^* from the mean normalized induced firing rate, has been derived from analysis of the background activity of KII sets in the bulb and cortex. The results in Fig. 5.18 suggest that the same amplitude-dependent characteristics may

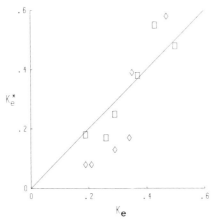

FIG. 5.18. Comparison of results of two independent methods for estimating the KI_P set feedback gain as a function of increasing input amplitude (Freeman, 1974f). □: Table 5.1 and Fig. 5.10; ◇: Table 5.2 and Fig. 5.14.

[†] The value for β can be obtained by using the sum of two basis functions to fit the PSTHs of periglomerular neurons

$$p(t) = p_o(e^{-\beta t} - e^{-bt}),$$

where b lumps into one term all of determinants of the rise time.

TABLE 5.3

ESTIMATION OF GAIN K_e^* FROM PULSE DENSITIES

Figure	P_o background (pulses/sec)	P_c crest (pulses/sec)	$\bar{P}$ mean (pulses/sec)	K_e^* average feedback gain
5.14a	9.4	11.9	14.5	.58
5.14b	9.6	26.1	18.5	.39
5.14c	11.4	42.6	31.5	.17
5.14d	13.9	85.1	41.8	.13
5.14e	12.1	119.6	42.6	.08
5.14f	12.9	173.9	45.4	.08
5.10a	13.2	35.2	22.9	.48
5.10b	14.4	39.6	23.2	.54
5.10c	12.7	59.9	25.0	.38
5.10d	12.4	71.5	29.5	.25
5.10e	13.4	92.6	37.3	.17
5.10f	15.3	108.6	41.7	.18

be common to the several KI sets in the bulb and cortex. This is a working hypothesis of considerable power that is used in Chapter 6.

Background activity is present in the KII sets of the bulb and cortex, which appears to be largely dependent, directly or indirectly, on the background or steady state output of the KI_P set. This feature is implicit in Sections 5.3 and 5.4 and explicit in Chapter 6. For the present, one of the principal functions assignable to the KI_P set is automatic gain control. Glomerular transmission attenuation is inferred to be similar to presynaptic inhibition, described in the brain stem and spinal cord by Eccles (1964) and Wall (1964) among others. It is not called "inhibition" here, because that term is restricted to an additive event mediated by a specific type of synapse, whereas glomerular transmission attenuation is a multiplicative event not mediated by axoaxonic synapses (see also Voronkov & Gusel'nikova, 1969).

The magnitude of attenuation is determined by a running time average of the active state of the KI_P set, which in turn is determined by a running time average of the input. By intuitive reasoning an important role of glomerular transmission attenuation is the control of PON input from the KO_R set to the KII_{MG} set. If the mean level of PON input is low, the forward gain through the glomeruli is relatively high, and conversely if the mean input is high, the forward gain is low. Considering the immense number of receptors sending axons to the bulb, an automatic control of the input amplitude is quite logical as the means for restricting the variation of the amplitude of input to the KII_{MG} set to a range that is optimal for its performance. In this respect it is similar to automatic gain control in the retina (Rushton, 1965) and probably in the spinal cord.

5.3. Reduction from the KII Level

5.3.1. TOPOLOGICAL ANALYSIS OF THE OLFACTORY BULB

It is inferred from anatomical and electrophysiological observations schematized in Fig. 4.25 that the olfactory receptors form a KO_R set which sends axons in the PON to the glomerular layer in the bulb (Fig. 4.23). The periglomerular KI_P set in the same layer receives input from the PON (Fig. 5.19a). The mitral–tufted KI_M and the granule KI_G set form the KII_{MG} set (see Figs. 1.1–1.3). There is PON input to the KI_M set but not to the KI_G set. There is an observable output for each of the three KI sets, consisting of pulse trains from neurons in the KI_P set and KI_M set and the surface EEG or AEP recording at the epicenter of a coherent domain in the KI_G set. The physiological output of the bulb to the cortex on mitral–tufted axons of neurons in the KI_M set in the LOT is not considered explicitly.

There is an artificial input to the bulb that is provided by electrical stimulation of the LOT, which sends an axon volley into the bulb anti-dromically, where it invades the neurons in the KI_M set and excites the neurons in the KI_G set synaptically. Additionally, there are several physiological channels into the bulb that are provided by centrifugal paths (tracts originating in the forebrain rather than the periphery, which end in the bulb). One of these originates in the anterior olfactory nucleus (N) crosses the midline in the anterior commissure and enters the contralateral bulb to end on the granule cells. In addition the same neurons in the nucleus (N) give axon collaterals into the ipsilateral bulb, which form synapses on the basal dendrites of the granule cells. Other centrifugal inputs not in the LOT to all three KI sets are not germane to the present analysis and are not shown. However, there is at least one feedback loop from KI_M axon collaterals through the anterior nucleus (N) back to the KI_G set shown by the arrow from M to N in Fig. 5.19a. There are probably others. The method for dealing with these loops is given in Section 5.3.3, so that they need not be considered explicitly. For a general discussion of this kind of problem, see Section 1.3.7.

In Fig. 5.19b the topological diagram is transformed on the premise that each KI set can be represented by a feedback loop between two KO subsets (Section 1.3.4). The diagonal pair of channels between M1 and G1 is used to represent the greater divergence of mitral–tufted neurons over the divergence of granule neurons, owing to the greater length of their dendrites in directions parallel to the surface (Section 4.3.1). The signs of action,

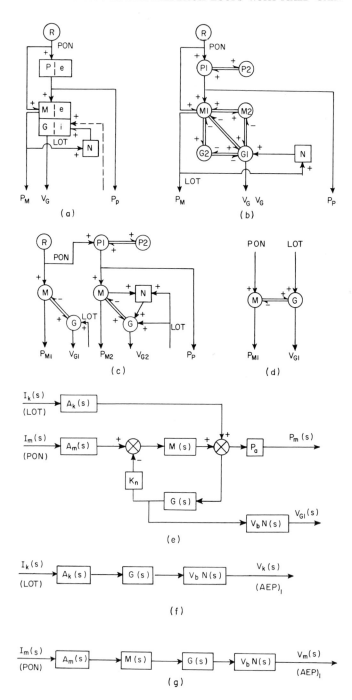

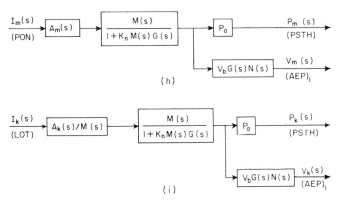

Fɪɢ. 5.19. Topological reduction of the olfactory bulb to a lumped, piecewise linear approximation.

+ for excitation and − for inhibition, are inferences based on preliminary electrophysiological analysis of responses to electrical stimulation of the PON and LOT (Section 4.5.2). The centrifugal inputs are reduced to a single channel to G1, on the premise that antidromic input on electrical stimulation to the mitral–tufted cells is delivered as an impulse by those cells to the granule cells, and the conduction delay for both inputs can be set to zero for computational purposes by taking zero time as the start of the surface AEP, following the mitral–tufted compound action potential.

Two simplifications are made for part (c) of the figure. The representation of the KII set in part (b) reflects the fact that subset M1 receives excitatory feedback from subset M2 and inhibitory feedback from subsets G1 and G2. By control of input amplitude, which varies the feedback gain in all three channels, it is possible (as described in detail in Chapter 6) to find an input amplitude at which the feedback from M2 is nulled by the feedback from G2. At this level the positive feedback loops can be deleted. Further, the input from R to M1 is both direct and through the periglomerular KI_P set. As described in Section 5.2.1, the impulse response of the whole system consists of a low-frequency transient and a high-frequency transient. As a simplifying approximation, the system is separated into two parallel channels, one consisting of the M1–G1 negative feedback loop and the other of the P1–P2 positive feedback loop in series with the M1–G1 loop. The high-frequency transient is assigned as the output of the first channel. The second channel is not considered at present. (See also Section 2.5.3 for the design of the adaptive filters used for the separation of components in the AEP.)

In part (d) consideration is restricted to input by electrical stimulation of the PON and LOT and to output in the form of impulse responses. The background input from the receptors R and from the nucleus N is assumed to be constant over any time ΔT of observation. This assumption is verified by including a prestimulus baseline segment in each AEP and PSTH and restricting consideration to those impulse responses with steady states over the prestimulus time range. The topology is reduced to a single negative feedback loop having two input channels and two output channels.

The transformation to part (e) is based on two premises. The spatial distributions of the active states are sufficiently uniform that the dynamics can be represented by a lumped circuit. For input amplitudes fixed at levels such that the positive feedback loops in the KII set are nulled, the amplitude-dependent gains are represented as fixed coefficients. The system is linearized by piecewise linear approximation (Section 5.1.2). A transfer function is assigned to each channel: mitral–tufted KI_M set $M(s)$, granule set $G(s)$, PON channel $A_m(s)$, LOT channel $A_k(s)$, KI_M pulse output channel P_a (there is no observed KI_M wave output channel—see Section 4.3.2), and granule wave output channel $V_b N(s)$ (there is no observed KI_G pulse output channel—see Section 4.3.2). The feedback gain is K_n, a positive real number (Section 5.1.2). The LOT input is an impulse $I_k(s) = I_k$, and the PON input is an impulse $I_m(s) = I_m$. The KI_M output in the pulse mode is $P(s)$, and the KI_G output in the wave mode is $V(s)$.

In part (f) the value of K_n is set equal to zero. In experimental conditions this represents the effect of giving a large dose of anesthetic that suppresses background pulse and EEG activity and reduces the AEP to a single surface-negative peak followed by a shallow surface-positive overshoot (Fig. 5.20), which closely resembles a PSP (Fig. 3.18d). This response form can be approached as a limiting case by incremental doses of anesthetic. With additional small doses it is unchanged, but with a large dose it disappears, and the animal dies. Induced pulse activity is reduced to a single compound action potential or to a short burst of pulses, both of which can be treated as impulse responses. In this condition the model has two input channels, a convergence point, and one output channel. The impulse response for LOT input is predicted by

$$V_k(s) = V_{bk} A_k(s) G_k(s) N_k(s). \tag{70}$$

The KI_G impulse response for PON input is predicted by

$$V_m(s) = V_{bm} A_m(s) M(s) G_m(s) N_m(s). \tag{71}$$

From the topology of the loop it is inferred that

$$G_k(s) = G_m(s) = G(s), \qquad N_k(s) = N_m(s) = N(s). \tag{72}$$

The input amplitudes, I_m and I_k, have been incorporated into the arbitrary forward gain constants, $V_{bk} = I_k V_b$ and $V_{bm} = I_m V_b$.

In part (g), the loop is represented as a forward element for $K_n \neq 0$.

$$C(s) = M(s)/[1 + K_n M(s) G(s)]. \tag{73}$$

For convenience the junction point for the LOT is moved before the loop, so that the transfer function is $A_k(s)/M(s)$, and the wave output branch point is moved outside the loop, so that the transfer function is $V_b G(s) N(s)$. The KI$_G$ impulse responses on LOT input are predicted by

$$P_k(s) = P_{uk} A_k(s) C(s)/M(s),$$
$$V_m(s) = V_{bm} A_m(s) C(s) G(s) N(s), \tag{74}$$

where $P_k(s)$ predicts the PSTH and $V_m(s)$ predicts the AEP. This completes the topological analysis for the designated experimental conditions.

5.3.2. DIFFERENTIAL EQUATIONS FOR THE OPEN LOOP CASES

As a guide in the construction of dynamic equations a set of open loop AEPs on LOT stimulation is measured (Section 2.5.2) with the sum of n exponential basis functions, where the optimal number $n = 5$ is determined experimentally as in Fig. 5.20a.

$$v_k(T) = \sum_{j=1}^{5} V_j e^{-a_j T}, \qquad \sum_{j=1}^{5} V_j = 0,$$
$$\hat{v}_k(T) = v_k(T) + \varepsilon(T), \tag{75}$$

giving 9 degrees of freedom in the curve-fitting process. The rate coefficients a_j are assigned positive real values increasing with j. The mean values of the parameters following nonlinear regression are

$$v_k(T) = -17 e^{-15T} + 46 e^{-104T} + 329 e^{-201T} - 531 e^{-573T} + 173 e^{-1014T}. \tag{76}$$

The Laplace transform of Eq. (75) is

$$V_k(s) = V_{bk} \prod_{j=1}^{3} (s + z_j) \bigg/ \prod_{j=1}^{5} (s + a_j) \tag{77}$$

where z_j and a_j are all positive real numbers. The existence of one zero $z_1 < a_1$ is inferred from the fact that V_1 is negative (Section 2.5.2). The mean value is near 0/sec. The second zero $a_2 < z_2 < a_3$ is deduced from the fact that V_2 and V_3 are both positive. The decay of the AEP from its crest is not exponential and must be fitted with the sum of two positive decaying exponential curves. The third zero $z_3 > a_5$ is deduced from the fact that $V_5 < |V_4|$ (see also Section 2.5.2).

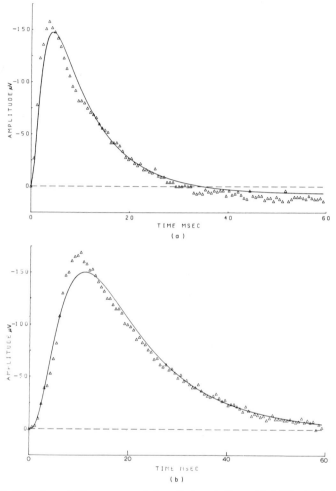

FIG. 5.20. Open loop AEP responses of the olfactory bulb to (a) LOT stimulation and to (b) PON stimulation (see also Figs. 2.19, 2.22, and 2.23) (Freeman, 1972b).

The open loop responses on PON stimulation cannot be fitted with the sum of any reasonable number of exponential curves, so a theoretical approach is used (see below). The transfer function for the KI_G set is approximated by third-order differential equation (Sections 2.5.2 and 5.1.1):

$$G(s) = bcd/(s+b)(s+c)(s+d), \tag{78}$$

where b represents the role of the mean passive membrane rate constant for the set, c represents lumped cable delay, and d represents lumped synaptic delay.

The transfer function for the output channel is

$$N(s) = as/(s+a). \tag{79}$$

The rate constant a is too large to represent the effect of the low-pass filter in the recording amplifier and too small to represent the passive membrane rate constant. Its range of values is consistent with the inference that the term $V_1 e^{-a_1 T}$ represents a dendritic afterpotential. This is substantiated by the finding that the experimental mean for a_1 is near zero. According to the ionic hypothesis (Section 3.2.3) the total charge exchanged over the entire response must be zero, so that $z_1 = 0$.

The impulse response of the LOT input channel is conceived as consisting of a unit impulse followed by dispersed volley resembling a one-dimensional diffusion process (Sections 2.3.3 and 5.2.2). The transfer function is

$$A_k(s) = 1 + K' \exp[-(sT_b)^{1/2}], \tag{80}$$

where K' is a positive real number. The irrational term is replaced by a rational approximation (Section 2.3.5) as in Section 5.2.2:

$$A_k(s) = (s+g)(s+h)/(s+e)(s+f), \tag{81}$$

where $e = (\pi/2)^2/T_b$, $f = (3\pi)^2/T_b$, and g and h are given by Eq. (45).

On substitution of Eqs. (78), (79), and (81) into Eq. (70),

$$V_k(s) = \frac{V_{bk}\,bcds(s+g)(s+h)}{(s+a)(s+b)(s+c)(s+d)(s+e)(s+f)}, \tag{82}$$

where $e - h$ depend on T_b and K' and V_{bk} is a real-valued constant. The form is compatible with Eq. (77).

The inverse Laplace transform of Eq. (82) gives

$$v_k(t) = \sum_{j=1}^{6} V_j e^{-a_j t}, \tag{83}$$

where the V_j are determined by partial fraction expansion (Section 2.2.3), and the a_j are determined by the poles in Eq. (82). This curve having 7 degrees of freedom is fitted to bulbar open loop AEPs (Fig. 5.20a) giving the typical values

$$\begin{aligned} v_k(t) = &-9.6\,e^{-6t} + 215\,e^{-123t} + 198\,e^{-192t} \\ &-585\,e^{-904t} - 109\,e^{-1110t} + 384\,e^{-1562t}. \end{aligned} \tag{84}$$

The evaluated transfer function is

$$V_k(s) = \frac{1.2 \times 2.7 \times 10^8 (1 + 0.25 \exp[-.019s]^{1/2})\,s}{(s+6)(s+192)(s+904)(s+1562)}. \tag{85}$$

The open loop responses on PON stimulation cannot be fitted with the sum of exponential curves, because two of the rate constants, a_2 and a_3, tend to converge to a common value on successive iterations of nonlinear regression (Section 2.5.1). It is assumed that the passive decay rates of the mitral–tufted and granule KI sets are equal, so that a double pole occurs in the transfer function for $V_m(s)$.

The functions for $A_m(s)$ and $M(s)$ are described by a single function

$$A_m(s) M(s) = \{1 + K' \exp[-(sT_b)^{1/2}]\}/(s+b). \tag{86}$$

in which the passive rate constant is explicit and the cable and synaptic delays in $M(s)$ are incorporated into the delay term for $A_m(s)$ from Eq. (81). Equations (78), (79), and (86) are substituted into Eq. (71), yielding

$$V_m(s) = \left[\frac{V_{bm}\, bcds(s+g)(s+h)}{(s+a)(s+b)^2(s+c)(s+d)(s+e)(s+f)}\right]. \tag{87}$$

The residue for the double pole is found by differentiating with respect to s:

$$R(s) = \frac{d}{ds}\left[\frac{(s+b)^2\, s(s+g)(s+h)}{(s+a)(s+b)^2(s+c)(s+d)(s+e)(s+f)}\right]$$

$$= \frac{D_1(s)}{D_2(s)} \quad \text{for} \quad s \to -b, \tag{88}$$

where $D_1(-b)$ and $D_2(-b)$ represent the polynomials in the numerator and denominator, respectively.

$$\begin{aligned}
D_1(-b) = &\, 2b^7 - [a+c+d+e+f+3(g+h)]b^6 \\
&+ 2[(g+h)(a+c+d+e+f)+2gh]b^5 \\
&+ [acd+ace+acf+ade+adf+aef+cde+cdf+cef+def \\
&- (g+h)(ac+ad+ae+af+cd+ce+cf+de+df+ef) \\
&- 3gh(a+c+d+e+f)]b^4 \\
&- 2[acde+acdf+acef+adef+cdef-gh(ac+ad+ae \\
&+ af+cd+ce+cf+de+df+ef)]b^3 \\
&+ 3[acdef+(g+h)(acde+acdf+acef+adef+cdef-hg \\
&\times (acd+ace+acf+ade+adf+aef+cde+cdf+cef+def)]b^2 \\
&- 2[(g+h)(acdef)]b + acdefgh, \tag{89}
\end{aligned}$$

$$D_2(-b) = [(a-b)(c-b)(d-b)(e-b)(f-b)]^2, \tag{90}$$

$$V_1 = \frac{(g-b)(h-b)(-b)}{(a-b)(c-b)(d-b)(e-b)(f-b)}, \tag{91}$$

$$V_2 = D_1(-b)/D_2(-b), \tag{92}$$

$$V_3 = \frac{(g-a)(h-a)(-a)}{(b-a)^2(c-a)(d-a)(e-a)(f-a)}, \tag{93}$$

$$V_4 = \frac{(g-c)(h-c)(-c)}{(b-c)^2(a-c)(d-c)(e-c)(f-c)}, \tag{94}$$

$$V_5 = \frac{(g-d)(h-d)(-d)}{(b-d)^2(a-d)(c-d)(e-d)(f-d)}, \tag{95}$$

$$V_6 = \frac{(g-e)(h-e)(-e)}{(b-e)^2(a-e)(c-e)(d-e)(f-e)}, \tag{96}$$

$$V_7 = \frac{(g-f)(h-f)(-f)}{(b-f)^2(d-f)(c-f)(d-f)(e-f)}, \tag{97}$$

$$v_m(t) = (V_1\,t\,e^{-bt} + V_2\,e^{-bt} + V_3\,e^{-at} + V_4\,e^{-ct} + V_5\,e^{-dt} + V_6\,e^{-et} + V_7\,e^{-ft})$$
$$\times\, V_{bm}\,b^2\,cd. \tag{98}$$

Equation (98) is fitted to bulbar open loop AEPs on PON stimulation. A typical example shown in Fig. 5.20b, yielding

$$v_m(T) = -13\,e^{-4T} + 164\,e^{-65T} + 103 \times 10^3\,T\,e^{-210T} - 468\,e^{-210T}$$
$$- 174\,e^{-571T} + 639\,e^{-747T} - 149\,e^{-1262T}. \tag{99}$$

The evaluated transfer function is

$$V_m(s) = \frac{0.5 \times 1.67 \times 10^{11}(1 + 0.46\exp[-(.039s)^{1/2}])s}{(s+4)(s+210)^2(s+747)(s+1262)}. \tag{100}$$

Measurements of open loop AEPs on PON and LOT stimulation give two sets of values for the rate constants in $G(s)$ and $N(s)$. The mean values and standard errors in units of reciprocal seconds for the comparable rate constants in $G(s)$ and $N(s)$ from the two sets of data are

$$\begin{aligned}
a_k &= 5.1 \pm .6, & a_m &= 4.0 \pm .3, \\
b_k &= 211 \pm 8, & b_m &= 226 \pm 11, \\
c_k &= 818 \pm 38, & c_m &= 775 \pm 11, \\
d_k &= 1430 \pm 58, & d_m &= 1212 \pm 51.
\end{aligned} \tag{101}$$

The means do not differ significantly for the two sets, so they are treated as two estimates of a common set of constants best evaluated from the overall means. The constraints set by Eq. (72) are considered fulfilled. In evaluated form,

$$A_k(s) = \frac{(s+171)(s+1116)(s-z_k)^2}{(s+128)(s+1156)}, \tag{102}$$

$$A_m(s)M_m(s) = \frac{219(s+112)(s+568)(s-z_m)^2}{(s+68)(s+219)(s+612)}, \tag{103}$$

$$G(s) = \frac{219 \times 796 \times 1321}{(s+219)(s+796)(s+1321)}, \tag{104}$$

$$N(s) = \frac{s}{(s+4.5)}. \tag{105}$$

The zeros at $s = z_k$ and $s = z_m$ are reintroduced from Eq. (164) in Chapter 2 as a reminder that although they are replaced by fixed constants in the open loop state, in which no complex conjugate poles appear, in the closed loop state they are introduced and evaluated explicitly. Alternatively, the zeros can be interpreted as representing the poles of the receiving subset $F_{1p}(s)$ which appear as zeros in the input channel $F_{fp}(s)$ of the lumped approximation for the closed loop transfer function of the KI set [Eq. (10) in part (c) of Section 5.1.2]. Further, the equivalence of Eqs. (103) and (104) to Eq. (179) and Eq. (197) in Chapter 2 should be noted.

5.3.3. DIFFERENTIAL EQUATIONS FOR THE CLOSED LOOP CASES

The closed loop topology is given in Fig. 5.19g. The transfer functions for the channels are evaluated in Eqs. (102)–(105). For a complete solution the transfer function $A_k(s)M(s)$ must be separated. The values for the zeros, z_m and z_k, and for K_n must be fixed. These are determined by measurements of the closed loop impulse responses on PON and LOT stimulation (Fig. 5.21).

Each AEP contains a relatively high amplitude damped sine wave which is identified as the impulse response of the negative feedback loop because there is an oscillation in the PSTH at the same frequency. This is called the *dominant transient*. There is a smaller transient at lower or higher frequencies that is considered to result from activity in some other feedback loop (see dashed line in Fig. 5.19a, for example). The subsidiary component must be measured to measure the AEP (Section 2.5.3), but its parameters are of no interest at present.

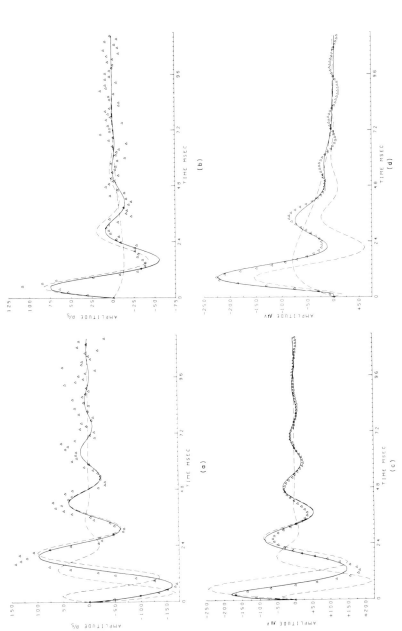

FIG. 5.21. (c, d) Closed loop AEP responses and (a, b) PSTH responses to (a, c) LOT and (b, d) PON electrical stimulation (Freeman, 1972c).

The AEPs in response to LOT stimulation (Fig. 5.21c) are fitted with the sum of two damped sine waves (see Fig. 5.7)

$$v(T) = \sum_{j=1}^{2} V_{kj}[\sin(\omega_j T + \varphi_j)e^{-\alpha_j T} - \sin(\varphi_j)\cos(\omega_j T)e^{-\beta T}], \quad (106)$$

in which V_{kj} represents initial amplitude in microvolts, ω_j the frequency in radians per second, φ_j the phase of onset in radians, α_j the decay rate in reciprocal seconds, and β represents the rate of rise of the first peak of the AEP.

This response pattern is that of a system containing two band-pass filters, $C_1(s)$ and $C_2(s)$ in parallel, each cascaded into poorly resonant band-pass filter, $B_1(s)$ and $B_2(s)$. Thus

$$V_k(s) = B_1(s)C_1(s) + B_2(s)C_2(s), \quad (107)$$

where

$$C_n(s) = \frac{V_{cn}}{(s + \alpha_n + j\omega_n)(s + \alpha_n - j\omega_n)}, \quad n = 1, 2, \quad (108)$$

and

$$B_n(s) = \frac{V_{bn}(s + z_n)}{(s + \beta + j\omega_n)(s + \beta - j\omega_n)}, \quad n = 1, 2. \quad (109)$$

The expression for $V_k(s)$, when reduced to a common denominator, contains two complex conjugate pairs of zeros. The existence and location of the pair nearest the $j\omega$ axis is shown by spectral analysis of the AEP (Section 2.5.3) and is strong evidence for the parallel arrangement specified by Eq. (107). Either parallel path can be treated independently of the other, so that calculation of the precise locations of the zeros is not needed here.

The transfer function for the dominant component of the KI_G set for LOT input is

$$V_{k1}(s) = \frac{V_b(s + z_1)}{(s + \alpha_1 + j\omega_1)(s + \alpha_1 - j\omega_1)(s + \beta + j\omega_1)(s + \beta - j\omega_1)}, \quad (110)$$

where z_1 is a real zero, for which the location on the real axis is determinable from the value for φ_1. The zero is a fictitious element that lumps in one value the effects of all higher-order poles and zeros not otherwise specified on the phase of the transient.

Equation (106) suffices also to measure bulbar PST histograms (Fig. 5.21a and b). To improve the accuracy of measurement of phase φ_1, the frequency ω_1 is fixed at the value for ω_1 in the concomitantly recorded AEP. The AEPs in response to PON stimulation (Fig. 5.21d) consist of a damped sine wave superimposed on a slowly changing surface-negative transient, which terminates in a prolonged shallow overshoot. The equation used to generate the curve fitted to these AEPs (see Section 4.3.3) is

$$v_1(T) = V_{m1}[\sin(\omega T + \varphi)e^{-\alpha T} - \sin \varphi \cos(\omega T)e^{-\beta T}],$$

$$v_2(T) = A_1 e^{-aT} + A_2 e^{-bT} + A_3 e^{-cT}, \tag{111}$$

$$v_m(T) = v_1(T) + v_2(T),$$

in which the rate constant c describes the rising phase of the baseline shift, b the decay rate, and a the rate of recovery from the overshoot.

Equation (111) has 11 degrees of freedom. The Laplace transform of $v_2(T)$ is taken:

$$V_2(s) = V_2 s/(s+a)(s+b)(s+c). \tag{112}$$

The zero at $s = 0$ in the numerator is inferred to exist (Section 2.5.2) from the fact that the sign of the amplitude coefficient a_1 of the term having the lowest rate constant a is always negative (downward being positive in potential but negative for analytic purposes). This step has the same rationale as that for the open loop responses (Section 5.3.2).

The inverse transform yields an equation for $v_m(T)$ with 9 degrees of

TABLE 5.4

OBSERVED AND PREDICTED PHASE

Frequency and decay rate	Observed[a]	Calculated
PON ω_m(rad/sec)	254 ± 11	254[b]
PON α_m(1/sec)	54 ± 8	54[b]
LOT ω_k(rad/sec)	275 ± 9	275[c]
LOT α_k(1/sec)	36 ± 7	36[c]
Phase φ (rad)[d]		
PON PST φ_{mp}	.86 ± .11	1.00
PON AEP φ_{mv}	−.58 ± .06	−.52
LOT PST φ_{kp}	2.06 ± .16	2.07
LOT AEP φ_{kv}	.55 ± .18	.55[e]

[a] Mean ± SE, $N = 8$.
[b] $K_N = 1.76$, $z_m = 2600$/sec.
[c] $K_N = 2.32$, $z_m = 3100$/sec.
[d] Positive value implies phase lead.
[e] $z_k = 5600$/sec.

freedom:

$$v_m(T) = V_{m1}\left[\sin(\omega T + \varphi)e^{-\alpha T} - \sin\varphi\cos(\omega T)e^{-\beta T}\right]$$

$$+ V_2\left[\frac{-ae^{-aT}}{(-a+b)(-a+c)} + \frac{-be^{-bT}}{(-b+a)(-b+c)} + \frac{-ce^{-cT}}{(-c+a)(-c+b)}\right].$$

$$(113)$$

This equation with 9 degrees of freedom is used to fit AEPs on PON stimulation. The damped sine wave transient $v_1(T)$ is inferred to be generated by the negative feedback loop. The nonoscillatory transient $v_2(t)$ is attributed to the response of the KII_{MG} set to the output of periglomerular KI_P set (Fig. 5.19c) in response to PON input. Consideration of $v_2(T)$ is deferred to Chapter 6.

The eight useful values (Table 5.4) from measurements on pairs of AEPs and PSTHs (4 values on LOT input and 4 values on PON input) are the 2 frequencies, ω_k and ω_m, and mean decay rates, α_k and α_m (averaged over the values for α_1 from AEPs and PST histograms) on LOT and PON stimulation, respectively, and the four mean values for phase: φ_{kp}, φ_{kv}, φ_{mp}, and φ_{mv}. Five of the values are used to fix K_n, z_m, and z_k.

The mean frequency and decay rate, ω_m and α_m are inferred to represent roots, $s = -\alpha_m \pm j\omega_m = -54/\text{sec} \pm j254$ rad/sec, of the loop transfer function,

$$C_m(s) = \frac{M(s)}{1 + K_n M(s) G(s)} . \tag{114}$$

In Section 5.3.2, $G(s)$ and $A_m(s)M(s)$ are evaluated in Eqs. (102) and (103). The combined transfer function is now divided into two parts on a trial basis,

$$A_m(s) = \frac{(s+112)(s+568)}{612(s+68)} , \qquad M(s) = \frac{219 \times 612(s-z_m)^2}{z_m^2(s+219)(s+612)} , \tag{115}$$

and

$$C(s) = \frac{219 \times 796 \times 1321}{(s+219)^2(s+612)(s+796)(s+1321) + 3.08 \times 10^{13}K_n(s-z_m)^2} . \tag{116}$$

The root locus plot for Eq. (114) is shown in Fig. 5.22, in which $z_m = 2600/\text{sec}$. For this value of z_m root loci pass through the experimentally determined points $s = -54/\text{sec} \pm j254/\text{sec}$. The value for K_n is 1.76. This is shown in finer detail in Fig. 5.23, which represents only the upper left quadrant near the origin of the s plane. When factored, Eq. (114) is

$$C_m(s) = (s-2600)^2(s+219)(s+796)(s+1321)$$

$$\div [(s+54+j254)(s+54-j254)(s+797+j495)$$

$$\times (s+797-j495)(s+1506)]. \tag{117}$$

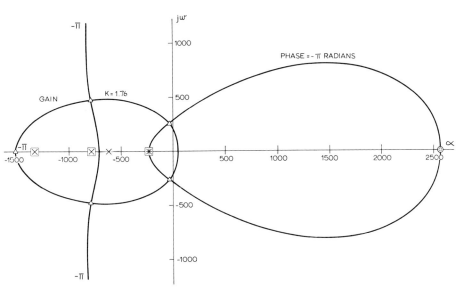

FIG. 5.22. Root locus plot for the reduced KII_{MG} set (Freeman, 1972c).

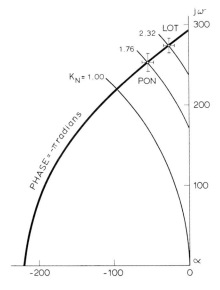

FIG. 5.23. Root locus plot as in Fig. 5.22 showing only the upper left quadrant of the s plane near the origin. The crosses show the means and standard deviations of $\alpha + j\omega$ from AEPs (Freeman, 1972c).

For approximately the same value of $z_k = z_j = 3100/\text{sec}$, the locus passes through the point in the s plane, where $s = -\alpha_k \pm j\omega_k = -36/\text{sec} \pm j275$ rad/sec, the mean values for frequency and decay rate on LOT stimulation. For a value of $K_n = 2.32$ in Eq. (114),

$$C_k(s) = (s - 3100)^2 (s + 219)(s + 796)(s + 1321)$$

$$\div \left[(s + 36 + j275)(s + 36 - j275)(s + 794 + j538)\right.$$

$$\times (s + 794 - j538)(s + 1497)\right]. \tag{118}$$

This completes the specification of the loop transfer function for PON and LOT input.

The results are tested by computing the predicted phase for each impulse response, from the topology given in Fig. 5.19g. For PON input and PST output,

$$P_m(s) = P_a A_m(s) C(s), \tag{119}$$

where $A_m(s)$ is given by Eq. (115) and $C(s)$ by Eq. (117). For $s = -54/\text{sec} \pm j254/\text{sec}$, by the inverse Laplace transform, $\varphi_{mp} = 1.00$ rad (Table 5.4). For PON input and PST output, from Eqs. (115) and (117),

$$V_j(s) = V_b A_m(s) C(s) G(s) N(s), \tag{120}$$

where $N(s)$ is given by Eq. (79). For $s = -54/\text{sec} \pm j254/\text{sec}$, $\varphi_{mv} = -0.52$ rad.

For LOT input and AEP output,

$$V_k(s) = V_b A_k(s) C(s) G(s) N(s)/M(s), \tag{121}$$

where $G(s)$, $M(s)$, and $C(s)$ are given by Eqs. (115) and (117), and $A_k(s)$ and $N(s)$ are given by Eqs. (102) and (105). The predicted value for φ_{kv} is set equal to the observed mean value $\varphi_{kv} = .55$ rad, by setting $z_k = 5600/\text{sec}$ in Eq. (101). For LOT input and AEP output,

$$P_k(s) = P_a A_k(s) C(s)/M(s). \tag{122}$$

When $s = -36/\text{sec} \pm j276$ rad/sec and $z_k = 5600/\text{sec}$, $\varphi_{kp} = 2.07$ rad.

The predicted values of the three unrestricted coefficients, φ_{mp}, φ_{mv}, and φ_{kp}, are within 1.3 standard errors of the observed means. The agreement implies that the rate coefficients of the neural sets in the bulb are invariant with respect to the change in the K_n from zero to the designated closed loop values.

The phase relations in Table 5.4 between the AEPs and PSTHs are estimates of the phase differences between the damped sinusoidal active states of the KI_M and KI_G sets in the KII_{MG} set. The values for phase should be compared with those in Table 3.1 (Section 3.3.4), which are estimates for the same phase differences between the active states of the

KI_M and KI_G sets during "spontaneous" EEG activity. The average phase lead for the KI_M set over the KI_G set is 1.44 rad on PON stimulation, 1.51 on LOT stimulation, and 1.40 for pulse probability waves. The correspondence in the average values support the feedback analysis. However, the wide variation in individual values of phase cannot be explained by the reduced KII set (see Example G in Section 1.3.1 and Sections 6.1.2 and 7.2.2).

The analysis serves to emphasize again the difference between the observable manifestation of an event such as $v_m(t) = \mathscr{L}^{-1}(V_m(s))$ and the lumped approximation $f_m(t) = \mathscr{L}^{-1}[V_m A_m(s) C(s) G(s)]$ for the active state $o_{Gv}(t, x, y, u)$ in the wave mode of the KI_G set in response to PON impulse input. That is, $N(s)$, which is derived from the open loop AEP analyses in Sections 2.5.2 and 5.3.2, has been taken out of the closed loop and has been placed in the wave output channel of the closed loop. The implication of this step is that $N(s)$ contributes significantly to the form of the observed output of the KI_G set but not to the form of the synaptic output of the KI_G set to the KI_M set. This step appears to be valid in respect to impulse input by way of the PON and LOT, but it has not yet been shown to hold for other types of input, particularly those having very low frequencies.

5.4. Reduction from the KIII Level

In each case of analysis of the dynamics of a neural mass the basic approach is the same: reduction of complexity by topological analysis; measurement of input–output functions; construction of a differential equation and solution of the equation to predict output for given input, and interpretation of the derived parameters. In each case there are particular difficulties in defining transfer functions, such as those for the input channels to the bulb, or limitations on the availability of observable output, such as the lack of pulse-trains from granule cells or of a well-defined field potential from the mitral–tufted KI_M set. To provide further insight into the variety of ways in which these difficulties and limitations can be handled, an analysis is given for the prepyriform cortex. The olfactory system comprising the bulb and cortex contains two KII sets with feedback between them so that the reduction to a single feedback loop is from the KIII level (Section 1.3.1).

5.4.1. TOPOLOGICAL ANALYSIS OF THE PREPYRIFORM CORTEX

A flow diagram summarizing the main proposed functional connections of the ipsilateral cortical mass is shown in Fig. 5.24a. The cortex contains two KI sets and possibly a third. Type A neurons are identified mainly

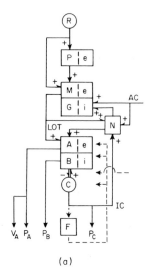

(a)

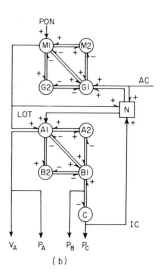

(b)

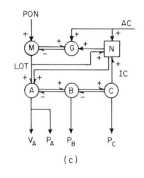

(c)

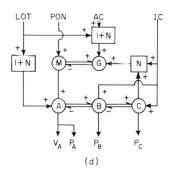

(d)

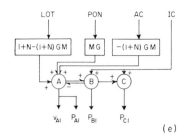

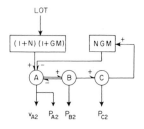

(e)

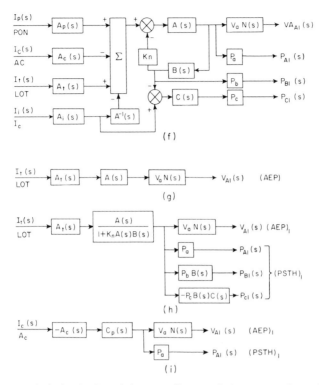

FIG. 5.24. Topological reduction of the prepyriform cortical mass to a lumped, piecewise linear approximation.

with superficial pyramidal cells (Section 4.4.1) and form the KI_A set. Type B neurons are deep pyramidal granule cells having short axons, which comprise the KI_B set. Their dense interconnection forms the KII_{AB} set. Some deep pyramidal and polymorphic neurons are identified as Type C neurons. There is electrophysiological evidence (Section 5.3.4) that they have interactions with the KI_B set, and it is reasonable to suppose that they have some synaptic interconnections between themselves. However, it is not yet known whether such interconnections exist, or whether they are sparse or dense, so the set of Type C neurons is classified tentatively as the KO_C set.

The primary input channel is from the KO_R set olfactory receptors through the PON, the bulbar KI_P and KII_{MG} sets (Section 5.3.1), and the LOT to the KI_A set. There are four directly observable electrophysiological outputs: the field of potential of the KI_A set, v_A (from area PC in Fig. 4.34, Section 4.4.1), and the pulse trains of neurons in the KI_A, KI_B, and KI_C

sets, respectively p_A, p_B, and p_C. There is synaptically mediated output from the KI_C through the internal capsule IC to several other masses in the forebrain F including the olfactory tubercle, the amygdaloid complex, and the thalamus. There is feedback from the KO_C set (and possibly also from the KII_{AB} set) to the anterior olfactory nucleus N and possibly to bulbar neurons. These possible connections are not included. The LOT axons also give collaterals to the nucleus, which sends many axons into the deeper half of the Layer Ib in the cortex (Section 4.4.1) to end on Type A neurons.

Two secondary or centrifugal input channels to the cortical mass are shown (Callens, 1967; Dennis & Kerr, 1968; Price, 1973). One is ipsilateral from other masses in the forebrain F through the internal capsule IC to various undetermined sets in the cortex with uncertain actions. The other is from the contralateral anterior olfactory nucleus and from the opposite forebrain by way of the anterior commissure AC. Some of the axons in the commissure go directly to the cortex, but most end in the ipsilateral nucleus N or in the bulb on the dendrites of the granule cells G.

This description is not complete. For example, the centrifugal connections of periglomerular and possibly of mitral-tufted cells, the interconnections within the nucleus, the probable differences between the terminations of mitral and tufted cell axons, the accessory bulb, etc., have all been omitted, because they are not needed for the present analysis.

In part (b) the two KII_{MG} and KII_{AB} sets are represented by interactions among KO subsets. The input on the primary channel is restricted to consideration of the effects of electrical stimulation of the PON, so the receptors are omitted. The periglomerular set KI_P, the direct centrifugal inputs to the cortex, and the physiological output channels through F, are not dealt with explicitly and are removed.

In part (c) it is assumed that the function of both KII sets can be maintained at the balance point by control of input, where the effects of positive feedback are nulled. In part (d) three other input channels are defined to represent the effects on the cortical mass of electrical stimulation of the LOT, the AC, and the IC.

In part (e) the four input channels are separated on the premise that they are usually stimulated singly and not in combination. The feedback channel from KO_C to KO_B is omitted, on the basis that the number of Type C units encountered is less than the number of Type B units, so that actions of KI_B on KO_C are dominant over reactions of KO_C on KI_B. The antidromic input from IC is extended to KI_B to replace this omission, so far as that input is concerned. The major change in part (e) is the separation of the long feedback channel from the short feedback channel between KI_A and KI_B. This is based on the premise that the negative feedback channel from KI_A through KI_B and KO_C and NGM to KI_A contains delay elements in series with those of KI_A and KI_B, so that its characteristic frequency must be much lower than the characteristic frequency of the negative feedback channel from KI_A through KI_B to KI_A. That is, the outputs of these two systems can be distinguished by spectral analysis of the AEP (Section 2.5.3), and low-frequency components can be tentatively assigned to the loop through NGM, or possibly to loops through F in part (a). It is assumed that the oscillatory components at very high frequency are due to the complex input channels (see Sections 2.5.3 and 7.1.3).

In part (f) the simpler subsystem is reduced by a piecewise linear lumped circuit approximation to a single negative feedback loop with four input channels and four output channels. A transfer function is assigned to each channel. Parts (g) and (h) represent three experimental situations in which the input is an electrical stimulus to a central tract, and the output conforms to the AEP or PSTH, or to the dominant component of the AEP or PSTH taken from the cortical mass. In part (g) the value for K_n is set equal to zero, corresponding to the effect of administration of a large dose of a general anesthetic such as ether or barbiturate. Unit responses are suppressed so that the output is restricted to v_A, corresponding to the AEP. The transfer function for LOT impulse input is

$$V_{A1}(s) = V_a A_t(s) A(s) N(s). \tag{123}$$

In part (h) the input is again electrical stimulation of the LOT for $K_n \neq 0$. For AEP output the transfer function is

$$V_{A1}(s) = V_a A_t(s) C_p(s) N(s),$$

where   (124,

$$C_p(s) = \frac{A(s)}{1 + K_n A(s) B(s)}.$$

For PSTH output on LOT stimulation,

$$P_{A1}(s) = P_a A_t(s) C_p(s),$$
$$P_{B1}(s) = P_b A_t(s) C_p(s) B(s), \tag{125}$$
$$P_{C1}(s) = P_c A_t(s) C_p(s) B(s) C(s).$$

For the responses to electrical stimulation of the anterior commissure AC

$$V_{A1}(s) = -V_a A_c(s) C_p(s) N(s),$$
$$P_{A1}(s) = -P_a A_c(s) C_p(s), \tag{126}$$

where $V_{A1}(s)$ and $P_{A1}(s)$ predict the output of the KI_A set, respectively, in the wave and pulse modes for impulse input. These outputs correspond only to the dominant component of the AEPs and PSTHs.

This completes the topological reduction of the cortical system to a level at which transfer functions can be constructed and evaluated with respect to observed impulse responses. As briefly given, the procedure consists in listing a set of statements about the mass, which are summarized inferences drawn from anatomical and electrophysiological data, and which are also hypotheses about the mechanism to be tested. The analysis consists in abstracting and deleting the properties that are unessential to a particular test in view.

5.4.2. DIFFERENTIAL EQUATIONS FOR THE CORTEX

An illustration of a cortical open loop surface AEP on LOT stimulation is shown in Fig. 2.22. The sum of basis functions from Eq. (190) in Chapter 2 is

$$v(T) = \sum_{j=1}^{4} B_j e^{-\alpha_j T}, \tag{127}$$

and its Laplace transform from Eq. (191) is

$$V(s) = K_f(s+z) \prod_{j=1}^{4} a_j/(s+a_j), \tag{128}$$

where K_f, z, a_j, and B_j are real numbers. The transfer function for topological analysis is from Eq. (123). The transfer function $A_t(s)$ in Eq. (123) for the LOT is inferred to include conduction delay T_a,

$$A_t(s) = a_4 e^{-sT_a}/(s+a_4), \tag{129}$$

on the premises that LOT conduction velocity is high, distances are short, and dispersion is minimal in comparison to PON dispersion (Section 5.3.2), and that transmission through the nucleus N and bulb GM is blocked in the open loop state. By choosing the time of onset of the AEP as the start of the wave response after the compound action potential of the LOT, $T_a = 0$ and

$$A_t(s) = a_4/(s+a_4). \tag{130}$$

From the relatively low value of a_1 and the negative sign of b_1 in Section 2.5.2, it is inferred that $z = 0$ and

$$N(s) = a_1 s/(s+a_1). \tag{131}$$

Therefore,

$$A(s) = a_2 a_3/(s+a_2)(s+a_3), \qquad V_a = K_f. \tag{132}$$

From the values in Section 2.5.2,

$$N(s) = \frac{92s}{s+92}, \quad A(s) = \frac{1.7 \times 10^5}{(s+223)(s+716)}, \quad A_t(s) = \frac{3164}{s+3164}. \quad (133)$$

Illustrations of oscillatory AEP from the cortex are shown in Figs. 2.23, 2.24, and 2.26. The equation of the dominant basis function in Section 2.5.3 is

$$v(t) = V_1[\sin(\omega_1 T + \varphi_1)e^{-\alpha_1 T} - \sin\varphi_1 e^{-\beta T}]. \quad (134)$$

The Laplace transform of Eq. (134) is

$$V(s) = K_1(s+\gamma_1)/(s+\alpha_1+j\omega_1)(s+\alpha_1-j\omega_1)(s+\beta). \quad (135)$$

Representative values for the parameters are given in Table 2.1, Section 2.5.3.

From Eq. (124) the expected transfer function for LOT input and AEP output in the closed loop state is

$$V_{A1}(s) = \frac{V_a A_t(s) A(s) N(s)}{1 + K_n A(s) B(s)}. \quad (136)$$

The transfer functions, $A(s)$ and $N(s)$, are inferred to be fixed over the transition from the open loop state to the closed loop state (Section 5.2.2). The transfer function for the LOT channel $A_t(s)$ is unknown, because activity in the closed loop state is transmitted to the nucleus and bulb and then back to the cortex. For the moment, $A_t(s)$ is arbitrarily set equal to 1, and $V_a = K_d$ with consequences which are analyzed in Section 5.4.3.

The transfer function for the feedback channel $B(s)$ is unknown, because no reliable output has yet been measured from the KI_B set in the open loop state in which activity in the pulse mode is suppressed or severely abridged. There is no reliably detectable output in the wave mode (Section 4.4.3).

The immediate aim of analysis is to evaluate the feedback gain of the loop K_n in Eq. (136). To this end the unknown impulse response of the feedback channel is modeled on a one-dimensional diffusion process (Section 2.3.5), which has only the properties of delay T_b and forward gain K_2. Let $K_n = K_1 K_2$. Then

$$K_1 A(s) = a_2 a_3/(s+a_2)(s+a_3),$$
$$K_2 B(s) = K_2 \exp[-(sT_b)^{1/2}]. \quad (137)$$

K_2 and T_b are evaluated from $s = -\alpha + j\omega$, where α and ω are taken from the dominant basis function of the AEP. At this value for s, the denominator of Eq. (136) is zero (Section 5.1.3) and

$$K_1 K_2 A(s) B(s) = -1. \quad (138)$$

The modulus and phase of the gain are separated:

$$K_1 = 1/|A(s)|, \qquad K_2 = 1/|B(s)|,$$

$$\varphi_1 + \varphi_2 = \pi. \tag{139}$$

From Eqs. (137) and (139)

$$K_1 = [(a_2 - \alpha)^2 + \omega^2]^{.5} [(a_3 - \alpha)^2 + \omega^2]^{.5}/a_2 a_3,$$

$$\varphi_1 = \tan^{-1}[\omega/(a_2 - \alpha)] + \tan^{-1}[\omega/(a_3 - \alpha)], \qquad \varphi_2 = \pi - \varphi_1. \tag{140}$$

From Eq. (137)

$$B(s) = \exp[-(sT_b)^{1/2}], \qquad \ln|B(s)| + j\varphi_2(s) = -(sT_b)^{1/2}. \tag{141}$$

Let $B = \ln|B(s)|$ and $\varphi_2 = \varphi_2(s)$. At $s = -\alpha + j\omega$, on squaring both sides of Eq. (141) and separating real and imaginary parts,

$$B^2 - \varphi_2^2 = -\alpha T_b, \qquad 2\varphi_2 B = \omega T_b, \qquad B^2 - \varphi^2 = -2\varphi_2 B\alpha/\omega . \tag{142}$$

By the quadratic formula there is one solution for B, because at $\omega = 0$, $B \neq \infty$:

$$B = \varphi_2[-\alpha/\omega + (\alpha^2/\omega^2 + 1)^{.5}]. \tag{143}$$

Let

$$\xi = -\alpha/\omega + (\alpha^2/\omega^2 + 1)^{.5}.$$

From Eqs. (142) and (143),

$$T_b = 2\varphi_2^2 \xi/\omega. \tag{144}$$

For convenience, T_b is expressed as T_2 in milliseconds ($\times 1000$), where T_2 is the delay time of the crest of the impulse response of $B(s)$, which is $T_b/6$:

$$T_2 = 333\varphi_2^2 \xi/\omega. \tag{145}$$

From Eq. (139),

$$\ln(K_2) = -B, \tag{146}$$

and from Eqs. (143) and (146),

$$K_2 = \exp(\varphi_2 \xi). \tag{147}$$

The negative feedback gain $K_n = K_1 K_2$ is determined directly from a_2, a_3, α, and ω by Eqs. (140), (143), and (147). For fixed values of a_2 and a_3 there is one-to-one correspondence between each point in the s plane and a point in $K_2 T_2$ coordinates (Fig. 5.25). The usefulness of this formulation lies in the fact that, even when little is known about a mass other than the existence of negative feedback interaction within it, the frequency and decay rate of its oscillatory impulse responses can be used to give numerical values to the essential parameters of the interaction, the loop gain, and delay.

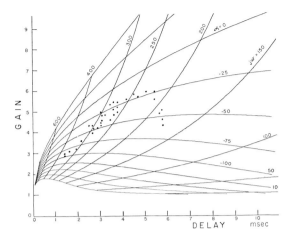

FIG. 5.25. Transformation of the coordinate system in the s plane to $K_2 T_2$ coordinates, where K_2 is the lumped feedback gain and T_2 is the lumped delay in a single negative feedback loop. The chief advantage of the transformation is that the experimental complex root locus in the s plane nearest the $j\omega$ axis ($\alpha = 0$) can often then be fitted with a straight line segment (Freeman, 1968c).

This is a step of major importance. The frequencies and decay rates of AEPs are epiphenomenal values that have little significance in themselves. The interaction strengths and transmission delays are primary functional parameters within the neural mass. Whereas studies of closed loop rate coefficients can never go beyond the level of appearances, studies of loop gains and delays can be expected to yield understanding of the constraints or invariant properties of the neural mass, and the nature of its variable parameters.

An empirical constraint on cortical (Fig. 5.25) and bulbar (Fig. 5.24) KII sets is linear covariation of K_2 and T_2, as defined in Eqs. (145) and (147). In cats, rabbits, and other mammals, when sets of AEPs are measured in constant experimental conditions and with fixed stimulus intensity, the frequency and decay rate of the AEPs vary from trial to trial. The calculated values for K_2 and T_2 covary as shown by the points in Fig. 5.25. The same linear relation holds in differing behavioral states (Freeman, 1968a) for part of the range of responses due to variation of stimulus intensity and for AEP changes following the administration of some pharmacological agents (Biedenbach, 1966). It holds for both the dominant and subsidiary basis functions (Figs. 6.2.4, 7.4, and 7.9), and there is provisional evidence that it holds for other neural masses in the brain, such as the hippocampus (Horowitz, 1972) and the superior colliculus (Pickering & Freeman, 1967). The analysis of this invariant property is given in Section 7.1.2.

5.4.3. TRANSFER FUNCTION OF THE LOT INPUT CHANNEL

When the LOT is stimulated in the lightly anesthetized animal, the cortical impulse response is oscillatory. If the LOT is cut at the site where it emerges from the bulb onto the brain surface, or if it is blocked at that site by the application to the surface of a local anesthetic, the same stimulus given to the LOT on the cortical side of the cut or block evokes an open loop response (Fig. 5.26a).

One interpretation of this result is that the oscillation is dependent on interaction between the bulb and the cortex. This possibility is ruled out by placing a second stimulating electrode on the LOT at some distance from the first electrode and delivering through it a tetanizing pulse train at a rate of 200 to 400 pps. The oscillation in response to single shocks is restored by

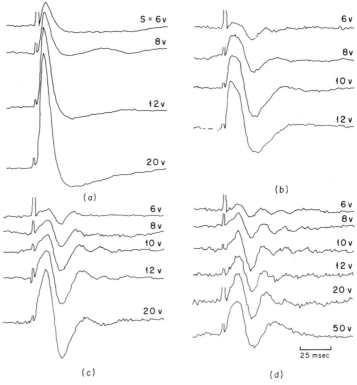

FIG. 5.26. Following surgical transection of the LOT, the prepyriform cortical AEP is reduced to the open loop state as in (a). When background input is supplied artificially by tetanizing the LOT, the oscillatory or closed loop form of the AEP is restored (Freeman, 1968c). (a) $T = 0\ V$; (b) $T = 25\ V$; (c) $T = 35\ V$; (d) $T = 45\ V$.

the tetanizing input (Fig. 5.26). There is oscillation at a single frequency, and the values for frequency ω and decay rate α of the AEP depend on the intensities of both the single pulse and the pulse train. The constraint holds for linear covariance of K_2 and T_2 calculated from ω and α. The oscillation under tetanization persists, moreover, when the deafferented cortex is undercut to sever all centrifugal and feedback connections with other neural masses in the forebrain (Freeman, 1968c). On cessation of tetanizing input, the AEP reverts to the open loop form within 30 sec.

These facts imply that a negative feedback loop does exist in the cortex as proposed in Fig. 5.24 and that it is responsible for the dominant oscillatory component of the AEP. The conversion to the open loop response in the absence of normal afferent connections or tetanizing input implies that the cortex normally receives a sustained depolarizing input through the LOT. When this is removed or blocked, the neurons in the cortical mass drop below their thresholds for pulse firing. Weak and even strong single-shock stimuli on the LOT induce dendritic responses from the KI_A set, but there is no feedback through the KI_B set, and pulse output from KI_A neurons is suppressed. This open loop state persists indefinitely unless an artificial background input is provided. That can only be done during the first 10–14 days after deafferentation before the cut ends of the LOT axons degenerate.

Unlike the prepyriform cortex the olfactory bulb is not reduced to the open loop state by deafferentation (cutting the PON) or isolation (additionally cutting the bulbar stalk including the LOT). The KII masses in the bulb and cortex are so similar in other respects that a source for sustained depolarizing input should be sought in the bulb, similar to the input from the anterior nucleus to the cortex. The obvious source is the KI_P set in the bulb (Section 5.2.3). This problem is considered further in Section 6.1.4.

The normal background input is not derived only from mitral–tufted cells in the olfactory bulb (Highstone, 1970). If a lesion is made in the anterior olfactory nucleus (Fig. 4.22) which destroys the rostral and external parts of the nucleus but spares the LOT, the amplitude of the first negative peak N1 of the AEP is not reduced on stimulation of the LOT, but the oscillation is greatly reduced. Antidromic conduction from the stimulus site over the lesion and into the bulb is not impaired, and the bulbar AEP is not changed in amplitude, frequency, or decay rate. This suggests that one source of the sustained depolarizing input to the cortex is the set of neurons comprising the rostral and external parts of the nucleus, which receive collaterals from mitral–tufted axons and send numerous axons into the cortex in Layer Ib. Removal of the ipsilateral bulb causes destruction of the anterior extremity of the nucleus but spares the remainder. The cortical open loop state persists indefinitely. This implies that a set of neurons in the nucleus requires input from mitral–tufted axons as a condition for transmitting sustained depolarizing activity to the cortex. The effect of LOT stimulation on the activity of neurons in the nucleus is to excite the neurons both orthodromically at various latencies and antidromically at a short fixed latency.

The effects on the cortex of activity transmitted antidromically to the bulb and retransmitted to the cortex are revealed in a different experiment. If the LOT is stimulated continually at a rate of 40 pps for 72 hr in a normal cat with implanted electrodes, the amplitude of the initial negative peak N1 gradually decreases nearly to zero (Fig. 5.27, curves A and B). The

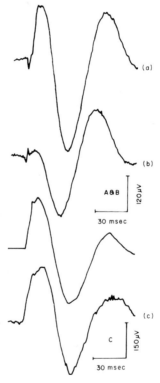

FIG. 5.27. The normal prepyriform AEP (curve A) consists of two components: an orthodromic response observed above after surgical removal of the bulb and restoration of background input by tetanizing the LOT (curve C) and a secondary response (curve B), which results from antidromically induced inhibition in the bulb, and which is unmasked by long-term LOT stimulation. This is shown by the similarity of curve C with curve A − B obtained graphically by subtracting curve B from A (Willey & Freeman, 1968). See also the AEP components in Figs. 2.25d, 2.27d, and 5.21c.

LOT compound action potential is unaffected and the latency and amplitude of the first positive peak P1 are changed only slightly (Willey & Freeman, 1968). Provided the intensity of the conditioning pulse train is not too high, the bulbar AEP is not altered.

The interpretation of this result is that transmission at the synapses of LOT axons with superficial pyramidal cell dendrites is greatly diminished by prolonged stimulation to the point where orthodromic transmission virtually fails. The persisting initially positive oscillatory AEP is not due to excitation of any slowly conducting inhibitory axons in the LOT for which there is no other evidence in any case (Willey & Freeman, 1968). It is due to antidromic input to the bulb, which activates granule cells (Section 5.3.1), transiently blocks the background excitatory output of mitral-tufted cells, and results in a transient drop in excitatory background input to the cortex. This disexcitation is equivalent to an inhibitory impulse input, because it initiates oscillation in cortical activity beginning with inhibition and not with excitation as normally occurs.

This conclusion implies that the cortical response to LOT impulse input (Fig. 5.27, curve A) consists of an orthodromic oscillatory impulse response which is initially excitatory (curve C), and a delayed antidromic oscillatory response which is initially inhibitory (curve B). The antidromic response is unmasked by long-term stimulation (curve B), and the orthodromic response is predicted by the difference which is curve A − B. The orthodromic response (curve C) is observed by cutting the LOT, tetanizing to replace the background input, and stimulating the distal cut end of the LOT.

In addition to the orthodromic excitatory volley to the cortex on LOT stimulation and the reflected inhibitory wave from bulb due to the antidromic volley, there is an excitatory reflected input from the bulb to the cortex. This is caused by mitral excitation among mitral–tufted cells in the KI_M set in the bulb (Green, Mancia & von Baumgarten, 1962; Nicoll, 1971). When an antidromic volley excites a subset of KI_M neurons, they excite another subset of KI_M neurons at the time of excitation of KI_G neurons, before the KI_G neurons exert their inhibitory effect. The secondary KI_M excitation is retransmitted to the cortex on the LOT and is estimated to arrive between 5 to 7 msec after the orthodromic volley. There is no detectable secondary compound action potential in the LOT because it is degraded by temporal dispersion (Section 2.3.3). The effects of the secondary volley can be predicted to take the form of producing a double crest in N1 of the prepyriform AEP and a double crest in the PSTH of Type A neurons during N1. Both phenomena occur, but they also occur after the bulb has been surgically removed, provided the cortex is given background tetanizing input to the LOT (Fig. 5.26). The tetanizing pulse train is required to overcome the open loop condition that follows removal of the bulb (Section 5.4.2). This means that the secondary excitation of the KI_A set during N1 on LOT single-shock stimulation has two causes: reexcitation in the KI_M set and reexcitation in the KI_A set. However, reexcitation in the KI_M set is generally less significant than in the KI_A set, because inhibition is more rapid in onset in the bulb on antidromic stimulation than in the cortex on orthodromic excitation. On very high-intensity LOT stimulation, however, reexcitation in the KI_M set is much more prominent than on low-intensity stimulation.

The transfer function for LOT input can be approximated by a set of two channels in parallel, each of which has a forward gain and a delay. This is done by neglecting dispersion:

$$A_t(s) = K_a e^{-sT_d} - K_b e^{-sT_b}. \tag{148}$$

If the frequencies of the two impulse responses are the same, the AEP appears to have one component at that frequency. The basis function fitted to that component has a phase and amplitude determined by the vector sum of the two components. If the frequencies are different, then two basis functions are required to fit the AEP. In either case the shape of N1 does not provide adequate information to evaluate the delay T_b in the channel through the bulb. The determinants of phase in the cortical oscillatory response due to $A_t(s)$ cannot be separated from the determinants of phase due to $C_p(s)$ within the KII_{AB} set. The cost of treating $A_t(s)$ as if it were unity, as is done in Section 5.4.2, is that the phase of the sinusoidal basis functions cannot be interpreted to yield information about the cortical mass, as is done in analyzing the bulbar mass (Section 5.3.3). However, the evaluation of K_n and K_2 from ω and α is not affected.

5.4.4. PULSE–WAVE RELATIONS IN CORTEX AND BULB

Spontaneous or background unit activity is easily observed in the prepyriform cortex of lightly anesthetized or waking, minimally restrained, animals. The pulses of single neurons occur at irregular intervals (see Section 3.3.2) and at average rates seldom exceeding 10 pps. There is a characteristic increase in rate with each act of inspiration, and when monitored with a loudspeaker the background unit activity often sounds like surf. Almost all cortical units are affected by a high level of LOT stimulation, but for a fixed stimulus electrode placement relatively few neurons are strongly affected by low level stimulation. Comparison of AEPs simultaneously recorded at the cortical surface with PSTHs from units in Layers II and III (Section 4.4.3) yield four types of unit responses to LOT stimulation (Figs. 5.24 and 5.28 and Section 4.4.1).

Units of Type A show two maxima of pulse probability during N1, the

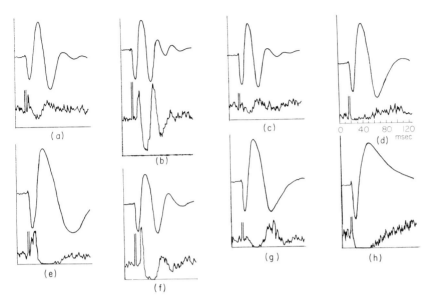

FIG 5.28. AEPs and PSTHs from 4 different types of cortical neuron, each at 2 stimulus durations. The AEP is recorded from the deep side of the prepyriform dipole field (Freeman, 1968b). Type A units for $180\,\mu m$ with (a) $N = 800$ at .012 msec and (e) $N = 220$ at .04 msec. Type B units for $450\,\mu m$ with (b) $N = 1600$ at .009 msec and (f) $N = 600$ at .015 msec. Type C units for $780\,\mu m$ with (c) $N = 2000$ at .01 msec and (g) $N = 400$ at .025 msec. Type D units for $200\,\mu m$ with (d) $N = 1200$ at .02 msec and (h) $N = 1200$ at .06 msec. Distances in μm are from zero isopotential surface.

first beginning within 1 msec of the LOT compound action potential, and the other about 4 msec later. The second peak is followed by inhibition and excitation, forming an oscillation in pulse probability at the frequency of and in phase with the dominant oscillatory component of the AEP. The first maximum is caused by LOT excitation of Type A neurons, and the second is due to reexcitation within the KI_A set, at the same time that inhibitory neurons are being excited but prior to the reaction of the inhibitory neural set onto the KI_A set.

Type B units have a single maximum in pulse probability that occurs at the time of the second maximum for Type A neurons. They also show cyclical inhibition and excitation at the dominant frequency of the AEP, but there is an approximate quarter-cycle lag in the oscillation. This is predicted for the output of a negative feedback loop (Section 5.3.3) in which the feedback set is inhibitory. On this basis the neurons generating Type B units are classified as inhibitory.

Type C units show no excitation during N1 for any intensity of LOT stimulation. The first sign of an effect is inhibition, which occurs at the time of inhibition of Type A neurons. Their pulse probabilities oscillate in phase with the dominant component of the AEP. Whereas Type A units are found mainly in Layer II and Type B units in Layer III, Type C units occur only in Layer III. They are inferred to be affected by LOT input only on transmission through the KI_A and KI_B sets.

Type D units occurring in Layers II and III show a very early pulse with high probability followed by a period of block or inhibition unrelated to the AEP. Their nature is uncertain. Possibly they are neurons sending axons into the LOT to the nucleus or to the bulb which are antidromically excited.

Neurons with strongly oscillatory PSTHs are less common in the cortex than in the bulb, and the phase relations between AEPs and PSTHs have not been quantitatively evaluated. This is a difficult problem in any case, because the effects of curvature and conduction delays and the complexity of the LOT transfer function make it difficult to define a reference phase for the AEP (Section 4.4.3). Some progress has been made by computing pulse probability waves for cortical neurons from simultaneous records of EEG waves and pulse trains (Section 3.3.3). The pulse probability waves for units identified by the AEP and PSTH as Type A neurons $P_A(T)$ have the same frequency as the cortical EEG, provided the spectrum of the EEG has a single peak near 40 to 60 Hz. If there are two spectral peaks in this range for the EEG, the frequency of $P_A(T)$ is at a value between the two peak EEG frequencies. On the average the phase of $P_A(T)$ with respect to the EEG autocorrelation function (Fig. 3.18b and e) is near zero $(0.17 \pm .34$ rad for 10 data sets), but the variation around the mean is high (Table 3.2 in Section 3.3.4).

The pulse probability wave for Type B units $P_B(T)$ has the same frequency as the EEG and, on the average, lags the EEG (Fig. 3.18c and f) by about one-quarter cycle $(-1.47 \pm .30$ rad for 12 data sets), but again the variation of individual measures is high (Table 3.3 in Section 3.3.5).

These phase relations differ from the phase relations in the bulb. In the cortex the EEG is generated by the KI_A set, which is excitatory and forms the forward channel of the feedback loop, whereas in the bulb the EEG is generated by the KI_G which is an inhibitory set forming the feedback channel. On the average, $P_A(T)$ is in phase with the EEG, $P_B(T)$ lags the EEG by a quarter cycle, and $P_M(T)$ from mitral–tufted cells in the bulb leads the EEG by a quarter cycle (Fig. 3.18a and d). The reasons should be clear.

In Sections 4.3.2 and 4.4.2 the bulbar and cortical fields are shown to consist of a dipole component generated by KI_G and KI_A sets, respectively, and a closed component generated by KI_M and KI_B sets, respectively. The intensity of both closed components oscillates at the same frequency as the dipole component but with an approximate quarter cycle phase difference. Both closed fields are expected to be maximally positive at the time of maximal excitation, because transmembrane current at the soma is outward. The polarity of the source or sink at the center of the field of each neuron determines the polarity of potential of the closed field, because the source–sink density is greatest there (Section 4.2.2). The field of KI_M is positive preceding each crest of the KI_G field (Sections 4.3.3 and 4.4.3), whereas the field of KI_B is positive following each crest of the KI_A field. That is, the phase relations between the closed fields and the dipole fields in the bulb and cortex are diametrically opposed, and this is predicted from the combination of field analysis and feedback analysis.

If the mean phase difference between $P_A(T)$ and $P_B(T)$ is precisely one-quarter cycle, then over an appropriate frequency range the rate coefficients in the forward channel must be equal to the rate coefficients in the feedback channel. Because the sources of delay are the same in both KI_A and KI_B neural sets, including synaptic and cable delays and the passive membrane, then $B(s) = A(s)$. The conditional premise cannot be justified on the basis of experimental measurements of phase. However, direct measurement of the rate coefficients in three neural sets, KI_M, KI_G, and KI_A, has given the virtually same value for the passive membrane rate constant, $a_2 = 220/\text{sec}$ and comparable values for lumped cable and synaptic delays near $a_3 = 720/\text{sec}$ and $T_c = .87$ msec. These constancies hold despite great differences in the geometry, synaptic microstructure, and transmitter chemistry of the three types of neurons. It is reasonable to postulate that $B(s) = A(s)$ as an extension of the observed constancy, supported by the observation that the predicted mean difference in phase of 1.57 rad is within the rather wide margin of experimental error.

Equations (125) are modified by setting $B(s) = A(s)$ and $A_t(s) = 1$:

$$P_{A1}(s) = \frac{P_a A(s)}{1 + K_n A^2(s)},$$

$$P_{B1}(s) = \frac{P_b A^2(s)}{1 + K_n A^2(s)}, \tag{149}$$

$$P_{C1}(s) = \frac{-P_c A^3(s)}{1 + K_n A^2(s)},$$

where

$$A(s) = 1.58 \times 10^5 \, e^{-sT_c}/(s + a_2)(s + a_3). \tag{150}$$

The solutions to these equations are found in the manner described in Section 5.3.2. They suffice to predict typical PSTHs of the three types related to the AEP, but they do not account for the observed range of variation. Further consideration is deferred to Chapter 6.

5.4.5. Channels for Centrifugal Input

The importance of background activity is further revealed by analysis of the effects of stimulation of the anterior commissure (AC in Fig. 5.24). Single-shock stimulation evokes a dipole field of cortical potential that begins with a latency of 8 to 10 msec with surface-positivity, followed by an oscillation similar to that on LOT stimulation (Fig. 5.29). It is superimposable

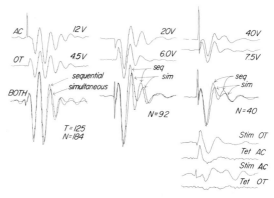

Fig. 5.29. AEPs from the surface of prepyriform cortex on stimulation of the anterior commissure (AC, see Fig. 4.22) or lateral olfactory tract (OT), or both (simultaneously or sequentially) to display the departure from superposition with increasing stimulus intensity. Time base is 125 msec for all traces.

with LOT responses and shows similar dependence of wave shape and amplitude on stimulus intensity. PST histograms of single cortical units show that some neurons undergo excitation during the rising phase of P1 of the AEP on AC stimulation, but the majority of units undergo inhibition during P1 without preceding excitation. Thereafter the pulse probabilities oscillate at the frequency of the AEPs.

These effects are similar to the effects of periamygdaloid (PA) stimulation of the cortex (Fig. 5.30) because a dipole field of potential is induced that is surface-positive at the onset of the oscillation, and whereas some units are initially excited during P1, most are inhibited. The PA-evoked potential, however, spreads from the posterior part of the cortex to the anterior part, whereas the AC-evoked potential spreads in the same anteroposterior direction as the LOT-evoked potential. An example is shown in Fig. 5.31 of the manner in which the zero isopotential surface during P1 rotates around the base of Layer Ib, in precisely the same way as it does during the response to LOT stimulation (Fig. 4.42). This can only occur if the axons carrying the inhibitory input travel in the LOT.

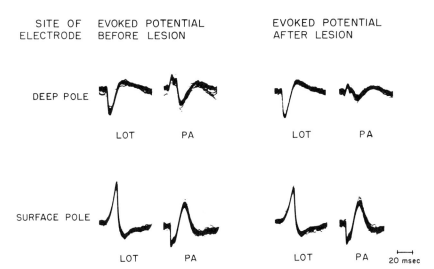

SITE OF   EVOKED POTENTIAL   EVOKED POTENTIAL
ELECTRODE   BEFORE LESION   AFTER LESION

DEEP POLE

         LOT   PA   LOT   PA

SURFACE POLE

         LOT   PA   LOT   PA   20 msec

FIG. 5.30. Surface-positive, deep-negative prepyriform dipole field responses also result from stimulation of the periamygdaloid cortex (PA), but the direction of spread is the reverse of the responses to AC stimulation. The effects of lesions made with the recording electrode show that the emf for responses to LOT input (and also AC input) are located in Layers Ia and Ib in the cortex, whereas the emf for responses to PA input are in Layer III (Freeman, 1959).

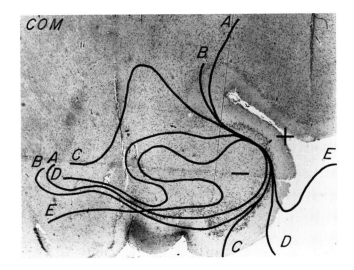

FIG. 5.31. The pattern of rotation of the prepyriform field of potential on AC stimulation is identical to that on LOT stimulation (see Fig. 4.42), showing that the initially inhibitory input to the cortex on AC stimulation is delivered through the LOT.

If the LOT is cut, or if the bulb is removed, the field potential evoked by commissural stimulation vanishes. It is not restored by tetanizing the LOT (Section 5.4.3). The same AC stimulus also excites neurons in the anterior olfactory nucleus within 2 to 3 msec, and it excites granule cells in the bulb at a latency of 4 to 5 msec. The mitral–tufted cells are thereafter inhibited, and the cortex is disexcited.

The effectiveness of this mechanism for commissural control of bulbar transmission is shown in Fig. 5.32. Single shocks are delivered to the PON, which cause a brief mitral–tufted cell response (recorded monopolarly in the upper part of the EPL), followed by a brief oscillation in the granule cell field potential (OB). The cortical response (PP recorded monopolarly on the surface of the cortex) to the PON input relayed through the bulb is seen to begin near the crest of N1 of the granule cell response. It consists of an oscillation in the amplitude of the field potential.

Each pair of traces consists of two superimposed single-shocked evoked potentials. The larger of the two is a control record, and the smaller is the result of delivering a tetanizing stimulus train to the AC at the indicated pulse rate, amplitude and pulse duration. With increasing intensity of tetanizing input there is at first a decrease in the amplitude of P1 and N2 of the cortical AEP (Fig. 5.32a), then a decrease in N1 of both the bulbar and cortical AEPs (b), and finally a block of transmission to the

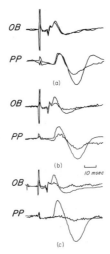

FIG. 5.32. Single-shock electrical stimuli are given to the PON, and evoked potentials are recorded from the olfactory bulb external plexiform layer (OB) and prepyriform cortex (PP) in Layer I. The effect of AC tetanization (250/msec) is to block transmission from the mitral–tufted cells (KI_M) to the bulbar granule cells (KI_G) and to the cortical superficial pyramidal cells (KI_A). (a) 5 V/.05 msec; (b) 5 V/.10 msec; (c) 5 V/.50 msec (amplitude/duration).

cortex (c), even though the mitral–tufted cell presumed apical dendritic action potential in response to PON input (see footnote in Section 5.2.1) is not significantly reduced. The result shows that AC input is sufficiently strong to block mitral–tufted output to the cortex, probably by reducing the transmembrane potential of the trigger zones of the neurons sufficiently below threshold. The remarkable feature is that single shock AC stimulation can cause a transient suppression of the output, which is indistinguishable at the cortex from an inhibitory impulse input. This gives further support to the use of Eq. (148).

The antidromic and commissural channels are only two of several centrifugal inputs to the bulbocortical system. Each neural set in the bulb, nucleus and cortex appears to have some form of such input. The analysis thus far suggests that the most prominent effects of centrifugal input on the cortex are likely to occur when the input is delivered to the bulb or especially to the nucleus, because these neural sets are critically placed in the topology (Fig. 5.24) for the regulation of cortical function.

For example, when the bulb and cortex on one side are undercut so that the PON, LOT, and blood supply are intact but all commissural and central connections are cut, the EEG shows that the bulb goes permanently into the waking state (Becker & Freeman, 1968). The intact bulb and cortex on the side opposite maintain the normal sleep–wake cycle. Undercutting removes a centrifugal input that normally acts to depress bulbocortical activity during sleep. It seems reasonable to suppose that the centrifugal input acts not on the whole cortex but on part of the anterior olfactory nucleus to suppress background input to the cortex. Similarly, undercutting[†] removes a dimension of variation of AEPs in relation to hunger (Section 7.1.2), for which the locus of cortical control might best be sought in the nucleus. These considerations are intended to suggest that, when the technical problems have been surmounted of determining which neural sets generate detectable signals and by what interactions, the analysis of the behavioral correlates of large-scale neural activity can be directed with more critical insight into the particular properties of the neural mechanisms involved.

[†] The bulb and prepyriform cortex have their main afferent inputs by way of afferent tracts which enter on the superficial aspects. The centrifugal afferent tracts enter from the deep aspects. The efferent tracts leave from the deep aspects. In this respect these paleocortical structures differ from the neocortex, in which all afferents as well as the efferents are on the deep aspect (Section 7.3.3). When neocortex is undercut so as to isolate it from all neural input, it loses its normal electrical activity and tends to become electrically "silent" (Burns, 1958). It is possible to isolate the bulb or the cortex from central and peripheral input, in which case the cortex becomes "silent" in the same way as the neocortex, though the bulb does not. The bulb and cortex offer the further option of selectively cutting either the peripheral afferent tracts (deafferentation), the centrifugal tracts (undercutting), or both (isolation).

CHAPTER 6

Multiple Feedback Loops with Variable Gain

6.1. Equilibrium States: Characteristic Frequency

6.1.1. DEFINITION OF THE THREE TYPES OF FEEDBACK GAIN

The KII set is formed by distributed interactions of excitatory and inhibitory neurons, which are themselves formed into internally interactive KI_e and KI_i sets. The KII set has a characteristic frequency at which the active states of both the KI_e and KI_i sets oscillate on impulse input. The characteristic frequency is displayed in the EEG and AEP generated by the interactive KI sets. Both the EEG and the AEP display oscillatory components at other frequencies. These arise either from the effect of a periodic input (such as respiration) or from interactions with other sets, with which the KII set is interconnected at the KIII or higher level. Each subset in the KII set, however, has only one characteristic frequency of oscillation.

The value for that frequency is time varying and depends on the levels of the active states of the KI_e and KI_i sets and on the nonlinear gain characteristics of the sets. The rate of change in the frequency with time commonly is sufficiently low that over a duration ΔT on the order of 100 msec the frequency can be treated as if it were constant. This condition holds for most AEPs and for many segments of the EEG. The value for the AEP frequency changes in relation to numerous experimental conditions, including the amplitude of electrical single shocks; the amplitude of the EEG; the presence of any of a variety of drugs, such as local and general anesthetics, or agents such as nicotine or picrotoxin applied locally; and a variety of behavioral conditions in waking animals, such as levels of arousal, selective attention, and motivation (see Chapter 7).

The dynamic properties of the KII set that determine the frequency are determined by the nonlinear stability characteristics of the KII set. As described in Section 1.3.5 there are at least three hierarchical stable states of the KII set. The lowest stable state is a zero equilibrium state in which the mean pulse rates of all subsets in the KII set are zero. The next stable state is a nonzero equilibrium state in which the mean pulse rates are nonzero. The higher stable state is characterized by a limit cycle in which the mean pulse rate oscillates at a certain frequency. The wave amplitudes are invariant in the first two states, and they are oscillatory about a zero mean at a fixed frequency in the third state.

Each state is stable only for a limited range of perturbation. That is, the stability is local and not global. For certain combinations of input or other disturbance the KII set is unstable. Correspondingly in certain experimental conditions the olfactory bulb and cortex display sustained oscillatory activity including certain EEG patterns and a high-amplitude pattern constituting a type of epileptic seizure.

In order to yield a measurable output frequency for a defined input and set of initial conditions, the KII set must be in a stable state. The amplitude-dependent nonlinearities of the interactions within the KII set that determine the frequency are analyzed with reference to measurements of the frequency ω and decay rate α of AEPs on electrical stimulation at each of a set of stimulus intensities. Any one AEP yields values for ω and α that can be plotted as a pair of points in the s plane representing a pair of conjugate complex roots. When the stimulus intensity is changed in small steps and an AEP is measured for each step, the sets of points constitute experimental root loci as a function of stimulus amplitude p_f. Alternatively, the root loci are treated as functions of wave amplitude v, and for each AEP an experimental estimate for v is based on the amplitude V_{k1} of the dominant damped sine wave fitted to the AEP with Eq. (203) in Chapter 2 or V_{j1} in Eq. (111) in Chapter 5. The analysis consists in constructing a differential equation in which the parameters representing gain coefficients are made to vary in accordance with the amplitude-dependent nonlinearities in the KI_e and KI_i sets. The equation is solved repeatedly for sets of values of the gain coefficients to give theoretical root loci. When the experimental and theoretical root loci converge, the model is considered to represent the dynamics of the KII set, and the gain values are interpreted in terms of the nonlinearities of the KII set.

The KII set has three types of interaction. The strength of interaction within the KI_e set is designated by K_e, and that within the KI_i set is designated by K_i. These two interactions each constitute positive feedback.

344   6 MULTIPLE FEEDBACK LOOPS WITH VARIABLE GAIN

The interaction between excitatory and inhibitory neurons constituting negative feedback is designated by K_n. K_n, K_e, and K_i are positive real numbers. The numerical values for K_n, K_e, and K_i all change with wave amplitude v so the analysis requires that all three quantities be defined on v. As in the case of evaluation of the gain in single feedback loops, the values for K_n, K_e, and K_i are determined from the values of the closed loop roots which most closely conform to the experimentally determined values of ω and α from AEPs. The topology of the lumped KII set is shown in Fig. 6.1a as equivalent to the interconnection of four KO sets (Section 1.3.1). The basic assumptions for the analysis have been listed and explained in Section 5.1.2. Three additional assumptions are introduced in order to simplify the descriptive equations.

(a)   The dynamics of each equivalent KO set in the KII set are described by a linear, time-invariant differential equation which is derived from and evaluated on the basis of evidence given in Sections 2.4.4 [Eq. (180)], 2.5.2, and 5.3.2, 5.4.2, and 5.4.4:

$$\frac{d^3v}{dt^3} + a_1\frac{d^2v}{dt^2} + a_2\frac{dv}{dt} + a_3 v = a_3 g_f i_f - a_4\frac{d}{dt}g_f i_f, \qquad (1)$$

$$a_1 = a + b + c, \qquad a_2 = ab + bc + ac, \qquad a_3 = abc, \qquad a_4 = ab.$$

The values of the parameters are $a = 220/\text{sec}$, $b = 720/\text{sec}$, and $c = 2300/\text{sec}$.

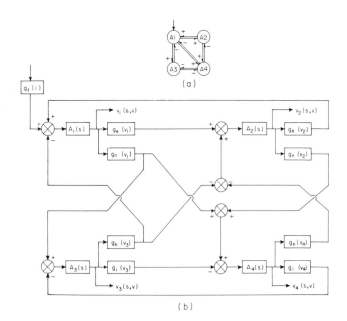

(a)

(b)

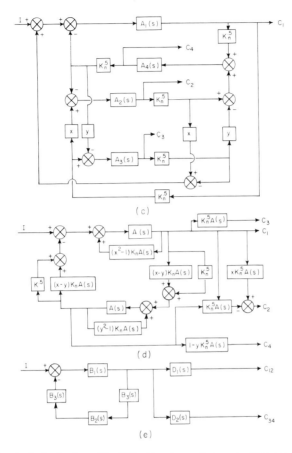

FIG. 6.1. Topological reduction of the KII set to a lumped piecewise linear approximation.

The input $g_f p_f$ is a linearized function of time (Section 3.3.6). For convenience the right side of Eq. (1) is written as $a_4[c-(d/dt)]g_f$. For AEPs and PSTHs, $p_f = I\delta(t)$, where I is a real number. The transfer function $A(s)$ of Eq. (1) as linearized is given by

$$A(s) = ab(c-s)/(s+a)(s+b)(s+c). \tag{2}$$

(b)   The amplitude-dependent nonlinearity is assumed to be the same for each equivalent KO set in the KII set. The input–output curve $G_2(v) \triangleq G(v)$ as defined in Section 3.3.6 of the nonlinear element in each KO set (Fig. 6.2) is given by the equations for wave to pulse conversion (Section 3.3.4):

$$p/p_o = \begin{cases} 3 - 2e^{-v}, & v \geqq 0, \\ e^{2v}, & v \leqq 0, \end{cases} \tag{3}$$

where v is the amplitude in dimensionless units of the empirical rate constant γ and p_o is the mean pulse rate of the KII set in pulses per second. Pulse to wave conversion is assumed to be linear, so that $G_v(p)$ is replaced by $g_v p$ and the input to the nonlinear element is in the wave mode v which is manifested in AEPs. The basis for estimating v is to be described.

The amplitude-dependent forward gain $g(v)$ of each equivalent KO set is given by the product of the derivative of Eq. (3) and the fixed coefficient $\tilde{v}_i < 0$, describing pulse to wave conversion in units of the empirical rate constants ζ/γ. That is, $\tilde{v}_i$ is given in units of reciprocal pulses per second (see Sections 1.2.4, 3.3.4, and 3.3.5 regarding specification of units for parameters):

$$g(v) = \begin{cases} g_o e^{-v}, & v \geq 0, \\ g_o e^{2v}, & v \leq 0, \end{cases} \tag{4}$$

$$g_o = -2p_o\tilde{v}_i.$$

(c)   The strength of interaction in each loop is assumed to be symmetric. That is, the gain of the forward channel from each equivalent KO set is equal to the gain in the feedback channel of each feedback loop, and feedback gain is the square of the gain of either channel.

On assumptions (a) and (b) the KII set is described by four simultaneous third-order nonlinear differential equations:

$$\frac{d^3v_1}{dt^3} + a_1\frac{d^2v_1}{dt^2} + a_2\frac{dv_1}{dt} + a_3v_1 = a_4\left(c - \frac{d}{dt}\right)[G_e(v_2) - G_n(v_3)$$
$$- G_n(v_4) + G_f(i)],$$

$$\frac{d^3v_2}{dt^3} + a_1\frac{d^2v_2}{dt^2} + a_2\frac{dv_2}{dt} + a_3v_2 = a_4\left(c - \frac{d}{dt}\right)[G_e(v_1) - G_n(v_4)],$$

$$\frac{d^3v_3}{dt^3} + a_1\frac{d^2v_3}{dt^2} + a_2\frac{dv_3}{dt} + a_3v_3 = a_4\left(c - \frac{d}{dt}\right)[G_n(v_1) - G_e(v_4)], \tag{5}$$

$$\frac{d^3v_4}{dt^3} + a_1\frac{d^2v_4}{dt^2} + a_2\frac{dv_4}{dt} + a_3v_4 = a_4\left(c - \frac{d}{dt}\right)G_n(v_1) + G_n(v_2) - G_i(v_3)].$$

The corresponding flow diagram is shown in Fig. 6.1b. The subscripts e, i, and n are used to distinguish the three types of channels. The sigmoid nonlinear functions are identical, $G = G_e = G_i = G_n$, but the channels carry activity at differing amplitudes.

The KII set represented by Eqs. (5) is linearized by replacing each $G(v)$ by a linear function. Usually the linearization is performed at an equilibrium point of the system. An equilibrium exists at $G_f(i) = 0$, $v = 0$, $p = p_o$. The nonlinear gain is replaced by the fixed gain g_o, which is given by a first-order

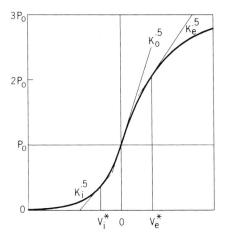

FIG. 6.2. The sigmoid input–output function is replaced by a straight line approximation. The slope of the line is given by the tangent to the curve at the effective operating amplitude v_e^* or v_i^*. See Fig. 3.20.

Taylor series expansion of the sigmoid curve. When all of the gains are equal, the KII set becomes a reduced KII set consisting of a negative feedback loop. The linearized form of the differential equations is

$$\frac{d^3 v_1}{dt^3} + a_1 \frac{d^2 v_1}{dt^2} + a_2 \frac{dv_1}{dt} + a_3 v_1 = -a_4\left(c - \frac{d}{dt}\right) g_o v_4 + g_p p_f,$$

$$\frac{d^3 v_4}{dt^3} + a_1 \frac{d^2 v_4}{dt^2} + a_2 \frac{dv_4}{dt} + a_3 v_4 = a_4\left(c - \frac{d}{dt}\right) g_o v_1. \tag{6}$$

We know, however, that the KII set is driven away from its equilibrium point by most inputs, and we want to determine its dynamic characteristics in nonequilibrium operating conditions. To do this we assert that there exists an effective operating value of the state variable v_e and v_i, of each KI set, that defines the operating point at which the system can be linearized. For the KI$_e$ set this value is v_e^* and for the KI$_i$ set it is v_i^*. By assumption (c),

$$v_1^* = v_2^* = v_e^*,$$

$$g_e(v_1^*) = K_e^{.5}, \qquad g_e(v_2^*) = K_e^{.5}, \tag{7}$$

in the KI$_e$ set, and in the KI$_i$ set,

$$v_3^* = v_4^* = v_i^*,$$

$$g_i(v_3^*) = K_e^{.5}, \qquad g_i(v_4^*) = K_e^{.5}. \tag{8}$$

A constraint is imposed such that

$$v_e^* \geq 0, \qquad v_i^* \leq 0. \tag{9}$$

From Eqs. (4),

$$K_e^{.5} = K_o^{.5} \exp(-v_e^*),$$
$$K_i^{.5} = K_o^{.5} \exp(2v_i^*), \tag{10}$$
$$K_o^{.5} \triangleq g_o.$$

Having defined the linearized gains $K_e^{.5}$ and $K_i^{.5}$ as the slopes of the nonlinear curve at the effective operating points, v_e^* and v_i^*, respectively, we now proceed to define the linearized gain $K_n^{.5}$, which represents the interaction strength between the KI_e and KI_i sets. $K_n^{.5}$ can be represented by a power function of $K_e^{.5}$ and $K_i^{.5}$ because of the exponential form of Eq. (3). Therefore let

$$K_e \triangleq K_n(K_n/K_o)^{\delta_e}, \qquad K_i \triangleq K_n(K_n/K_o)^{-\delta_i}. \tag{11}$$

Then

$$K_e = x^2 K_n, \qquad K_i = y^2 K_n, \tag{12}$$

where x and y are abbreviated notations defined by

$$x^2 \triangleq (K_n/K_o)^{\delta_e}, \qquad y^2 \triangleq (K_n/K_o)^{-\delta_i}. \tag{13}$$

In the following investigations, we will frequently use δ_e, δ_i as well as x and y. By assumption (c),

$$G_e(v_j) \propto K_e^{.5} v_j, \quad G_i(v_j) \propto K_i^{.5} v_j, \quad G_n(v_j) \propto K_n^{.5} v_j, \quad j = 1, \ldots, 4. \tag{14}$$

The input nonlinearity is replaced by

$$G_f(i) \propto K_f p_f. \tag{15}$$

Then the KII set represented by Eqs. (5) is linearized[†] at the effective

---

[†] The point is reiterated that linearization is effected at a point far from equilibrium. Usually the equations are linearized at equilibrium by assuming the steady state, so that Lyapunov stability theory can be applied. Here we wish to describe the operation of neural sets when they have been driven far from equilibrium by transient or steady input. The "proof" of the existence of stable steady state or limit cycle activity is experimental and not analytic. For example, a model representing a neural mass is here considered valid if it predicts limit cycle activity for conditions in which the corresponding EEG activity is observed. In this procedure the constant in the first-order Taylor series expansion representing the displacement from equilibrium of the effective operating amplitude v_e^* or v_i^* is implicit in the gain and is not evaluated. The sets of root loci that depend on selected values v_e^* and v_i^* may be called *describing functions*. For a full discussion of the theoretical basis for this approach, see Chapter 13 in Smith (1958).

operating point (v_e^*, v_i^*):

$$\frac{d^3v_1}{dt^3} + a_1\frac{d^2v_1}{dt^2} + a_2\frac{dv_1}{dt} + a_3v_1 = a_4\left(c - \frac{d}{dt}\right)[K_e^{.5}v_2 - K_n^{.5}(v_3 + v_4) + K_f p_f],$$

$$\frac{d^3v_2}{dt^3} + a_1\frac{d^2v_2}{dt^2} + a_2\frac{dv_2}{dt} + a_3v_2 = a_4\left(c - \frac{d}{dt}\right)[K_e^{.5}v_1 - K_e^{.5}v_4],$$

$$\frac{d^3v_3}{dt^3} + a_1\frac{d^2v_3}{dt^2} + a_2\frac{dv_3}{dt} + a_3v_3 = a_4\left(c - \frac{d}{dt}\right)[K_n^{.5}v_1 - K_i^{.5}v_4],$$

$$\frac{d^3v_4}{dt^3} + a_1\frac{d^2v_4}{dt^2} + a_2\frac{dv_4}{dt} + a_3v_4 = a_4\left(c - \frac{d}{dt}\right)[K_n^{.5}(v_1 + v_2) - K_i^{.5}v_3],$$

$$(16)$$

where $K_e^{.5} = xK_n^{.5}$ and $K_i^{.5} = yK_n^{.5}$.

6.1.2. SOLUTION OF THE DIFFERENTIAL EQUATIONS

The set of linearized[†] equations is solved by use of the Laplace transform. The system topology in Fig. 6.1b is redrawn in a topologically equivalent flow diagram (Fig. 6.1c), which is reduced by block substitution to a major negative feedback loop containing two minor positive feedback loops and two minor forward loops (Fig. 6.1d). The equations for the two minor feedback loops are

$$B_1(s) = \frac{A(s)}{1 - (x^2 - 1)K_n A^2(s)}, \tag{17}$$

$$B_2(s) = \frac{A(s)}{1 - (y^2 - 1)K_n A^2(s)}, \tag{18}$$

and the equation for the minor forward loops is

$$B_3(s) = K_n^{.5}[1 + (x - y)K_n^{.5}A(s)], \tag{19}$$

where $A(s)$ is evaluated by Eq. (2). The equation for the major feedback loop (Fig. 6.1e) is

$$C_1(s) = \frac{F(s)}{1 + B_3^2(s)B_2(s)B_1(s)}. \tag{20}$$

In expanded form

$$C_1(s) = \frac{A(s)[1 - (g^2 - 1)K_n A^2(s)}{[1 - (x^2 - 1)K_n A^2(s)][1 - (y^2 - 1)K_n A^2(s)]}. \tag{21}$$
$$+ K_n A^2(s)[1 + (x - y)K_n^{.5}A(s)]^2$$

[†] See footnote on preceding page.

When $A(s)$ is given by Eq. (2), the polynomials in s in the numerator (10th order) and denominator (12th order) are factored to give

$$C_1(s) = \frac{ab(s+a)(s+b)(s+c)(c-s)\prod_{b=1}^{6}(s+z_b)}{\prod_{j=1}^{12}(s+\beta_j)}. \tag{22}$$

The transfer function of the KII set on input to an excitatory subset and output from the KI_e set is (Fig. 6.1e)

$$C_{12}(s) = D_1(s)C_1(s), \tag{23}$$

where

$$D_1(s) = 1 + xK_n^{;5}A(s) - K_n^{;5}A(s)B_2(s)B_3(s). \tag{24}$$

When $\delta_e = \delta_i$, Eq. (24) simplifies to

$$B(s) = \frac{1 + xK_n^{;5}A(s) - y^2 K_n A^2(s)}{1 - (y^2 - 1)K_n A^2(s)}. \tag{25}$$

After evaluation of Eq. (25) with Eq. (2) and factoring,

$$B(s) = \frac{\prod_{j=1}^{6}(s+z_j)}{\prod_{b=1}^{6}(s+z_b)}, \tag{26}$$

where the z_b are identical to the z_b in Eq. (22). Then

$$C_{12}(s) = \frac{ab(s+a)(s+b)(s+c)(c-s)\prod_{j=1}^{6}(s+z_j)}{\prod_{j=1}^{12}(s+\beta_j)}. \tag{27}$$

Equation (27) is an approximation for Eq. (23) when $\delta_e \neq \delta_i$. Then for impulse input to the KI_e set, $c_{12}(t) = v_e(t)$, and

$$v_e(t) = \sum_{j=1}^{12} B_j e^{-\beta_j t}, \tag{28}$$

where B_j and β_j are real or complex.

The transfer function of the KII set for input to an excitatory subset and output from the KI_i set is (Fig. 6.1e)

$$C_{34}(s) = D_2(s)C_1(s), \tag{29}$$

where

$$D_2(s) = K_n^{;5}A(s)[B_3(s)B_2(s)(1 - yK_n^{;5}A(s))]. \tag{30}$$

When $\delta_e = \delta_i$, Eq. (30) simplifies to

$$D_2(s) = \frac{2K_n^{;5}A(s)[1 + (\tfrac{1}{2}x - y)K_n^{;5}A(s)]}{1 - (y^2 - 1)K_n A^2(s)}. \tag{31}$$

After evaluation of Eq. (31) with Eq. (2) and factoring,

$$D_2(s) = \frac{sK_n^{;5}ab(c-s)\prod_{j=1}^{3}(s+z_j)}{\prod_{b=1}^{6}(s+z_b)}, \tag{32}$$

so that

$$C_{34}(s) = \frac{a^2b^2K_n^{;5}(c-s)^2\prod_{j=1}^{3}(s+z_j)}{\prod_{j=1}^{12}(s+B_j)}. \tag{33}$$

Equation (33) is an approximation for Eq. (29), when $\delta_e \neq \delta_i$. For impulse input to the KI_i set, $c_{34}(t) = v_i(t)$, and the output is given by Eq. (28), in which the values for β_j are the same as for $v_e(t)$, but the values for B_j are different from those for $v_e(t)$.

This completes the specification of the topology of the KII set in analytic form. That is, the nonlinear differential equation describing the interactions among excitatory and inhibitory neurons is lumped and piecewise linearized, and it is solved through the forms of Eq. (27) for the output of the KI_e set and Eq. (33) for the output of the KI_i set.

Example A. The computations required to solve Eq. (20) are shown for a simple case in which the linear part of the open loop transfer function for each set is approximated by a first-order differential equation. The Laplace transform is given by

$$A(s) = 200/(s+200). \tag{34}$$

The values for the strengths of interaction are postulated to be

$$K_o = 4.0, \qquad K_n = 2.0, \qquad \delta_e = 0, \qquad \delta_i = 0. \tag{35}$$

From Eqs. (11) and (15),

$$\begin{aligned} x^2 &= 1, & K_e &= 2, \\ y^2 &= 1, & K_i &= 2. \end{aligned} \tag{36}$$

Equations (17)–(19) become

$$B_1(s) = A(s), \qquad B_2(s) = A(s), \qquad B_3(s) = K_n^{;5}. \tag{37}$$

Equation (20) is reduced to that of a single negative feedback loop:

$$C(s) = \frac{A(s)}{1 + K_n A^2(s)}. \tag{38}$$

Equation (34) is substituted into Eq. (38) and after clearing of fractions,

$$C(s) = \frac{200(s+200)}{(s+200)^2 + 2(200)^2}. \tag{39}$$

The denominator is factored to give

$$C(s) = \frac{200(s+200)}{(s+200+j280)(s+200-j280)}.$$ (40)

The inverse transform yields

$$c(t) = 200\cos(280t)e^{-200t}.$$ (41)

The impulse response of the KII set for the designated strengths of interaction is predicted to consist of a damped cosine wave. In this condition where $\delta_e = \delta_i = 0$, the three types of interaction are equal in magnitude, and the KII set can be treated as a single negative feedback loop (Section 5.2.1).   ☐

Example B.   As in Example A, let

$$A(s) = 200/(s+200),$$ (42)

and let

$$K_o = 4.0, \qquad K_n = 2.0, \qquad \delta_e = -.5, \qquad \delta_i = -.5.$$ (43)

From Eqs. (11) and (15),

$$x^2 = 1.4, \qquad K_e = 2.8,$$
$$y^2 = .7, \qquad K_i = 1.4.$$ (44)

From Eqs. (17)–(19),

$$B_1(s) = A(s)/[1-0.8A^2(s)],$$
$$B_2(s) = A(s)/[1+0.6A^2(s)],$$ (45)
$$B_3(s) = 1.4[1+.5A(s)].$$

On substitution of Eq. (42) into Eqs. (45) and clearing of fractions,

$$B_1(s) = 200(s+200)/[(s+200)^2 - 0.8(200)^2],$$
$$B_2(s) = 200(s+200)/[(s+200)^2 + 0.6(200)^2],$$ (46)
$$B_3(s) = 1.4(s+300)/(s+200).$$

Equations (46) are factored and substituted into Eq. (20) to give

$$C(s) = \frac{\dfrac{200(s+200)}{(s+20)(s+380)}}{1 + \dfrac{2(200)^2(s+300)^2}{(s+20)(s+380)(s+200+j155)(s+200-j155)}}.$$ (47)

On clearing fractions,

$$C(s) = \frac{200(s+200)(s+200+j155)(s+200-j155)}{(s+20)(s+380)(s+200+j155)(s+200-j155)+2(200^2)(s+300^2)}. \tag{48}$$

The root locus plot for Eq. (48) is shown in Fig. 6.3. The open loop poles are shown as crosses at $s = -20$, $s = -380$, and $s = -200 \pm j155$. The open loop zeros are shown as circles at $s = -300$. The closed loop poles are shown as triangles at the intersections of the root loci with the gain contour for $2(200)^2$. The closed loop zeros are shown as squares at $s = -200$ and $s = -200 \pm j155$. The transfer function is

$$C(s) = \frac{200(s+200)(s+200+j155)(s+200-j155)}{(s+200)(s+361)(s+117+j296)(s+117-j296)}. \tag{49}$$

The inverse transform of Eq. (49) gives the impulse response, which is the sum of a damped sine wave and a rapidly decaying exponential.

$$c(t) = 67 \sin(296t - 1.57)e^{-117t} + 67e^{-361t}. \tag{50}$$

The exponentials determine the rise time at the onset. □

Example C. Let

$$A(s) = 200/(s+200), \tag{51}$$

and

$$K_o = 4.0, \qquad K_n = 2.0, \qquad \delta_e = 0.4, \qquad \delta_i = 0.4. \tag{52}$$

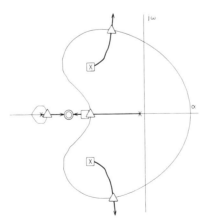

FIG. 6.3. Root locus plot for the KII set, using a first-order delay element for $A(s)$, and with $\delta_e < -\frac{1}{3}$.

From Eqs. (11) and (13),

$$x^2 = 0.76, \qquad K_e = 1.52,$$
$$y^2 = 1.32, \qquad K_i = 2.64. \tag{53}$$

From Eqs. (17)–(19),

$$B_1(s) = \frac{200(s+200)}{(s+200)^2 + 0.48(200)^2},$$

$$B_2(s) = \frac{200(s+200)}{(s+200)^2 - 0.64(200)^2}, \tag{54}$$

$$B_3(s) = 1.4\left(1 - .4\frac{200}{s+200}\right).$$

The roots are found by use of the quadratic equation, and the expressions are introduced into Eq. (20). Following rearrangement, we have

$$C(s) = \frac{200(s+200)(s+40)(s+360)}{(s+200+j140)(s+200-j140)(s+40)(s+360) + 2(200)^2(s+120)^2}. \tag{55}$$

The roots of the denominator are found by the root locus technique (Fig. 6.4),

$$C(s) = \frac{200(s+200)(s+40)(s+360)}{(s+60)(s+200)(s+272+j296)(s+272-j296)}. \tag{56}$$

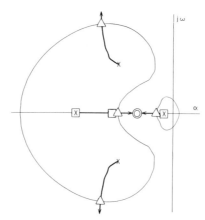

FIG. 6.4. Root locus plot for the K II set, using a first-order delay element for $A(s)$, and with $\delta_e > -\frac{1}{3}$.

The inverse transform yields

$$c(t) = 213 \sin(296t + 1.32) e^{-272t} - 11 e^{-60t}. \tag{57}$$

For the designated strengths of interaction, the impulse response of the KI_e set receiving an excitatory impulse in the KII set is predicted to consist of a damped sine wave, which is initially upward or excitatory. It is super-imposed on a small monotonic baseline shift $20e^{-60t}$ which is downward or inhibitory. □

These examples are unrealistic because the first-order approximation for $A(s)$ is an inadequate representation for the delay characteristics of KO sets. In realistic cases where $A(s)$ is represented by a third-order approximation such as Eq. (2), the 12th-order polynomial in the denominator of Eq. (20) must be factored either by root locus techniques or by use of a general purpose computer. However, the main features appearing in the solutions using the first-order approximation hold for the more complex analyses. These are the existence of a complex pair of poles not far from the $j\omega$ axis for all the designated values of δ_e and δ_i, and a real pole and real zero between the open loop pole and the $j\omega$ axis for positive values of δ_e (see Example C). The real pole or the real zero may appear in the right half of the s plane, but only for certain combinations of K_n, K_e, and K_i, which do not occur in the physiological range of KII operation in the bulb and cortex. They are of interest in connection with the development of epileptiform seizure activity (Freeman, 1973), but this is not discussed here.

6.1.3. Experimental and Theoretical Root Loci

The AEPs from the olfactory bulb and prepyriform cortex contain a dominant damped sine wave component. The frequency, decay rate, and amplitude of the component change in characteristic patterns when the stimulus intensity is varied over an appropriate range. The frequency ω and decay rate α are measured for each AEP by techniques described in Section 2.5.3, and the values from sets of AEPs are used to plot sets of points in the upper half of the s plane. Each set forms an experimental root locus.

Equation (2) is substituted into Eqs. (17)–(20), and after clearing of fractions the denominator is expanded into a 12th-order polynomial. The polynomial is evaluated by assigning values to four coefficients: $K_o, K_n, \delta_e, \delta_i$. It is factored, and the complex root nearest the $j\omega$ axis is plotted in the upper half of the s plane. The procedure is repeated for an ordered sequence of values of K_n, on the premise that increasing wave amplitude of either or both KI sets must result in decreasing negative feedback gain. This results in a theoretical root locus for the KII set as a function of decreasing K_n. Families of root loci are computed for selected fixed values of K_o, δ_e and δ_i, which represent hypothetical constraints on the dynamics of the KII set. The theoretical locus is selected that corresponds most closely to each experimental locus, and the required gain parameters are interpreted in terms of their physiological significance.

The varieties of experimental root loci depending on stimulus intensity fall into two general classes which reflect dynamic *modes* of the KII set with differing constraints. The constraints are introduced through specification of the relation between δ_e and δ_i. In the *first mode* the peak to peak amplitudes of the single-shock evoked potentials comprising the AEP are at or above the amplitudes of the background EEG. In the *second mode*, which is described in Section 6.1.5, the reverse relation of amplitudes holds. The two modes are fundamentally different for the following reason. In the first mode the response amplitude depends on the input, and there is an orderly relation between stimulus amplitude and the feedback gains. In the second mode amplitude depends largely on the amplitude of background EEG activity which, with respect to the stimulus input, is a random variable, and there is a random relation between stimulus amplitude and the feedback gains. In the first mode an experimental root locus is obtained by varying the input amplitude, whereas in the second mode the input amplitude may be fixed or varying in a small range.

Some examples of experimental root loci in the first mode now follow.

Example A.   Single shocks are given to the LOT, and AEPs are constructed from responses evoked antidromically in the olfactory bulb of an anesthetized cat. The stimulus pulse duration is fixed at .1 msec, and the current amplitude is monitored with an oscilloscope. The stimulus current is increased in small steps over a range from threshold to an upper level between 2 to 4 times threshold. Threshold is the stimulus amplitude at which the single-shock evoked potential is just clearly visible without averaging against the background EEG and has approximately the same peak to peak amplitude as the EEG. The AEPs are measured by means of curve-fitting (Fig. 6.5). The values for the frequency ω and decay rate α are plotted as open triangles in the upper left quadrant of the s plane (Fig. 6.6a). At low intensity, the value for ω is relatively high, and the value for α is relatively low. The AEP is poorly damped and oscillates at a high frequency. At high intensity, the AEP is heavily damped and has a lower frequency. The decay rate α has increased and the frequency has decreased. The set of values for ω and α form an experimental root locus with variation of input intensity that runs downward and away from the $j\omega$ axis with increasing intensity and with increasing response amplitude (see arrow). The curves are the regression line and the 95% confidence intervals.   □

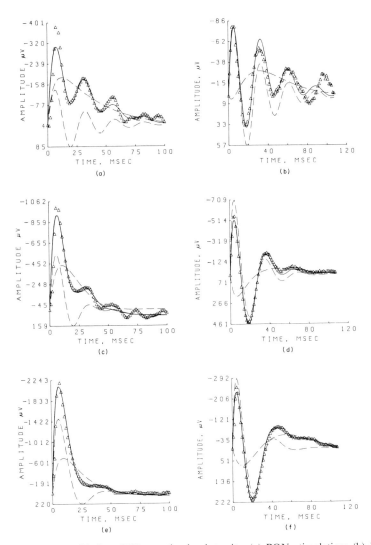

FIG. 6.5. Relation of bulbar AEPs to stimulus intensity. (a) PON stimulation; (b) LOT stimulation.

Example B. An array of 64 electrodes is placed on the surface of the olfactory bulb in an anesthetized cat, and single shocks are given to the PON. A set of 64 AEPs is constructed (Fig. 4.27a), and each AEP is measured by curve-fitting as described in Section 5.3.3. The amplitude V_1 of the damped sine wave component increases in all directions toward the epicenter of the response focus. The frequency ω is independent of amplitude, and the decay rate α increases with increasing amplitude. The

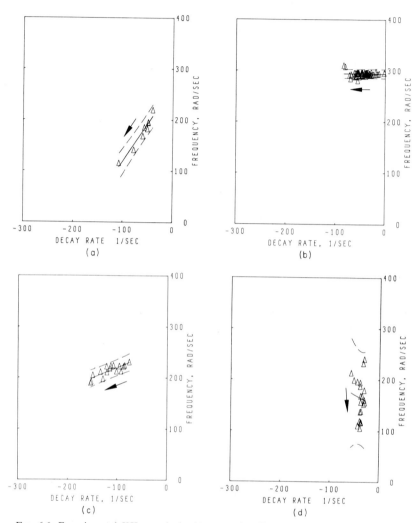

FIG. 6.6. Experimental KII root loci with regression lines and 95% confidence intervals. Arrows show direction of increasing stimulus intensity and AEP amplitude.

experimental root locus with variation of AEP amplitude (Fig. 6.6b) runs perpendicular to the $j\omega$ axis, in the direction of increasing decay rate with increasing amplitude.   □

Example C.   The observations in Example B are repeated 20 min after a small supplemental dose of pentobarbital is given intravenously (Fig. 6.6c).   □

Example D.   Single shocks are given to the LOT, and AEPs are constructed from transcortical bipolar recordings in the prepyriform cortex of a
waking cat for different levels of stimulus intensity as in Example A. The
values for frequency ω and decay rate α of the dominant damped sine wave
are plotted in Fig. 6.6d. The response frequency decreases with increasing
input and AEP amplitudes, but the decay rate does not. The experimental
root locus is roughly parallel to the $j\omega$ axis and runs downward with increasing response amplitude.   □

These four examples suffice to illustrate the chief characteristics of experimental root loci of KII sets in the first mode, in which the response
amplitudes are greater than the amplitude of background EEG activity. In
this mode the wave amplitude is determined by input intensity. This constraint is introduced into the equations by setting

$$\delta_i = \delta_e. \tag{58}$$

This implies that when the average response amplitude is greater than
background activity, the gains during each evoked potential are determined
mainly by the evoked activity and not by the background activity. (In the
second mode, of course, the converse is true.) The value for $K_e^{.5}$ is determined
by the effective operating amplitude of evoked activity in the KI_e set v_e^*
and the value for $K_i^{.5}$ is determined by the effective operating amplitude of
evoked activity in the KI_i set v_i^* by Eqs. (10). Each half cycle of oscillatory
activity consists in successive activity of each kind in one passage around
the negative feedback loop, so the product of the two sequential gain
factors suffices to determine the loop gain K_n.
By Eqs. (12)–(13), it follows immediately from Eq. (58) that

$$K_n = (K_e K_i)^{.5} \tag{59}$$

in the first mode. Further, when $\delta_e = 0$ as in Example A in Section 6.1.1,
then from Eqs. (11) and (13),

$$K_e = K_n, \qquad K_i = K_n, \qquad x = y = 1. \tag{60}$$

Equation (20) reduces to the form for the reduced KII set (Section 1.3.1),

$$C(s) = A(s)/[1 + K_n A^2(s)], \tag{61}$$

for which the theoretical root locus in the upper left quadrant of the s plane
is shown in Fig. 6.7a. This is almost identical to the root locus for the
negative feedback loop shown in Fig. 5.23. The small square on the locus
in Fig. 6.7a represents a convenient value for $K_o = 2$. The slash marks
represent the locations of the root on the locus for different values of K_n.
At the square, $K_n = 2$. Above the square, $K_n = 2.5$, 3.0, etc., and below the

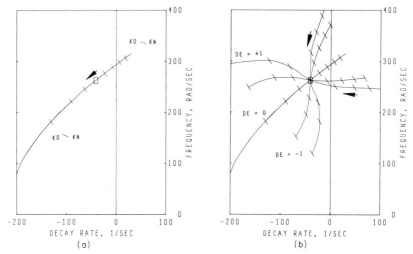

FIG. 6.7.   (a) Root locus for the reduced KII sets with $\delta_e = \delta_i = 0$ and □: $K_o = K_n = 2.00$. (See Figs. 5.22 and 5.23). (b) Root loci for the KII set in the first mode with fixed K_o, and with 5 representative values for δ_e. From extreme left in counterclockwise direction, $\delta_e = 1, .5, 0, -.5, -1$. Arrows show direction of increasing wave amplitude and decreasing K_n (in steps of 0.5).

square, $K_n = 1.5, 1.0,$ and 0.5, changing in each direction by steps of 0.5. The arrow gives the direction of decreasing K_n. These conventions are adhered to in subsequent root locus plots.

The effect of changing $\delta_e = \delta_i$ is shown in Fig. 6.7b. For $\delta_e > 0$ the locus becomes more horizontal, and for $\delta_e < 0$ it becomes more vertical. A family of root loci is computed for each value of $\delta_e = \delta_i$ by fixing K_o at each of an ordered sequence of values. Each experimental root locus is superimposed on an appropriate family at the appropriate value for $\delta_e = \delta_i$, depending on the angle formed between the experimental locus and the $j\omega$ axis. The value for K_o is determined from the position of the experimental locus.

In Example A (Fig. 6.6 and 6.8), $\delta_e = -.30$. In Example B, $\delta_e = +.40$, and in Example C, $\delta_e = +.20$. In Example D, $\delta_e = -1.00$. In each example, there are theoretical root loci for values of K_o differing by steps of .5. For Example A, $K_o = 2.5$. In Example B, $K_o = 3.0$, and in Example C, $K_o = 1.0$. In Example D, $K_o = 2.3$. The value for K_n for each AEP is determined from the position of the pole on or nearest the theoretical root locus, and the values for K_e and K_i are computed from Eqs. (11).

The values for K_n, K_e, and K_i all decrease in varying proportions with increasing stimulus intensity and wave amplitude. The logarithm of K_n is found to decrease linearly (Fig. 6.9) with increasing wave amplitude (V_1

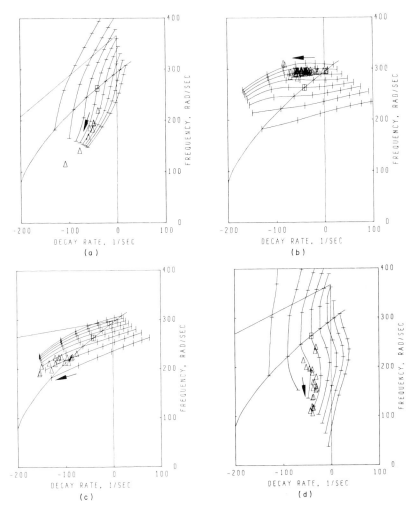

FIG. 6.8. Root loci for KII set in the first mode, with values for δ_e determined by experimental data (see Fig. 6.6). Each curve is a locus for fixed K_o, differing in steps of 0.5 and increasing upward and to the right. (a) $\delta_e = \delta_i = -.30$; (b) $\delta_e = \delta_i = .40$; (c) $\delta_e = \delta_i = +.20$; (d) $\delta_e = \delta_i = -1.00$. $\square$: $K_o = K_n = 2.00$.

of the dominant damped sine wave component in the equation fitted to the AEP). This is predicted by Eqs. (10)–(13).

An alternative method for reducing K_n is to administer a general anesthetic that reduces the level of background activity, specifically the mean background pulse rate p_o on which g_o and K_o depend [Eq. (4) and Section 3.3.6]. Under very deep anesthesia both p_o, K_o, and K_n are reduced to zero,

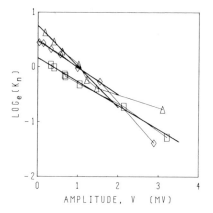

FIG. 6.9. Relation between amplitude of the dominant component (V_1 in the equations fitted to the AEPs, see Sections 2.5.3 and 5.3.3) and the values for K_n derived from Fig. 6.8. □: LOT, slope = −.46/mV; ◇: PON-L, slope = −.53/mV; △: PON-M, slope = −.78/mV. L: baseline shift present; M: baseline shift absent (see Fig. 5.11).

which constitutes the open loop state. If small doses are given incrementally and an AEP is taken at each level, the measured values for ω and α are found to change in the same patterns as for increasing stimulus intensity at the same site.

Example E. Single-shock stimuli are given to the PON in a cat already anesthetized with pentobarbital. Small supplemental doses of pentobarbital are given intravenously at intervals of 3 min. Just preceding each dose, an AEP is taken. The AEPs (Fig. 6.10b) show decreasing frequency and amplitude with successive doses. The root locus is shown in Fig. 6.11a with $\delta_e = -1.0$ and K_o between 2.0 and 1.5.   □

Example F. The effect of the cumulative doses of pentobarbital abates after 1 to 2 hr. Characteristically the oscillatory component of the AEPs on either PON or LOT stimulation returns rapidly, but the baseline shift on PON stimulation may return much more slowly or remain minimal or absent. The pattern of change in AEP with increasing stimulus intensity is shown in Fig. 6.10a. The root locus is shown in Fig. 6.11b. The locus resembles that in Example A rather than Example B with $\delta_e = -.40$ and $K_o = 2.5$.   □

Example G. The effect of increasing the stimulus rate is to decrease the AEP amplitude with no effect on frequency or decay rate. This is attributed to glomerular transmission attenuation (Section 5.2.3). The attenuation effect is detectable by using steady state stimulus pulse trains at the designated rates,

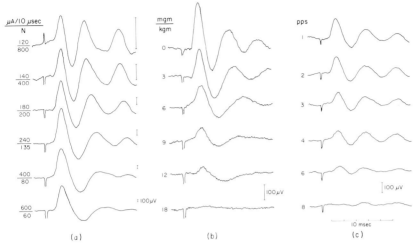

FIG. 6.10. Comparison of the effects on the bulbar AEP from PON stimulation of (a) increased stimulus intensity, (b) supplemental pentobarbital and (c) increased stimulus rate.

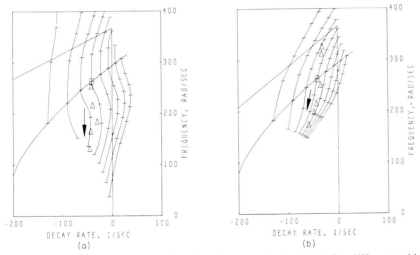

FIG. 6.11. (a) Root locus plot for the effect of pentobarbital on the bulbar KII_{MG} set with $\delta_e = \delta_i = -1.00$. $\square$: $K_o = K_n = 2.00$. (b) Root locus plot for increasing stimulus intensity for PON stimulation of the KII_{MG} set, following presumptive depression of the KI_P set with $\delta_e = \delta_i = -.40$.

but its magnitude is considerably less in the absence of a well-developed AEP baseline shift than when a shift is present. The attenuation effect (Section 5.2.3) and the baseline shift are both attributed to periglomerular neurons. $\square$

To avoid confusion we note that the baseline shift in the bulbar AEPs on PON stimulation (nonoscillatory dashed curves in Figs. 6.5 and 6.12a–c) is generated by the KI_G set; just as the oscillatory component is (oscillatory dashed curves). The oscillatory component is the impulse response of the KI_G set for impulse input to the KII_{MG} set. The baseline shift is the response of the KI_G set to input from the KI_P set. That input consists of the impulse response of the KI_P set (Fig. 6.12d–f) on PON stimulation. The KI_P set does not contribute to the field potential recorded at the surface of the bulb (Section 4.3.2). Therefore the baseline shift in the AEPs is caused by periglomerular activity, but it is not a direct manifestation of that activity.

It is intuitively obvious that the feedback gains depend on the ratio of the amplitudes of test activity to background activity and not on either alone. If test response amplitude is raised (Example F) or if background activity is reduced (Example E) K_n is decreased. If both change together, K_n is unchanged (Example G). Conversely, if the test response amplitude is lowered or if background activity is increased, K_n is raised.

Example H. Single-shock stimuli are given to the LOT in a cat so deeply anesthetized with pentobarbital that the AEP from the prepyriform cortex is reduced to a single cycle of oscillation (Fig. 6.13). A stimulus train at 250/sec is given to the LOT through a second stimulating electrode pair

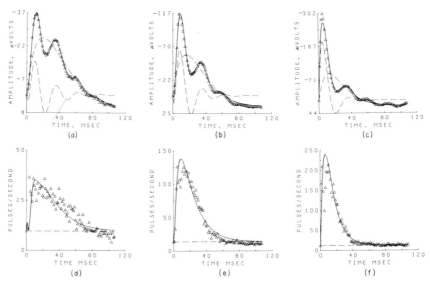

FIG. 6.12. (a)–(c) Bulbar AEP on PON stimulation and attributed to the KI_G set. (d)–(f) PSTHs attributed to a periglomerular neuron in the KI_P set. Moving from left to right increases stimulus intensity.

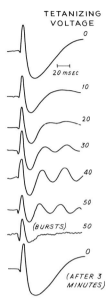

FIG. 6.13. Suppression of oscillation in prepyriform AEP on LOT stimulation and temporary restoration by LOT tetanization (see Fig. 5.26) (Freeman, 1968c).

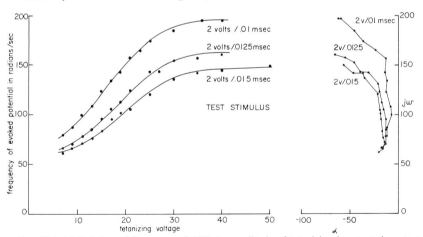

FIG. 6.14. (a) Relation of frequency of AEP to amplitude of tetanizing input at three test input amplitudes. (b) Root locus plots for frequency and decay rate of AEPs with increasing tetanizing input (upward) (Freeman, 1968c).

which provides an artificial source of background activity in the cortex. The test stimulus intensity is held constant. The frequency of the AEP increases monotonically with increasing tetanizing voltage, which implies that K_n increases with an increase in background activity in the cortex.   □

The effect of background activity on AEP frequency is described in Section 5.4.3 for experiments in which normal cortical background activity is suppressed by cutting the LOT. The dependence of response frequency on tetanizing input is shown in Fig. 6.14a, and some experimental root loci are shown in Fig. 6.14b. The relations between K_n, K_e, and K_i required to generate matching theoretical root loci have not yet been found, so the gains cannot yet be evaluated.

6.1.4. BIAS CONTROL OF CHARACTERISTIC FREQUENCY

The physiological significance of the parameter $\delta_e = \delta_i$ is revealed by combining Eqs. (11) to give

$$\frac{1}{1+\delta_e}\ln\left[\frac{K_e}{K_o}\right] = \frac{1}{1-\delta_i}\ln\left[\frac{K_i}{K_o}\right] \tag{62}$$

and substituting Eqs. (10) into Eq. (62) to give

$$-2v_e^*/(1+\delta_e) = 4v_i^*/(1-\delta_i). \tag{63}$$

Equation (63) is solved for the ratio v_e^*/v_i^* in terms of δ_e:

$$v_e^*/v_i^* = 2(\delta_e+1)/(\delta_e-1). \tag{64}$$

By Eq. (64), if $\delta_e = -.33$, then $v_e^* + v_i^* = 0$. This means that the KII set is symmetrically balanced about the equilibrium point at $v = 0$, because the operating point of the KI_i set is equal and opposite in sign to the operating point of the KI_e set. If $\delta_e > -.33$, then $v_e^* + v_i^* > 0$. This means that the operating points are not symmetrically located with respect to the equilibrium point at $v = 0$ of the KII set and are displaced toward the excitatory side $v > 0$. If $\delta_e < -.33$, then $v_e^* + v_i^* < 0$, which means that the operating points are displaced toward the inhibitory side.

The interpretation is that the value for δ_e in the first mode reflects a bias in the operation of the KII set: When $\delta_e > -.33$, the bias is excitatory; when $\delta_e < -.33$, the bias is inhibitory; when $\delta_e = -.33$, the bias is zero.

The term "bias" as used here denotes an internal operating bias, which is a displacement of the effective operating points with respect to the equilibrium. It should not be confused with input bias, which is one determinant of the operating bias.

In each of the foregoing examples the test stimulus provides an impulse. The measured response contains a damped sine wave, for which the mean amplitude is near zero. However, in two of the examples (B and C) the PON input to the KII set is not merely an impulse. On PON stimulation the afferent volley initiates oscillation in the bulbar KII_{MG} set, and it simultaneously triggers prolonged excitatory activity in the KI_P set of periglomerular neurons, which excites the KII_{MG} set (Section 5.4.3). The prolonged KI_P excitation (Fig. 6.12d–f) constitutes an excitatory bias that shifts v_e^* and v_i^* in the excitatory direction (Fig. 6.12a–c). The bias is seen in the form of the baseline shift of AEPs, on which the oscillation is superimposed for PON stimulation (Fig. 6.5a), but not for LOT stimulation (Fig. 6.5b) because LOT input does not go to the KI_P set. In Examples B and C, $\delta_e > 0$.

The contribution of excitatory bias by the KI_P set to the KII_{MG} set is further revealed by comparing Examples B and F. The level of periglomerular output in Example B is high, as shown by the prominent baseline shift (Fig. 6.12 or Fig. 6.5a). The value for $\delta_e = \delta_i$ is .4, which implies the existence of strong excitatory bias (Fig. 6.8b). The level of periglomerular output in Example F is low, as shown by the near absence of a baseline shift. The value for $\delta_e = \delta_i$ is $-.4$ (Fig. 6.11f), which implies the near absence of operating bias. The locus in Example F is very similar to that in Example A in which the KII_{MG} set is activated antidromically, bypassing the KI_P set.

An intriguing aspect of KI_P excitatory bias of the KII_{MG} set is that, during the impulse response, the bias effect appears mainly in the output of the KI_G set, the AEP, and not in the output of the KI_M set, the PSTH (see Figs. 5.21b and 6.15). During the surface negative baseline shift the mitral–tufted cells

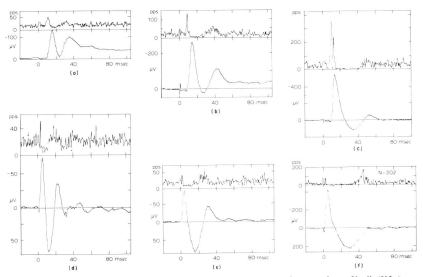

FIG. 6.15. PSTHs of single mitral-tufted cell (KI_M set) and AEPs from surface of bulb (KI_G) set on PON (a–c) or LOT (d–f) stimulation. Moving from left to right increases stimulus intensity (Freeman, 1972c). (a) $N = 400$ at 22 V; (b) $N = 400$ at 30 V; (c) $N = 178$ at 50 V; (d) $N = 1500$ at 20 V; (e) $N = 800$ at 2.5 V; (f) $N = 202$ at 60 V.

are inferred to receive prolonged excitation from the periglomerular cells and prolonged inhibition from the granule cells. The two bias effects virtually cancel, which suggests that a zero in the KII_{MG} transfer function for KI_M output cancels the pole representing the KI_P input. A zero in the appropriate location on the negative real axis has been shown to exist for KI_M output and not to exist for KI_G output by Eqs. (27) and (33) (see also Example C in Section 6.1.2 with $\delta_e = \delta_i = .40$ and Fig. 6.6b).

On LOT stimulation in Example D the orthodromic volley initiates oscillation in the cortical KII_{AB} set, and it also initiates oscillation in the bulbar KII_{MG} set antidromically. The bulbar activity is retransmitted to the cortex (Section 5.4.3) as an initially inhibitory damped sine wave. Its first inhibitory peak arrives during N1 and extends into P1 of the cortical AEP. The retransmitted input consists in the reduction of background excitatory input during the period of maximal saturation of pulse formation by threshold. It is equivalent to an inhibitory bias superimposed on the orthodromic excitatory impulse input. Therefore, $v_e^* + v_i^* < 0$ and $\delta_e < -.33$. (For an alternative explanation, see Section 6.2.5).

On LOT stimulation in Example A the oscillation in the bulbar KII_{MG} set is initiated by the antidromic volley, but the KI_P set is not affected. There is no excitatory bias as in Example B. The examples of bulbar AEPs in Fig. 6.5b show small transients which are initially inhibitory. These reflect an event that is still unexplained. It may result from retransmission into the bulb of activity evoked by the orthodromic volley to the cortex. That is, LOT stimulation excites neurons in the bulb, the cortex, and the anterior olfactory nucleus (Section 5.4.3). The neurons in the nucleus have axon collaterals which return to the bulb and end on granule cells. The small transient in the AEPs may reflect secondary excitation of the KI_G set through the nucleus on LOT stimulation. Alternatively, it may result from excitation of centrifugal fibers running to the bulb in the LOT (Section 5.31). In any case the secondary transient is relatively small in comparison to the dominant component, so that Examples A and F can be considered to be close approximations to the performance characteristic of a KII set with zero operating bias at which $v_e^* + v_i^* = 0$ and $\delta_e = \delta_i = -.33$.

Comparison of Examples A and B (Fig. 6.8) shows that the effect of excitatory bias as in Example B. The examples of bulbar AEPs in Fig. 6.5b dependent of wave amplitude. In the unbiased KII set both frequency and decay rate change with amplitude. When a spatially nonuniform input evoked by electrical stimulation is delivered to the KII set through the LOT, the wave amplitudes differ over the set, and so also does the characteristic frequency. An example of frequency dissociation in a KII_{MG} response to LOT input is shown in Fig. 6.16. On the other hand when a spatially non-uniform input is given to the KII_{MG} set by PON stimulation, the bias

LOT

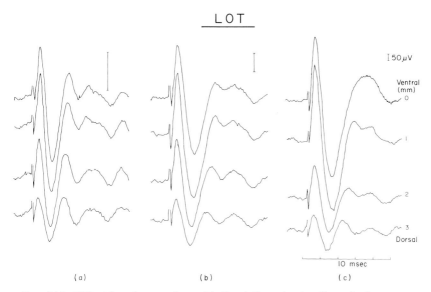

(a)   (b)   (c)

FIG. 6.16. AEPs taken from surface of bulb at the epicenter (0 mm) of a response domain on LOT stimulation and at points spaced 1 mm apart on the surface toward the ventral edge of the domain. Note the frequency dissociation of the AEPs that is seldom seen on PON stimulation of the bulb (see Fig. 4.27). (a) $N = 1000$ at 500 $\mu A/10$ μsec; (b) $N = 500$ at 600 μA; (c) $N = 340$ at 800 μA.

contributed by the KI_P set converges the frequency, so that oscillation occurs at the nearly same frequency over the entire response focus independently of local amplitude. Moreover the decay rate is high in local regions with high amplitude (Fig. 4.32 in Section 4.3.3), so the response focus tends rapidly toward uniform amplitude as well as uniform frequency, due to the excitatory bias determined by the KI_P set.

The effect of inhibitory bias is shown in cortical AEPs in response to LOT stimulation, where it accentuates the dependence of response frequency on response amplitude and makes the decay rate relatively independent of amplitude (Figs. 6.6d and 6.8d).

For both types of bias the strength of the bias usually increases with increasing stimulus intensity in the same proportion as the amplitude of the damped sine wave, at least over the lower range of stimulus intensity. This implies that the ratio v_e^* to v_i^* is constant, and, by Eq. (64) $\delta_e = \delta_i$ is constant. In the absence of bias $\delta_e = \delta_i = -.33$. The constancy is the principal basis for the effectiveness of defining δ_e and δ_i by Eqs. (11).

Because K_o is defined as maximal gain in Eqs. (10), then in the first mode where $\delta_e = \delta_i$ and AEP amplitude > EEG amplitude,

$$K_n \lesseqqgtr K_o. \tag{65}$$

This constraint is reflected in comparing the experimental and theoretical root loci in Figs. 6.8 and 6.11. These experimental root loci are characteristic types that reflect the designated constraints on the dynamics of the KII set. Departures from these types occur in this mode and show that different constraints hold in different experiments. For example, in Fig. 6.17a, the experimental locus from data taken in the same way as in Example B conforms to a theoretical locus for $\delta_e = \delta_i = -.20$, and for $K_o = .7$. However, the constraint that $K_n \leqq K_o$ is violated, so the loci cannot be convergent. In Fig. 6.17b, the experimental points do not form an identifiable locus. These and similar departures can be explained for example by assuming that $\delta_e = \delta_i$ is not constant, but the explanations are not very helpful at present in furthering understanding of the KII mechanism.

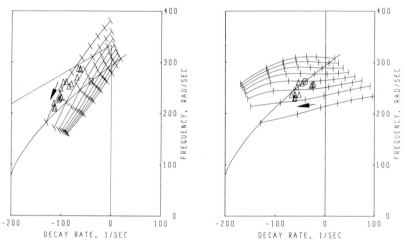

FIG. 6.17. Root locus plots for the KII$_{MG}$ set on PON stimulation with recording of AEPs at different locations in the response domain. (a) $\delta_e = \delta_i = -.20$; (b) $\delta_e = \delta_i = .40$. □: $K_o = K_n = 2.00$.

6.1.5. Root Loci Dependent on EEG Amplitudes

In the second mode of KII operation the peak to peak amplitudes of single-shock evoked potentials are less than those of the background EEG amplitudes. The effective excitatory inhibitory wave amplitudes, v_e^* and v_i^*, during each impulse response are determined more by the EEG than by test input. The phase of the oscillatory dominant component of each evoked potential is at random with respect to the phase of the EEG, so on some trials saturation is accentuated and on others it is minimized or reversed. The constraint that $K_n \leqq K_o$ no longer holds. The AEP gives information about mean wave amplitudes of the test response, but it does not show directly the wave amplitudes which determine K_e and K_i, so the constraint that $K_n = (K_e K_i)^{.5}$ no longer holds.

From the analysis of experimental data (Section 7.1.2) the following constraint is imposed:

$$\delta_i = -2\delta_e - 1. \tag{66}$$

Several important relations immediately follow. From Eqs. (11),

$$K_e/K_o = (K_n/K_o)^{\delta_e + 1},$$
$$K_i/K_o = (K_n/K_o)^{2(\delta_e + 1)}, \tag{67}$$
$$K_i/K_o = (K_e/K_o)^2.$$

From Eq. (10),

$$v_e^* = -v_i^*. \tag{68}$$

That is, the effective operating points of the KI_e and KI_i sets are symmetrically displaced from the equilibrium point. By combining Eqs. (67) and solving for K_n, we have

$$K_n = (K_e K_i K_o^{3\delta_e + 1})^{1/(3\delta_e + 3)}. \tag{69}$$

Whereas in the first mode K_n is the geometric mean of K_e and K_i, in the second mode K_n depends on K_o as well (Fig. 6.2). The degree of dependence is reflected in the value of δ_e, which in turn reflects the degree to which the EEG or background activity determines the KII characteristics in respect to a given input. When $\delta_e = -.33$, then $\delta_i = -.33$ and

$$K_n = (K_e K_i)^{.5},$$

as in the first mode, Eq. (58). When $\delta_e = 0$, then $\delta_i = -1$ and

$$K_n = (K_e K_i K_o)^{.33}.$$

When $\delta_e = .33$, then $\delta_i = -1.67$ and

$$K_n = (K_e K_i K_o^2)^{.25}.$$

The sequence shows that higher values of δ_e reflect an increasing importance of K_o in determining K_n, as compared with the importance of K_e and K_i.

Theoretical root loci as a function of K_n for $K_o = 2$ and for differing values of δ_e are shown in Fig. 6.18a. For $\delta_e = -.33$, the locus is identical to that for the KII set in the first mode at $\delta_e = \delta_i = -.33$ (see Fig. 6.8a). With increasing values of δ_e, the root locus rotates counterclockwise about the point at $K_o = 2$. The direction of each locus is decreasing frequency with decreasing values of K_n and increasing wave amplitude.

Experimental root loci of this type are commonly observed in the conditions specified for bulbar and cortical KII operations in the second mode.

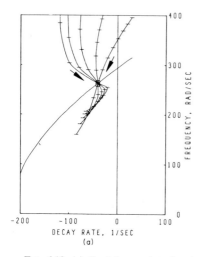
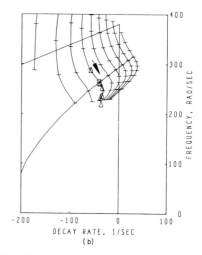

FIG. 6.18. (a) Root locus plots for the KII set in the second mode with fixed K_o and selected values of δ_e. From right to left at top, $\delta_e = -.33, -.17, 0, +.17, +.33$. Arrows show direction of decreasing K_n and increasing wave amplitude (see Fig. 6.7 for first mode). (b) Root locus for KII_{MG} responses in the second mode on PON stimulation at low intensity with $\delta_e = 0$ and $\delta_i = -1.00$. $\square$: $K_o = K_n = 2.00$.

Values for δ_e are estimated from the angle formed by each experimental locus and the $j\omega$ axis. Values for K_o are estimated by calculating families of theoretical root loci for sets of values of K_o at selected values of δ_e. For each experimental locus K_o is determined by extrapolation. Values for K_n, K_e, and K_i are estimated for each AEP as described in Section 6.1.3.

Example A.   Single-shock stimuli are given to the PON at each of a set of amplitudes, and a set of AEPs is taken from surface recording on the bulb of an anesthetized cat. The input amplitudes range from threshold for single-shock responses, as in Example A in Section 6.1.2, downward to just above threshold for the AEP on prolonged averaging (e.g., $N > 1000$). The frequency ω and decay rate α are measured by fitting a curve to each AEP from Eq. (111) in Chapter 5. The experimental locus is shown for 6 AEPs in Fig. 6.18b. A family of theoretical root loci is calculated in the second mode for $\delta_e = 0$ and $\delta_i = -1$. The inferred value for K_o is 2.0, and the range for K_n is 2.5 to 1.5. The sequential order of the points is not strictly dependent on the sequence of change in stimulus amplitude. $\square$

Example B.   An array of 64 electrodes is placed on the surface of the bulb, and single shocks are given to the LOT at an intensity 2.5 times threshold for single responses. The AEP consists of a heavily damped, low-frequency sine wave with little detectable baseline shift (Fig. 6.19a). There

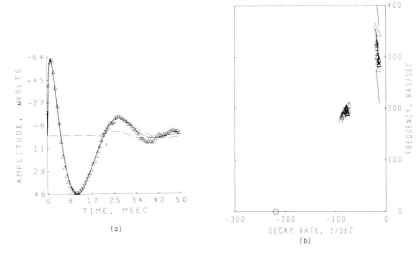

FIG. 6.19. (a) Average AEP from 12 surface sites over a response domain in the bulb on LOT stimulation, with variation in response amplitude with site. (b) Experimental root loci for dominant (lower left) and minor (upper right) components.

is a higher-frequency oscillation which is triggered by the second negative peak N2 of the primary event. The equation fitted to the AEP is

$$v(T) = V_1[\sin(\omega_1 T + \varphi)e^{-\alpha_1 T} - \sin\varphi\cos\omega_1 T\,e^{-\beta T}] \tag{70}$$
$$+ V_2\sin[\omega_2(T - T_n)]\,e^{-\alpha_2(T - T_n)},$$

where $V_2 = 0$ for $t < T_n$, and T_n is the delay in onset of the secondary oscillation with frequency ω_2 and decay rate α_2. A set of 12 AEPs is selected with amplitudes varying from a high value at the epicenter to low values in the surround. The experimental root loci for the two components are shown in Fig. 6.19b. The dominant component displays KII operation in the first mode, with $\delta_e = \delta_i = -.3$, $K_o = 1.5$, and K_n ranging from 1.0 to .5 (Fig. 6.20a). The secondary component displays KII operation in the second mode, with $\delta_e = -.17$, $\delta_i = -.67$, $K_o = 2.8$, and K_n ranging from 4.4 to 2.3 (Fig. 6.20b). The range of variation in wave amplitude for the dominant component is above the range of the EEG, whereas that of the secondary component is below it. □

Example C. The prepyriform cortex in a cat is undercut to remove all centrifugal input to the bulb and cortex, but the PON, bulb, and LOT are intact. Electrodes are implanted in the LOT for stimulation and in the cortex for recording, and the cat is allowed to recover. Single shocks are given to the LOT at levels ranging from threshold for single evoked

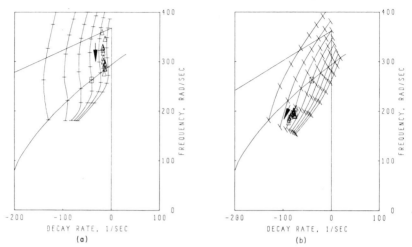

FIG. 6.20. (a) Root locus of minor components in the second mode; $\delta_e = -.17$, $\delta_i = -.67$. (b) Root locus of the dominant component in the first mode of operation of the KII_{MG} set; $\delta_e = \delta_i = -.30$. □: $K_o = K_n = 2.00$.

potentials downward to minimally detectable responses with prolonged averaging and upward to about 4 times threshold. AEPs are collected and measured with Eq. (203) in Chapter 2. The experimental root locus in the lower part of the wave amplitude range (Fig. 6.21a) demonstrates KII operation in the second mode, with $\delta_e = +.33$, $K_o = 2.0$ and K_n ranging from 2.5 to 1.5. The upper part of the wave amplitude range (Fig. 6.21b) demonstrates

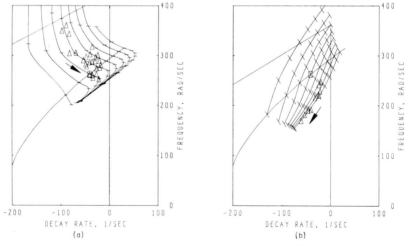

FIG. 6.21. Root locus plots in the s plane for KII operation in the (a) second mode and (b) first mode. (a) $\delta_e = .33$; $\delta_i = -1.67$. (b) $\delta_e = \delta_i = -.30$.

KII operation in the first mode, with $\delta_e = \delta_i = -.30$, $K_o = 3.0$, and K_n ranging from 2.0 to 0.7. The transition from the second to the first mode occurs when the single responses and the EEG have about the same amplitudes. For both sets of experimental and theoretical root loci the frequency decreases with increasing wave amplitude.

These same data are shown in Fig. 5.25 in Section 5.4.2, in which the cortical KII set is described in terms of an equivalent single negative feedback loop. The feedback gain K_2 and lumped feedback delay T_2 are both variable. Experimental root loci from KII operation in the second mode, when transformed from the s plane to $K_2 \cdot T_2$ coordinates, are commonly found to take approximately the form of straight lines. The same property holds for theoretical root loci in the second mode (Fig. 6.22a), over a range of variation in K_n in the vicinity of K_o. The transformation is useful, because it offers a simple, direct method for determining whether a neural mass is operating in the KII first mode (Fig. 6.22b) or second mode (Fig. 6.22a). Moreover, the parameters tend to be normally distributed after the transformation, which is useful in statistical analysis (Section 7.1.2). □

A change in the AEP also may result from interaction between the AEP in response to a fixed stimulus and the changing EEG. The clearest instance is "spontaneous" variation of the AEP, when the stimulus intensity of the LOT is fixed at a level near threshold for single responses observed against the EEG. Sets of AEPs are collected from waking, minimally restrained animals at rest. Each AEP differs slightly from the others on successive

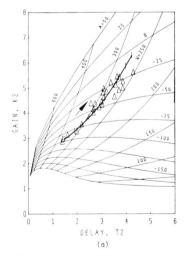
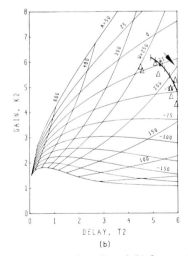

FIG. 6.22. Root locus plots for KII operation in the (a) second mode and (b) first mode following transformation of the data in Fig. 6.21 into $K_2 \cdot T_2$ coordinates (see Fig. 5.25).

trials, and the measurements of frequency ω and decay rate α vary seemingly at random from trial to trial. There is covariance of ω and α, such that sets of values serve to define an experimental root locus for "spontaneous" variation. The phenomenon is present in both the bulb and the cortex, but it is more prominent in the cortex.

Example D. A waking cat with implanted electrodes is given single shocks to the LOT at a rate of 7/sec and at threshold for single responses recorded in the prepyriform cortex. AEPs are summed over 100 shocks. A set 30 AEPs is measured with Eq. (203) in Chapter 2, and the values for ω and α are plotted as points in the upper left quadrant of the s plane (Fig. 6.23a). The slope of the experimental root locus in comparison to those in Fig. 6.18a suggests that a value for $\delta_e = .33$ in the second mode is appropriate. From the family of curves in Fig. 6.23a, the value for K_o is 2.5, and values for K_n ranges from .6 to 2.0. The same data are shown in Fig. 6.23b, following transformation of the values for ω and α into $K_2 \cdot T_2$ coordinates, as in Example C. Again, there is almost linear covariance between K_2 and T_2 for the theoretical and experimental root loci. □

Example E. The covariation of K_2 and T_2 is observed in the prepyriform cortical AEPs on LOT stimulation in many differing behavioral states and over a wide range of stimulus intensities in all animals thus far observed. A composite set of data is shown in Fig. 6.23c, in which the covariation of $K_2 \cdot T_2$ from 30 AEPS in each of 9 cats is represented by a regression line and 95% confidence intervals. The regression parameters (mean $\pm$SE) are

$$K_2 = 1.03(\pm.36) + 1.06(\pm.11)\,T_2. \tag{71}$$

The mean and 95% confidence intervals are

$$K_2 = 5.2 \pm .56, \qquad T_2 = 3.9 \pm .51. \tag{72}$$

Theoretical root loci in $K_2 \cdot T_2$ coordinates are shown in Fig. 6.23d for $\delta_e = .33$, $\delta_i = -1.67$, and $K_o = 2.0\pm.5$. The implied means and 95% confidence ranges are

$$
\begin{aligned}
K_n &= 1.80 \quad (1.40\text{--}2.20),\\
K_e &= .96 \quad (.89\text{--}1.04),\\
K_i &= .83 \quad (.55\text{--}1.20),
\end{aligned}
\tag{73}
$$

by Eqs. (11).

Because the stimulus intensity is fixed, the pattern of "spontaneous" variation must reflect a randomly changing state of the bulb or cortex with respect to its gain parameters. The congruence of theoretical and

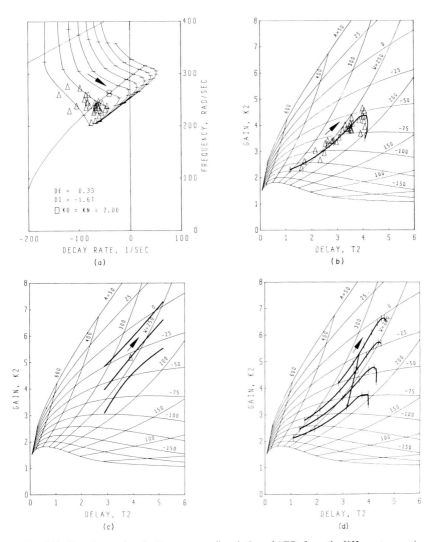

FIG. 6.23. Root locus plots for "spontaneous" variation of AEPs from the KII_{AB} set operating in the second mode on LOT stimulation. (a) Example of experimental values of ω and α from 30 AEPs of a cat during a standard behavioral state (working in an ergometer, Section 7.1.2) and of theoretical root loci with $\delta_e = .33$ in the second mode. (b) Transformation of data in (a) into $K_2 \cdot T_2$ coordinates; theoretical root locus (thick curve) is for $K_o = 1.25$, $\delta_e = .33$, K_n from 2.0 to .5. (c) Regression line from Eq. (71) for average "spontaneous" covariation of K_2 and T_2 from AEPs of 9 cats; upper and lower curves denote 95% confidence intervals; $\triangle$ denotes means in Eq. (72). (d) Transformation of selected theoretical root loci from (a) into $K_2 \cdot T_2$ coordinates with $\delta_e = .33$ in second mode; arrow shows direction of decreasing K_n; $\square$ denotes $K_o = K_n = 2$; slash marks show K_n in steps of .2; near-vertical curve is the locus for the reduced KII set.

experimental root loci in Figs. 6.23c and d implies that the variation is attributable to random variation in the degree of saturation due to EEG activity in the KII set. Equations (73) indicate that if the negative feedback gain K_n varies randomly, the standard deviation of the distribution of values is about $\pm 11\%$ of the mean value of K_n.   □

Example F.   The procedure in Example D is repeated for fixed stimulation of either the PON or the LOT, while taking the AEPs from the olfactory bulb. The data are shown in $K_2 \cdot T_2$ coordinates in Fig. 6.24. The same covariance is observed in bulbar AEPs irrespective of stimulus site.   □

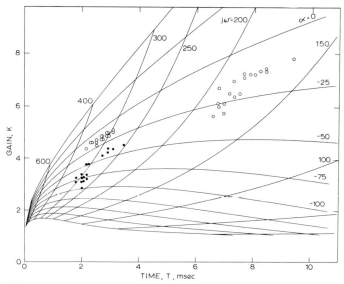

Fig. 6.24. Experimental root locus for "spontaneous" variation of the KII$_{MG}$ set operating in the second mode on LOT (○) or PON (●) stimulation in $K_2 \cdot T_2$ coordinates. (Freeman, 1972c).

The almost linear covariance between K_2 and T_2 is observed in "spontaneous" variation of AEPs from the bulb and cortex of anesthetized cats and rabbits, but the range of variation is much smaller. The amplitude of the EEG is also much lower in anesthetized animals than in waking animals.

6.2. Limit Cycle States: Mechanisms of the EEG

6.2.1. STABILITY PROPERTIES OF KII SETS

The experimental data we have considered thus far consist mainly of AEPs and PSTHs, which invariably decay to the prestimulus baseline, provided the time base for averaging is long enough. In most conditions the EEGs of the bulb and cortex decay to very low amplitudes in a few seconds, if one blocks the air flow over the olfactory mucosa by pinching the nostrils shut, thus forcing the animal to breathe through the mouth. It is appropriate then to use an explanatory model in which the equations have a stable equilibrium. However, in some conditions the EEG of the bulb or cortex displays high-amplitude sustained oscillation, which may continue for hours independently of respiration, and which is clearly the manifestation of stable limit cycle behavior of the bulb or cortex. To investigate these conditions we must analyze the stability properties of the KII set to determine how it may become unstable and whether it can display limit cycle behavior.

The nonlinear equations (5) describing the KII set have an equilibrium point at $v = 0$, $p = p_o$. The system linearized at the equilibrium point consists of a single negative feedback loop. For increasing values of K_o in the linearized system there are two complex root loci which cross the $j\omega$ axis into the right half of the s plane at about $\omega = 290$ rad/sec (the locus curving upward to the right in Fig. 6.22a and preceding figures). The value for K_o at the crossing is about 3.3. For $K_o < 3.3$ the linearized system is stable, and for $K_o > 3.3$ it is unstable.

If the system linearized at equilibrium is stable, then the nonlinear system is locally stable for small perturbations. But if it is linearized instead at the operating points, the stability of the nonlinear system cannot be directly inferred from the stability of the linearized system. In the first mode the maximal gain in every loop is K_o, and input driving the system away from equilibrium can only decrease the feedback gains. Therefore, the local domain of stability of the nonlinear system must include most operating points in the first mode. However, the stability is not global for two reasons. First, the transfer function of the KII set contains zeros in the right half of the s plane. Second, in the second mode the maximal values of K_e, K_i, or K_n may exceed K_o. That is, even with the constraint that $K_o < 3.3$, we can expect the KII set to become unstable under certain conditions. The problem is how to determine those conditions.

If $K_o > 3.3$, the KII set linearized at equilibrium is unstable, but the distributed nonlinear reduced KII set is stable, in the sense that it has a locally stable nonzero equilibrium for $K_o < 3.3$ and a locally stable limit cycle for $K_o > 3.3$ (Ahn & Freeman, 1974a, b). Proof has not yet been devised for the existence of a stable limit cycle for the full KII set. Intuitive reasons have been given for expecting nonlinear stability of KI sets (Section 5.1.4). Essentially for the same reasons the KII set is nonlinearly stable. If the KII system linearized at the operating point $v_e = v_e^*$, $v_i = v_i^*$ has a complex pole pair in the right half of the s plane, oscillatory activity must increase in amplitude until the gains are reduced by saturation, and the poles move to the $j\omega$ axis.

In the absence of proof, the following rules are conjectured in terms of the root locus plots of the KII set linearized at the effective operating points.

(1)   If the roots all lie in the left half of the s plane, the nonlinear KII set has a stable equilibrium to which the active states return when input is terminated.

(2)   If complex conjugate poles lie on root loci in the right of the s plane, the poles move on the root loci in the direction of decreasing K_n to the $j\omega$ axis and stay there, and the KII set has a stable limit cycle.

(3)   If two conjugate root loci cross the $j\omega$ axis from the left half into the right half of the s plane with decreasing K_n, the KII set has an unstable limit cycle.

The basis for these rules is the set of experimental findings that in the left half of the s plane, where experimental root loci are observable, they conform to theoretical root loci. Both types of root loci are functions of wave amplitude. We then infer that the same conformance holds in the right half of the s plane, in which experimental root loci are not observable, but in which there is the same theoretical relation between wave amplitude and complex frequency as in the left half. According to these rules stable limit cycle activity is expected (though not proven) of a KII set in at least three conditions. They are increased K_e in the first mode, decreased K_i in the first mode, and increased K_o in either mode. Each of these predicted limit cycle states is found to correspond to an experimental condition, in which limit cycle activity is observed in the olfactory bulb or cortex.

In addition to complex root loci crossing the $j\omega$ axis the KII set has a root locus on the real axis of the s plane (Figs. 6.3 and 6.4). For certain high values of $K_n > K_o$ in the second mode (which are forbidden in the first mode) the root locus crosses into the right half of the s plane with increasing K_n and decreasing amplitude v. As in the case of the KI$_P$ set (Section 5.2.3) there is a stable nonzero equilibrium for values of v and of K_n that gives a pole at the origin of the s plane. If K_n is sufficiently high to give a pole on the right real axis, activity should increase in the KII set until K_n is reduced and the pole moves to the origin. The resulting value of K_n constitutes an upper limit on the range of stable values for K_n, which is reflected in an upper limit on the values that ω and α of complex pole pairs can take in the s plane. For different values of K_o there is a boundary in the s plane, which is shown in Figs. 6.8, 6.11, 6.18, 6.20, 6.21, and 6.23 as a diagonal line between 300 and 400 rad/sec. Then according to the KII model linearized at the operating point (v_e^*, v_i^*), the values for $(\alpha, j\omega)$ from AEPs should not occur above the diagonal line. This suggested constraint is sometimes violated but not commonly.

Of course, not all EEG patterns suggest limit cycle operation, though many patterns do. The proposal to be described is that in waking or anesthetized animals the bulb and cortex are at some times in the nonzero equilibrium state and at other times in the limit cycle state. They often switch between the two states. Switching to either state can occur in either mode 1 or mode 2 and either with or without deliberate stimulation. That is, at times oscillations occur in the EEG because the bulb or cortex is "ringing" in response to random pulse input and at other times the oscillation is due to limit cycle activity, which a naive observer might call "spontaneous."

6.2.2. LIMIT CYCLE STATES IN THE FIRST MODE

In Section 6.1.4 the value for $\delta_e = \delta_i$ in the first mode is interpreted as manifesting an operating bias in the KII set, which is a displacement of the effective operating points toward the excitatory or inhibitory sides. If the bias is excitatory and $\delta_e > -.33$, the displacement increases the saturation (gain reduction) in the KI_e set and decreases it in the KI_i set. Then some other condition that decreases K_e might give a value for $\delta_e > -.33$. Conversely if the bias is inhibitory and $\delta_e < -.33$, the displacement increases the saturation (gain reduction) in the KI_i set and decreases it in the KI_e set, so that some other condition causing a decrease in KI_i might give a value for $\delta_e < -.33$.

Values for $\delta_e = \delta_i$ of $+1$ and -1 have special significance when seen from this point of view. From Eqs. (11), when $\delta_e = \delta_i = 1$,

$$K_n = (K_e K_o)^{.5}, \qquad K_i = K_o. \tag{74}$$

In this case the forward gain of the inhibitory subsets is fixed, and the change in K_n is due solely to variation in $K_e^{.5}$, the forward gain of the excitatory subsets. Conversely, when $\delta_e = \delta_i = -1$,

$$K_n = (K_i K_o)^{.5}, \qquad K_e = K_o. \tag{75}$$

In this case the excitatory forward gain is fixed, and variation in the negative feedback gain depends solely on changes in the inhibitory forward gain. Therefore, the model provides the basis for predicting the effects on the KII set of changing selectively the level of forward gain of either the KI_e set or KI_i set.

Example A. Stimulating and recording electrodes are placed on the exposed surface of the PON to record the bulbar EEG and evoked potentials in an anesthetized cat. Preliminary records are obtained of the EEG and the AEP. A cotton pledget soaked in 4% picrotoxin in Tyrode's solution is applied to the surface of the bulb around the monopolar recording electrode.

The effect within the first 5 min is to abolish the AEP and EEG. If the stimulus intensity is approximately doubled, the AEP reappears, but the surface-negative baseline shift is diminished, and the decay rate is greatly increased (Fig. 6.25, upper trace). After 5 to 15 min the EEG reappears as a sustained sinusoidal oscillation at high amplitude (several millivolts, which is 10–20 times the normal EEG amplitude), and at a frequency of 125 to 150 rad/sec (20–24 Hz). The AEP has the same frequency as the EEG and a very low decay rate (Fig. 6.25, middle trace). The oscillation persists as long as the picrotoxin is applied, and it terminates within a few minutes after removing the drug and washing with Tyrode's solution. The AEP frequency returns to a higher value, but the baseline shift does not return (Fig. 6.25, lower trace).   □

The effects shown in Fig. 6.25 are achieved by the surface application of 4% nicotine or 2% strychnine in Tyrode's solution as well as by use of picrotoxin. These three agents are believed to block the actions of inhibitory neurons (Eccles, 1964). From Eq. (75) the effect on KII operation of a selective reduction in the forward gain of neurons in the KI_i set is described by operation in the first mode with $\delta_e = \delta_i = -1$. The theoretical root loci in Fig. 6.8d show that for values of K_o from 3.0 to 3.5, the complex poles

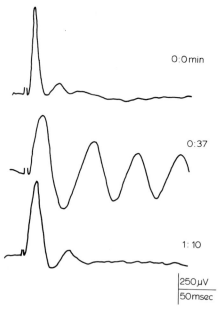

FIG. 6.25. Effect on bulbar AEP from PON stimulation of the local application of 4% picrotoxin with $N = 100$.

lie in the right half of the s plane. With increasing wave amplitude the values for K_n decrease, and the poles move in the direction of decreasing frequency. Between 120 to 150 Hz the root loci cross back to the left half of the s plane. This crossing represents a stable limit cycle, because with further increase in wave amplitude, the poles must move into the left half of the s plane and wave amplitude must decrease and increase K_n. This explanation is incomplete because it is uncertain how the required increase in K_o can occur, and the effects of the drugs on the KI_P set manifested in the disappearance of the baseline shift are not accounted for.

Example B. In Example E in Section 6.1.3 it is shown that the effect of pentobarbital on the bulbar AEP from PON stimulation is to decrease the frequency with little effect on the decay rate. The theoretical root locus (Fig. 6.11e) that conforms to the experimental root locus is for $\delta_e = \delta_i = -1$. In Section 6.1.3 the effect is interpreted as manifesting an inhibitory bias during the reduction in background activity by pentobarbital. Here it is interpreted as the effect of selective reduction in K_i in the KI_i set on the bulbar AEPs, because while pentobarbital does in fact reduce background activity, it is thought to act by suppressing the actions of inhibitory neurons (Eccles, 1957). Pentobarbital has virtually the same effect on prepyriform cortical AEPs on LOT stimulation. This is not the only effect of the anesthetic on the bulb and cortex. In some experiments there is a marked decrease in the decay rate of AEPs in the low frequency range of 50 to 100 rad/sec (8 to 16 Hz), and a selective increase in sensitivity of the cortex to LOT stimulus rates of about 10/sec (Freeman, 1960b). The change in the cortex can be represented (Fig. 6.11e) by a concomitant decrease in K_n to 0.7 and increase in K_o to 4.0. The physiological basis for the required increase in K_o is unclear. However, under moderately deep pentobarbital anesthesia there are characteristic short bursts of near-sinusoidal wave activity at about 12 Hz (Gault & Leaton, 1963), which occur at irregular intervals. That is, the experimental data show that an instability of the cortex occurs in the conditions and with the properties suggested by the root loci in Fig. 6.11e (see also Libet & Gerard, 1939; Yamamoto & Yamamoto, 1962).   □

Example C. A hypodermic needle cannula is inserted into Layer I of the prepyriform cortex for the injection of microgram amounts of drugs in crystalline form (Biedenbach, 1966). The cannula is electrically insulated on its shaft, which ends 1 or 2 mm above the tip, so that bipolar recordings are made from the site of injection across the prepyriform dipole zero isopotential surface (Section 4.4.2). A stimulating electrode is placed in the LOT, and after the several leads and the cannula are cemented to the skull, the animal is allowed to recover for two weeks.

The injection of crystalline acetylcholine chloride has no detectable effect on the AEP. When it is combined with prostigmine sulfate which blocks the hydrolysis of acetylcholine by cholinesterase, there is a short-lasting change in the wave form of the AEP, consisting of a decrease in frequency ω and decay rate α with no significant change in amplitude V_1. The same change in the AEP (Fig. 6.26a) is caused by injection of 2 to 7 μgm of a cholinomimetic drug, carbaminoylcholine (carbachol), but they are greater and last longer (carbachol is not hydrolyzed by cholinesterase). The EEG shows high amplitude bursts with each inspiration, which in 15 to 40 min become continuous and independent of respiration (Fig. 6.26b).

The pattern of change in ω and α from 7 cats is shown in the s plane in Fig. 6.27c. The same data are shown in $K_2 \cdot T_2$ coordinates in Fig. 6.27d. From Eq. (74) it is inferred that the effect of the drugs is to increase the values of K_e. That is, cholinomimetic agents can be inferred to enhance the forward gain of the KI_A set of superficial pyramidal cells in the prepyriform cortex. This of course does not prove that acetylcholine is the transmitter substance of these neurons (for a review see Pradhan & Dutta, 1971), but it shows that substances which either block cholinesterase or mimic the effects of acetylcholine appear to increase the forward gain of the neurons in the set. Theoretical root loci for $\delta_e = \delta_i = +1$ are shown in Figs. 6.27a and b.

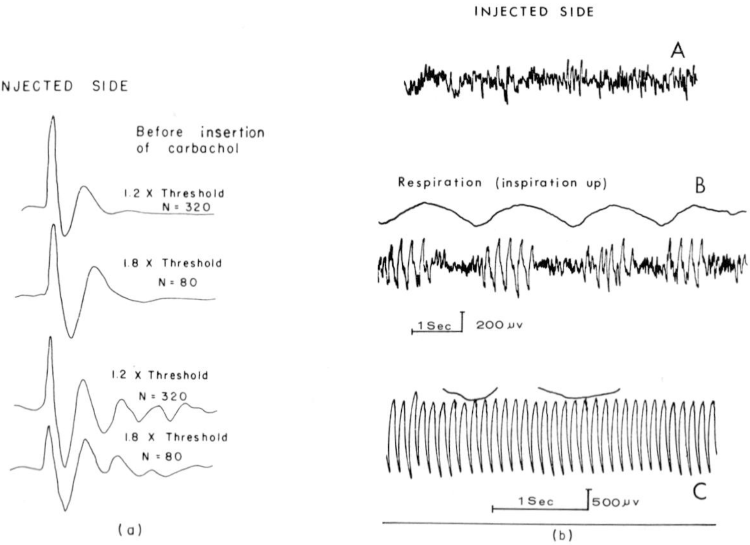

FIG. 6.26. (a) Prepyriform AEPs at two levels of LOT stimulation before insertion (upper pair) and 45 min after insertion of carbachol into the recording site. (b) Prepyriform EEG activity before insertion of carbachol (A) ±45 min later (B), and 85 min later (C) (Biedenbach, 1966).

This holds for the AEPs. The limit cycle activity in the EEG cannot be explained by a unitary change in the KII_{AB} set, because the frequency is too low. It is possible to explain it by assuming in addition that K_o is reduced significantly by carbachol, but it is more likely that complex changes occur involving feedback loops between the KII_{AB} set and other sets at the KIII level (see Section 6.2.4). □

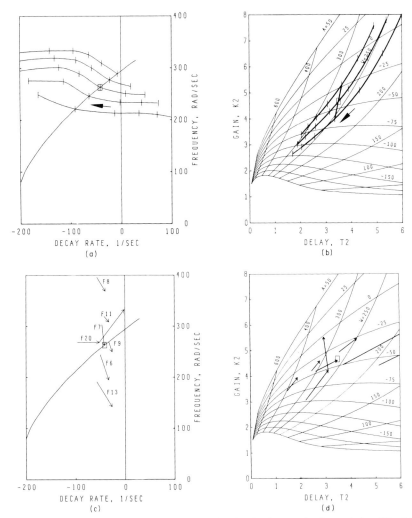

FIG. 6.27. (a) Root locus plot for KII operation in the first mode, $\delta_e = +1$ (see Fig. 6.7). (b) Transformation of the lower three curves in (a) into $K_2 \cdot T_2$ coordinates. (c) Changes in AEP from before to after insertion of carbachol (data from Biedenbach, 1966). (d) Transformation of (c) into $K_2 \cdot T_2$ coordinates. □: $K_o = K_n = 2.00$.

These examples show that limit cycle activity can be induced in the bulb and in the cortex by drugs that are known to alter the chemistry of synaptic transmission. The KII model linearized at the operating points gives reason to expect stable limit cycle behavior either for sufficient increase in K_e or for sufficient decrease in K_i. The model does not prove the existence of limit cycles and does not allow calculation of the limits of the domains of stability. It can suggest the nature of drug actions, but it cannot predict them with sufficient precision to specify main effects and side effects. Before the field of the pharmacology of neural masses can be adequately explored, the nonlinear equations should be thoroughly explored, which is a very difficult task. However, the linearized model can provide guidelines to the structure of the nonlinear equations, in preparation for the work of obtaining particular solutions.

6.2.3. LIMIT CYCLE STATES IN THE SECOND MODE

The characteristic property of the EEG both of the bulb and of the cortex is the occurrence of bursts of sinusoidal activity with each inspiration (Fig. 6.28). The frequency of oscillation in each burst is centered at 40 Hz. The burst phenomenon was first observed by Adrian (1950) who called it the "induced wave" to distinguish it from the low-amplitude EEG activity ("intrinsic wave") between bursts (Fig. 6.29). The bursts ("induced waves") can be interpreted as manifesting limit cycle behavior of the KII set in the second mode.

The families of theoretical root loci shown in Figs. 6.18b and 6.23a imply that if K_o exceeds 2.6 to 3.0 and δ_e exceeds 0 to .33, the theoretical root loci cross into the right half of the s plane with decreasing values of K_n, and then cross back into the left half at a lower frequency on the $j\omega$ axis. The remarkable feature is that for widely ranging values of K_o and δ_e above the designated levels, the second crossing occurs in a relatively narrow frequency range from 245 to 263 rad/sec (39 to 42 Hz). This range is virtually identical to the range of frequencies (40 ± 3 Hz) observed in the sinusoidal bursts of bulbar and cortical EEG, which accompany inspiration in waking, unrestrained animals (Section 3.3.1). The correspondance is evidence that the KII_{MG} set operates in the second mode in generating these bursts.

The inferred mechanism is as follows. With each inspiration there is a sustained volley of impulses delivered from the receptors to the glomeruli by way of the PON. The mean activity in many parts of the bulb increases (Fig. 6.29), both in respect to the pulse mode p_o and the wave mode $\tilde{v}_i$ as defined in Sections 3.3.4–3.3.6. The maximal forward gain of each KO set is defined [Eq. (4)] as

$$g_o = -2p_o\tilde{v}_i, \tag{76}$$

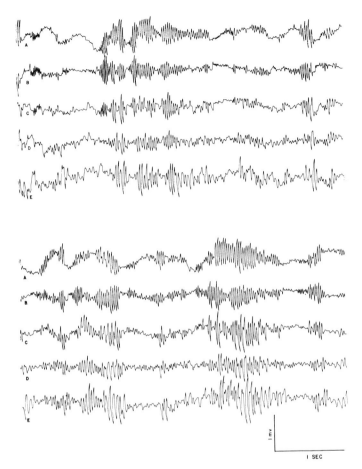

FIG. 6.28. Bursts of EEG activity from olfactory bulb (A) and prepyriform cortex (B–E) in a waking cat (Freeman, 1960a).

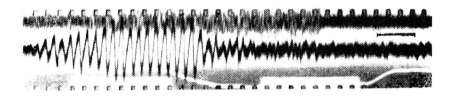

FIG. 6.29. Induced wave begins after the onset of pulse activity. Inspiration marked by upper white line. Upper tracing is a surface EEG recording, and lower tracing shows pulse activity in the white matter. Time mark is 0.1 sec (Adrian, 1950).

where p_o is KII mean pulse rate and $\tilde{v}_i$ is the linearized pulse to wave conversion factor. Both the slope of the sigmoid input–output curve (Figs. 3.20 and 3.21) and the maximal loop gain, $K_o = g_o^2$, in each KI set increase.

The input also contains a transient which initiates oscillatory activity in subsets in many parts of the bulb, and which can be treated as a set of impulses (Section 2.3.1). It is likely that the afferent surge to the bulb is not spatially uniform so that the operating characteristics of the KII_{MG} set are not spatially uniform. The effective amplitude of local transient input determines local wave amplitudes and the local value for K_n. The level of sustained local PON input determines the new local values of p_o, $\tilde{v}_i$, and K_o. The ratio of sustained input to transient input determines the local bias which specifies δ_e.

At the onset of inspiration the evoked activity is greater than the pre-existing activity, so the KII_{MG} mass is operating in the nonzero equilibrium stable state in the first mode with $\delta_e = \delta_i$. Due to the activity of peri-glomerular neurons it is likely that $\delta_e > 0$, so that, in respect to local variations of the effective amplitude of PON transient input, the frequencies of local subsets converge to values in the vicinity of 300 rad/sec (50 Hz). In respect to local variations in K_o, there is likely to be a distribution of frequencies around 50 Hz. If $K_o > 3.3$ and $K_n > 3.3$ in the first mode, the closed loop poles for some local subsets must lie to the right of the $j\omega$ axis, and the amplitudes of oscillatory activity in those subsets must increase exponentially (Fig. 6.30). The KII set enters the stable limit cycle state in the first mode.

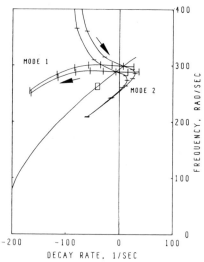

FIG. 6.30. It is suggested that the 40-Hz burst in the EEG arises when a previously stable limit cycle near 50 to 60 Hz becomes unstable, as the KII set switches from the first mode to the second mode. $\square$: $K_o = K_n = 2.00$.

If the KII_{MG} set continues to operate in the first mode, the increase in wave amplitude causes K_n to decrease, and the closed loop poles move to the $j\omega$ axis and remain there for as long as the values for K_o remain high. The dynamics of each local subset enter a limit cycle (Ahn & Freeman, 1974a, b), and the frequencies of oscillation remain dispersed. This is a mechanism for the "intrinsic" bulbar EEG at a relatively high mean frequency and low amplitude as described by Adrian (1950) and shown in Fig. 6.29 from his work.

The onset of exponentially increasing oscillation may, however, cause a change in KII operation to the second mode, in which the closed loop poles move away from the $j\omega$ axis downward, and then to a range of convergence near $j\omega = 250$ rad/sec (Fig. 6.30). If the poles move past this point into the left half of the s plane with increasing wave amplitude and decreasing K_n, the decay rates become negative, and the amplitude decreases. Then K_n increases and the poles move again toward and across the $j\omega$ axis. Intuitively, it is seen that the convergence range contains stable limit cycles, and as long as K_o is held at a high value, the activity of all local subsets oscillates at nearly the same frequency, irrespective of local variations in K_o, δ_e, δ_i, and the amplitude of initial input. When the afferent surge terminates after the end of inspiration, and when its effects have dissipated in the KI_P set, the value for K_o decreases, and the burst terminates. The KII set returns from the stable limit cycle state to the stable equilibrium state.

This is the proposed mechanism for the "induced wave" of Adrian. The activity of the bulbar KII set does not oscillate at 40 Hz in response to an impulse or a collection of impulses. The frequencies of the impulse responses are distributed around 50 Hz. Instead, the KII set is induced by sustained PON input and by the input from the KI_P set into an unstable state in which local oscillations increase and converge to stable limit cycles with narrowly distributed frequencies and high amplitudes. The process is observed by direct inspection of the EEG in which bursts characteristically begin at low amplitude and high frequency and evolve rapidly to oscillation at high amplitude and low frequency (Figs. 6.28, 6.29, and 3.12).

This result is fundamentally important in respect to the nature of bulbar and cortical operation. The EEG is the manifestation of summed dendritic currents from large numbers of neurons. High-amplitude EEG waves can only occur at high frequencies, if the oscillatory activities of the neurons generating the EEG have common or nearly common frequencies. Shared frequencies can arise either because the local subsets of neurons in KII sets have common characteristics, in which case the frequencies converge, or because the local subsets of neurons are coupled by interconnections, in which case the oscillations are pulled together or entrained. Entrainment implies further that the phase of the oscillation of each local subset becomes fixed or is locked to the oscillation of the response domain.

Whereas local interaction is the basis for the existence of oscillation, there is no evidence that the interaction required for global entrainment across response foci is sufficiently strong. The phase gradients found to exist over the bulbar (Fig. 4.32) and cortical (Fig. 4.43) surfaces for evoked activity, and over the cortical surface of the EEG (Boudreau & Freeman, 1963) are evidence against entrainment. The theoretical root loci shown in Figs. 6.18b and 6.21b show that there is no need to resort to the mathematics of coupled nonlinear oscillators (Dewan, 1964) to describe the bulbar and cortical EEG frequency convergence. This result further justifies the assumption that the nonlinear operations of KI and KII sets can be described by piecewise linear approximations, because the nonlinearities are solely of the saturation kind. That is, they are amplitude dependent and not time dependent. Further implications from this result are discussed in Sections 7.2.1–7.2.3.

6.2.4. Sources of Error and Limitation

Errors of measurement arise from the fitting of sums of damped sine waves to AEPs, partly because the background EEG is never completely averaged out, and partly because strictly linear functions do not conform ideally to the bulbar and cortical impulse responses. The deviations are apparent in the residual least mean squares deviations. The extent of error can be estimated for any one AEP in the presence of "spontaneous" variation by measuring the distance from its point in the s plane to the regression line between ω and α, or by measuring pairs of AEP taken concomitantly from two different sites in a response focus. The error is smallest with high values of ω and low values of α, which derive from prolonged damped sine waves. As a general rule the 67% confidence interval for values of ω is ± 6 rad/sec; for α it is ± 3/sec; and for φ it is .1 rad. The 67% confidence intervals for single AEPs at low amplitude and without correction for "spontaneous" variation are about 5 times greater.

There is a systematic error in the measurement of α which is introduced by random variation of ω during averaging to obtain the AEP. If the frequency is a random variable with mean ω_o and standard deviation σ_ω, the sum of a set of impulse responses given by $\sin(\omega t)e^{-\alpha t}$ empirically (Freeman, 1963) can be approximated by

$$v(T) = \sin(\omega_o T)e^{-(\alpha + \sigma_\omega)T}. \qquad (77)$$

For example, if $\omega_o = 250$ rad/sec, $\sigma_\omega = \pm 25$ rad/sec and $\alpha = 0$, the sum of the distributed undamped sine waves diminishes with time in a Gaussian curve, which can be fitted with the curve

$$v(T) = \sin(250T)e^{-25T}. \qquad (78)$$

The ranges of variation of EEG and AEP frequencies suggest that σ_ω may be commonly 5–10% of ω_o, so that the estimates for α from AEPs may exceed the true average values for α by up to 30/sec.

This systematic error implies that the experimental root loci are displaced to the left of the $j\omega$ axis from their true positions by the averaging process. This does not alter the interpretation of the dynamics of the KII set in a significant way, but it results in estimates for K_o or K_n that are lower than their true values, depending on the orientation of the experimental root locus with respect to the $j\omega$ axis.

In making estimates for ω and α in order to evaluate the closed loop transfer functions for the bulb and cortex (Sections 5.3.3 and 5.4.2), we assume that the KII set is in the reduced state. This assumption is justified by asserting that when the stimulus intensity is fixed at or near the threshold for single responses against the EEG, the "spontaneous" variation causes the values for K_n to fluctuate randomly about the mean at K_o at which, in the second mode, $K_e = K_i = K_n$. The variations between animals in the estimates for ω and α in this state may be due either to failure of the assumption to hold, or to variation in the open loop rate constants between animals (see Sections 2.5.2 and 5.3.2). For convenience the composite values from the bulb and cortex are used to evaluate the open loop transfer function for the KII set, and to compute theoretical root loci. If there are variations in open loop rate constants between animals, the effect is to distort the values estimated for the feedback gains, but the basic dynamics are not altered.

The use in the computations of the same asymmetric nonlinear gain characteristic for all sites of wave to pulse conversion in both KII_{AB} and KII_{MG} set (Section 6.1.1) is feasible for two reasons. First, the bulbar and cortical outputs in the first and second modes are taken from only one KI set in each KII set, so that differences between the performance characteristics of the KI_e and KI_i sets cannot be detected by concomitant measurements. Second, differences between KI_e and KI_i operations may be incorporated into the values for δ_e and δ_i. For example, the nonlinear gain characteristic displayed in the pulse probability gradients for background activity of KI_B neurons imply that the dominating nonlinearity in that set is for pulse to wave conversion (Fig. 3.19 in Section 3.3.6), and not for wave to pulse conversion as assumed in Section 6.1.1 (Fig. 3.19b). The asymmetry between the curvatures and asymptotes of the two sigmoid input–output curves (A and B) is greater for pulse to wave conversion (a) than for wave to pulse conversion (b) by a factor of three. The assumption that the 2 to 1 asymmetry of wave to pulse conversion holds throughout the KII_{AB} set may in part give rise to the apparent inhibitory bias, which is inferred from the values for $\delta_e = \delta_i$ of $-.60$ to -1.0 for cortical AEPs during KII_{AB} operation in the first mode (Section 6.1.4 and Fig. 6.8d).

The assumption that the same wave to pulse nonlinearity holds in the KII_{MG} set for both mitral–tufted cells and granule cells is justified only by the conformance of theoretical and experimental root loci, because the granule cells do not generate extracellularly detectable action potentials. The dendritic spines of the granule cells are indistinguishable from axonal boutons in electromicrographs, and the narrow stalks might serve to electrically uncouple all-or-none discharges of neighboring spines while permitting the main dendritic stem to transmit steady bias currents into the boutons, so desynchronization of the activity in spines can account for the absence of detectable extracellular action potentials. In mass actions the KI_{MG} set operates as if the KI_G and KI_M neurons maintain the same amplitude-dependent nonlinear transformations.

In order to show that the nonlinear input–output curves of the excitatory and inhibitory neurons in a KII set are different, it will be necessary to find a KII set in which outputs are observable in the wave and pulse modes for both KI_e and KI_i sets. The nearest approach to this goal is the KII_{AB} set in which the KI_A set has observable output in the wave and pulse mode, and the KI_B set has observable output in the pulse mode only (Section 5.4.1).

In this case it is possible to estimate $g_o = K_o^{.5}$ for the KII_{AB} set from $g_o = -2p_o\gamma\zeta\tilde{v}_i$. The mean value $p_o = 12.7$ pulses/sec in Table 3.2 gives the mean firing rates of Type A units. The empirical rate constant for wave to pulse conversion is the mean of $\gamma = 1.64/mV$. In Table 3.3 the mean value for $\zeta = 0.42/$pulses/second, the empirical rate constant for pulse to wave conversion, and $\tilde{v}_i = -3.06\sigma$, where $\sigma = -.0444$ mV is the standard deviation of the EEG amplitude. The estimate for $K_o^{.5}$ from the conditional pulse probabilities is 2.37. The estimate for $K_o^{.5}$ from KII_{AB} analysis in Example D in Section 6.1.5 is 1.41.

The two estimates should have the same values because the conditions in which observations are made are similar, except with respect to the conditions of test input. The most likely reasons that the estimates differ are that the value estimated for K_o is too low due to variation of frequency during averaging the AEPs, and that the value for p_o is too high. This is due to a bias in the observer to pick units for analysis that are firing at relatively high rates. Due to the difficulty in determining unbiased values for p_o or in defining an equivalent value for p_o in the KI_G set, p_o is treated as a single parameter for the entire KII set. This is consistent with the assumption that the gain curve is the same for every equivalent KO set.

These considerations show that the techniques of measurements of AEP have sufficient precision to delineate the experimental root loci with enough clarity to fit theoretical root loci to them, and the simplifying assumptions used in computing theoretical root loci are not critical for the results. The estimated values for the feedback gains are less important than the dependence or nondependence of the values on physiological, pharmacological, and behaviorable variables.

There are three present deficiencies with respect to experimental data. The first is the present requirement for simultaneous recording of segments of EEG and pulse trains lasting 20 sec and more as the basis for constructing conditional pulse probability tables (Section 3.3.3). As stated by Elul (1972) it is most likely that the EEG is the gross result of a collection of nonstationary processes in neural masses, and that it is likely that the statistical properties of subsets of neurons undergo changes at intervals of at most a few hundred milliseconds. The first demonstration of the existence of pulse probability waves in the bulb and prepyriform cortex (predicted on the properties of AEPs and PSTHs, Sections 5.3.3 and 5.4.4) was based on segments of the EEG lasting 200 sec or more. With improvements in methods based on better understanding of the neural mechanisms this time interval has been decreased by an order of magnitude, and with foreseeable improvements may be decreased by yet another order of magnitude. We should strive ultimately to examine pulse–wave relations in single bursts lasting only a few hundred milliseconds, but the techniques for doing this are not in hand.

The second is the lack of measurements on transbulbar and transcortical steady potentials. Such measurements require special electrodes and preamplifiers. They are needed as the basis for further analysis of the bias controls postulated to be generated by KI sets and to influence the performance of KII sets (see Section 7.3.2).

The third is the failure of the analysis of KII sets to account for the existence of experimental root loci in the frequency range of 120 to 180 rad/sec (19 to 28 Hz). These frequencies are present in the cortical AEPs of naive cats as subsidiary components, and they usually become the dominant component in the AEPs of attentive cats (see Section 7.1.3). The experimental root loci in this frequency range are very similar to those in the frequency range near 250 rad/sec. Examples are shown in $K_2 \cdot T_2$ coordinates in the right side of Figs. 6.24 and 7.9.

Frequencies of oscillation in this range can be accounted for by assuming low values of K_i for KII operation in the first mode (Fig. 6.8d and Section 6.2.2). However, the experimental root loci cannot be replicated by this means. Moreover, the EEG from the posterior prepyriform cortex commonly shows oscillation at frequencies near 40 and 22 Hz (Figs. 3.1 and 6.28), which implies that two pairs of complex poles exist simultaneously in these frequency ranges. This is not consistent with the properties of the KII set. Cortical AEPs also commonly show the existence of at least 2 spectral peaks (Section 2.53). which implies the coexistence of 2 pairs of complex poles.

Example A. Sets of AEPs are taken with cortical electrodes from cats trained (see Section 7.1.1) to press a lever for milk on LOT stimulation. The stimulus intensity is changed in small steps from below the threshold to well above the threshold, and an AEP is taken at each step. The Fourier transform is taken by numerical integration of each AEP, and the amplitude is plotted as a function of frequency for each spectrum. The spectra are normalized to unit peak amplitude (Fig. 6.31). The lowest spectral curve is the amplitude spectrum (the square root of the power spectrum) from the autocovariance of the EEG recorded from the same electrodes in the same behavioral state. At subthreshold stimulus intensity the AEP activity is concentrated above the upper spectral peak of the EEG. At threshold for trains of evoked potentials, both for the cat and for the observer, there are two spectral peaks in the AEP activity, which correspond approximately to the two peaks in EEG activity. At suprathreshold stimulus intensity the activity in the lower spectral peak for the AEP predominates.   □

The multiple spectral peaks observed in Fourier transforms of AEPs (Section 2.5.3) can be accounted for by the interaction of subsets in the KII$_{AB}$ set with other neural sets at the KIII level. One possibility is that a KII$_{AB}$ subset in the posterior prepyriform interacts with a KI or KII set in the amygdaloid nucleus. Another possibility is that the KO$_C$ set of cortical deep pyramidal cells, which is described in Section 5.4.1 as a noninteractive excitatory set, may transiently become sufficiently interactive in attentive cats to constitute a KI$_C$ set. These and other possibilities have not yet been explored, but they seem to offer considerable promise for further clarification of the cortical mechanism, particularly in regard to the properties of its outflow tracts to adjacent forebrain structures.

Example B. The operation of the KII set has been predicted by solving a 12th-order linear differential equation, and that of the KI set has been predicted by an 8th-order equation. The series topology of a KII set in a negative feedback loop with a KI set need not require a solution of a 20th-order equation, because all of the higher-order poles can be lumped into a single equivalent pole for lumped delay in each set (see Sections 2.3.4 and 2.3.5).

Let the KII set be in a stable state limit cycle with poles at $s = \pm j250$ and $s = -100$. The transfer function is approximated by

$$C(s) = \frac{6.25 \times 10^6}{(s+j250)(s-j250)(s+100)}. \tag{79}$$

Let the KI set be in a stable equilibrium state (Section 5.2.3) with poles at

$s = 0$ and $s = -100$. The transfer function is approximated by

$$P(s) = 10^2/s(s+100).$$ (80)

The transfer function $D(s)$ for output for the KIII set from the KII set

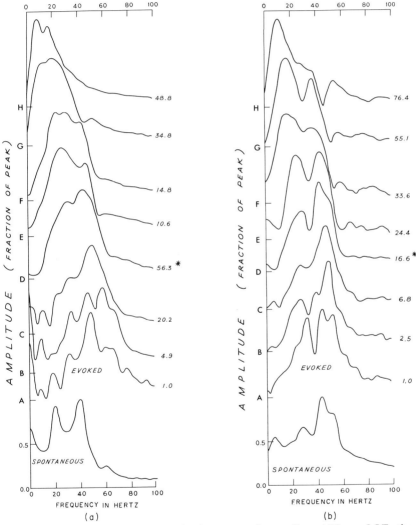

FIG. 6.31. Two example of changes in the spectra of prepyriform AEPs on LOT stimulation with increasing stimulus intensity (see Fig. 2.24). Lower curve in each case is the amplitude spectrum of the EEG (Freeman, 1970). * Transition from mode 1 to mode 2.

with negative feedback from the KI set is

$$D(s) = \frac{C(s)}{1 + K_c C(s) P(s)},$$ (81)

where K_c is the loop gain between the KII set and the KI set. In expanded form,

$$D(s) = \frac{6.25 \times 10^6 s(s+100)}{s(s+j\omega)(s-j\omega)(s+100)^2 + 6.25 \times 10^8 K_c}.$$ (82)

The root locus plot for variation in K_c is shown in Fig. 6.32. For a value of $K_c = 4.2$, there is a pair of complex poles at $s = \pm j140$. The KIII frequency is slightly greater than half the KII characteristic frequency, which is the common property of cortical AEPs and the EEG. □

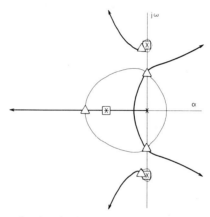

FIG. 6.32. Root locus plot for the interaction at the KIII level of the KII set in the stable limit cycle of the second mode with a KI_e set in the stable nonzero equilibrium mode. For an appropriate level of gain, stable limit cycle activity is predicted at a frequency near 20 Hz.

6.2.5. COMPARISONS WITH RELATED MATHEMATICAL MODELS

Earlier mathematical models of neural mass actions dealt mainly if not exclusively with excitatory interactions (e.g., Beurle, 1956). Recently several models have been developed with the KII set as their starting point. In each model the subsequent development differs from that given here, and the differences are instructive.

Wilson & Cowan (1973) postulate a distributed set of excitatory and inhibitory neurons in a sheet, in which each neuron has input from itself and both other types and output to itself and both other types (Fig. 6.33a and b).

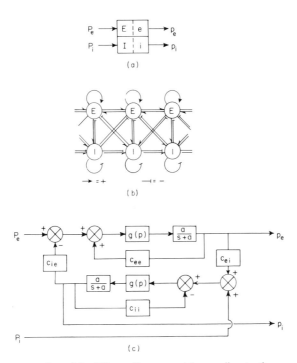

FIG. 6.33. Representation of the Wilson–Cowan model according to the conventions used in the text.

The connection densities of each neuron with others diminish exponentially with distance. Each set of neurons sums the input on all its input channels and operates on the sum by a nonlinear sigmoid input–output function. The sum is passed through a linear filter and excites the fraction of neurons in its set that are not refractory, to give the output of the set. The mathematical description consists of two coupled nonlinear integrodifferential equations. They are solved by use of simplifying approximations and computer techniques. They yield several interesting spatial properties, such as Mach bands, hysteresis effects, and spreading waves of activity for selected inputs and combinations of parameters. However, we have no experimental data here on which to base comment on these spatial properties.

In a preceding report (Wilson & Cowan, 1972) they describe a simpler model that results from reducing the distributed model to a point on the surface. Their point approximation is different from the lumped approximation of the KII set given here in several ways, relating to the topology, the time dependence, and the amplitude dependence.

In regard to topology, the Wilson–Cowan model includes channels for autoexcitation and autoinhibition (Fig. 6.33b), as well as for mutual excitation and mutual inhibition. The autoexcitatory and autoinhibitory channels become insignificant on spatial integration in the distributed model. For this reason they are omitted in the KII set (see Sections 1.3.4 and 6.1.1, Fig. 6.1a). In the point approximation of Wilson and Cowan, the channels for mutual excitation and inhibition disappear, and those for self-effects remain. When the topology is given according to the conventions used here (Fig. 6.33c), we see that the major negative feedback loop contains two minor loops, one positive (for autoexcitation) and the other negative (for auto-inhibition). The positive feedback property of mutual inhibition has been deleted. For this reason the Wilson–Cowan point approximation is not a lumped approximation of the distributed KII set.

The open loop time-dependent transfer function of each set of neurons in the Wilson–Cowan model is approximated by a single pole $A(s) = a/(s + a), a > 0$. The omission of higher-order delays contributed by synapses and dendritic cable properties means that quantitative comparisons are difficult to make between experimental and theoretical results. For example, a model with a first-order approximation for $A(s)$ with $a > 0$ in a reduced KII set cannot enter a limit cycle state (Fig. 5.5), whereas with a second-order approximation it can (Fig. 5.7). In order to obtain limit cycle behavior from the model with the first-order approximation, the several connection densities must be given arbitrarily chosen compensatory values (see Example B in Section 6.1.2 and Fig. 6.3), and they lose their anatomical and physiological quantitative significance.

The amplitude-dependent nonlinearity is introduced into the Wilson–Cowan equations on the basis of the threshold property of wave to pulse conversion. In their topology it precedes the linear filter property of passive membrane operating on dendritic current. The pulse to wave nonlinearity here postulated to precede the linear transfer function is not considered by them. When expressed according to the conventions used here [see Eqs. (5)], their equations are

$$\frac{dp_e}{dt} + ap_e = a(1 - r_e p_e) G(c_{ee} p_e - c_{ie} p_i + P_e),$$

$$\frac{dp_i}{dt} + ap_i = a(1 - r_i p_i) G(c_{ei} p_e - c_{ii} p_i + P_i),$$

(83)

where p_e and p_i are the active states in the pulse modes of the sets of excitatory e and inhibitory i neurons, a is the passive membrane rate constant, r_e and r_i are refractory period coefficients, c_{ee}, c_{ei}, c_{ie}, and c_{ii} are coupling coefficients, and P_e and P_i are inputs. The operator G denotes a nonlinear function for which they have used the logistics curve as the basis for obtaining numerical solutions to Eqs. (83):

$$G(p) = 1/[1 + e^{-\gamma(p - p_r)}].$$

(84)

The form of the curve is sigmoid and is interpreted as resulting from a unimodal distribution of neural thresholds in each set, where p_r is the mean value of threshold. This curve is symmetric and has fixed asymptotes, whereas the input–output function used here is asymmetric and has state-dependent asymptotes. The effects of the variable asymptotes are incorporated by them into their treatments of inputs and refractory periods. As Wilson & Cowan (1972) state, the precise form of the input–output curve does not influence the qualitative properties of the KII set, but in experimental analysis the curve must be specified in detail.

The terms relating to refractory period, r_e and r_i, are omitted here because the channels for autoexcitation and autoinhibition are deleted as insignificant, and the effects of the absolute and relative refractory periods are expressed in the value for the upper asymptote of the sigmoid input–output curve.

Grossberg (1973) begins his analysis with the KII set and then suppresses it by assuming that the excitatory and inhibitory neurons have uniform properties and uniform inputs. His neural elements become mixtures of excitatory and inhibitory neurons in a sheet. He then assigns to each element an autoexcitatory feedback channel, a set of channels for inhibitory output, and a set of channels for inhibitory input. Interaction is solely by mutual inhibition, and there is no negative feedback. The topology according to the conventions used here is shown in Fig. 6.34 for three elements

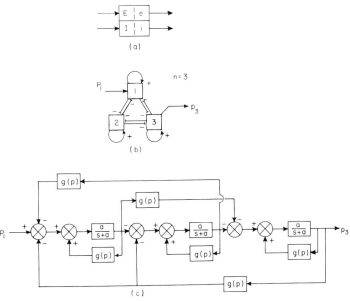

FIG. 6.34. Representation of the Grossberg model according to the conventions used in the text.

(not K sets). The differential equation for each element is

$$dp_j/dt + \left[a + \sum_{k \neq j}^{n} G(p_k) \right] p_j = (b - p_j) G(p_j) + P, \qquad j = 1, 2, ..., n. \quad (85)$$

Here p_j is the state variable of the jth element, a is a first-order rate constant, $b - p_j$ represents the number that are not refractory, and P is input. Then G is a nonlinear function relating output to input in each channel. As in Eqs. (5) used here, the summation follows rather than precedes the nonlinear operation in his topology.

Grossberg derives a sigmoid input–output curve from the analysis of the properties his system must have, if it is to have the desirable features for information processing that are inferred to exist in visual systems. The main difference between his sigmoid curve and that used here is that the central segment of his curve is linear or nearly so. The curve used here (and by Wilson and Cowan as well) has maximal rate of change in gain with change of input at the central point of inflexion of the curve. Grossberg emphasizes an important property shared by all these systems, which is signal normalization. That is, the inhibitory feedback activity increases with the input activity, so that the output activity varies over a narrower amplitude range than the input activity does. Then the activity delivered to the sigmoid nonlinearity is compressed into the central range of the nonlinearity and away from the asymptotes.

Zetterberg (1973) has deduced the form of the sigmoid nonlinearity by using probability theory, but has applied it only to a network resembling the reduced KII set, in which the feedback channel contains an unexplained double pole. Harth, Csermely, Beek & Lindsay (1970) and Anninos, Beek, Csermely, Harth & Pertile (1970) describe the interactions of mixed sets of excitatory and inhibitory neurons in "netlets," but without distinguishing the outputs of the two types. Their concern is with the existence of stable and unstable equilibria and with hysteresis phenomena, rather than with limit cycles.

Despite the relatively small number of reports concerning it, the main outline of a theory of KII sets is now reasonably clear. Interactions of all three kinds must be allowed for among interconnected excitatory and inhibitory neurons or else be excluded for specific reasons. The time, distance, and amplitude dependencies of the two minimal state variables can be separated. The linear open loop transfer function of subsets of neurons must be approximated minimally (for physiological modeling) by a second-order differential equation. The connection densities should decrease with distance from each subset, the excitatory more rapidly than the inhibitory. Autoexcitation and autoinhibition may be neglected. The nonlinear input–output curve must be monotonically increasing and have slopes approaching zero for both input extremes.

Each of the coupled nonlinear partial integrodifferential equations describing the KII dynamics is closely related to the heat equation, which by itself is familiar and has many solutions. The coupling of two or more such equations causes formidable difficulties. There are no general solutions, only particular solutions. The value of the solutions to the linearized equations is that the conditions for setting up particular cases can be carefully evaluated in advance with respect to experimental data, so that the solutions, when found, can reasonably be expected to conform to the data.

CHAPTER 7

Signal Processing by Neural Mass Actions

A neural signal is defined here as a space–time pattern of neural activity in a KO or KI set that is both an apparent effect and a representation of a stimulus to the nervous system. The stimulus can be in one or several sensory modalities, and there is no limit on the time interval or on the distance within the nervous system between the time and location of the stimulus and the time and location of the signal. The representation may be found after an unspecified number of transformations, so that, for example, the pattern of action potentials in a pool of spinal motorneurons during the execution of a movement constitutes a signal. If the pattern consists in the activity of one or a few neurons in a KO set (e.g., Barlow, 1969), the representation is discrete, and the concepts of pulse logic apply (Freeman, 1972e, f). If the pattern consists in the cooperative activity of a KI set, the concepts of mass action apply. In either case the identification of neural signals is based on the correlation of neural activity patterns with behavioral patterns.

7.1. Behavioral Correlates of Wave Activity in KII Sets

7.1.1. The Operational Basis for Correlation

The neural signal is a pattern of neural activity and is therefore a value or set of values taken by a state variable of activity (Sections 1.2.3 and 1.3.2).

The state variables of mass actions in the nervous system are the active states of KO and KI sets. When certain precautions are taken as described in Chapter 4, the pulse trains and EEG waves recorded in neural masses can be treated as observable electrical correlates of the active states of KO and KI sets. Most KI sets are interactive with other KI sets, and their pulse and EEG wave activities reflect the properties of KII sets and higher-order sets, up to and including the whole brain. For this reason, it is essential in observing the electrical activities of KO and KI sets to stipulate the global state of an animal with respect to a set of broadly conceived central and peripheral states and conditions.

Due to the open-ended nature of this task, the behavioral correlates of the EEG are determined by an inductive process. The main attributes of the EEG are listed, including the principal frequency components, their amplitudes, their spatial distributions, and significant qualitative features such as bursts or spike complexes. Then a broad variety of stimuli is given in the several sensory modalities. The state of arousal (Lindsley, 1960) is manipulated through the types of sleep and the waking state. A representative sample of reflex behavior is elicited (flexion, righting, locomotion, etc.), and a wide range of motivated behavior (Stellar & Corbit, 1973) is induced (searching, eating, attack, escape, copulation, etc.). The relation of each type of behavior to a property of the EEG is tabulated.

In general, the EEG is the best available source of information about KII sets, because it establishes the domain of normal function including the significant variables and their dynamic ranges. The EEGs of the bulb and cortex are continually changing, both randomly and in relation to a broad variety of behavioral states in waking and sleeping animals. Two nonspecific correlates are found for the waking EEGs. The amplitude of the dominant frequency component at 40 Hz is correlated with the degree of motivation (hunger, thirst, fear, rage, sexual excitement, etc.). With increasing food deprivation, for example, there is a monotonic increase in the amplitude of the EEG without change in frequency. With increasing arousal or generalized excitability there is an increase in the amplitude and a decrease in the dominant frequency of the EEG, irrespective of the cause. The principal specific correlate is the occurrence of the 40 Hz activity in bursts synchronized with inspiration and superimposed on an irregularly shaped wave, which recurs at the frequency of respiration. Oral activity (chewing, licking, sneezing, yawning, biting, etc.) is accompanied by a transient decrease in EEG amplitude, largely but not solely due to the alteration in respiratory pattern. There is no established relation between the frequency, amplitude, or (so far as is yet known) spatial distribution of the bulbar and cortical EEGs and the odors to which the animals are deliberately or unavoidably exposed (Freeman, 1962a–e, 1963).

Example A.   The combination of motivation and arousal is shown in Fig. 7.1. A cat with electrodes implanted in the prepyriform cortex for recording its EEG has been deprived of food for 48 hr. It has been placed in a sound proof box for 2 hr, until it has settled into a waking but inactive state. At the arrow below the upper EEG trace an odor of fish is introduced into a steady air stream entering the box. There is an increase in EEG activity and the onset of searching behavior. During recording of the lower EEG trace the same procedure is repeated after feeding the cat to satiety on fish. There is no overt behavioral response, and there is little change in the EEG. The results show that the development of a state of increased arousal requires an antecedent state of increased motivation.   □

Example B.   Waking cats with implanted electrodes are encouraged to sniff odorous substances (Fig. 7.2), either natural (e.g., catnip, dog feces) or artificial. In some instances the bursts at 40 Hz are accentuated, in others depressed, and in yet others unchanged. Mouth breathing, particularly prolonged expiration during vocalization, is accompanied by a decrease in the EEG activity. In a quiescent cat a single tug on the tail sufficient to induce a righting reflex does not cause 40-Hz bursts to appear, but repeated tugs do so, whether or not retaliation occurs.   □

Example C.   The quantitative relationships between the two nonspecific behavioral correlates and the amplitude of the prepyriform EEG is established as follows. Cats are trained to work in an ergometer (Freeman,

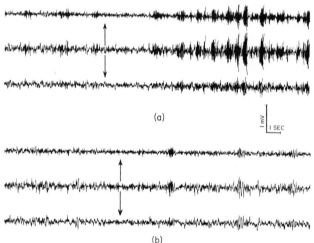

(a)

1 SEC

(b)

FIG. 7.1. EEG from prepyriform cortex of cat. At arrows the odor of fish was introduced into an air stream flowing into the box. (a) Cat deprived of food for 48 hr. (b) Same cat shortly after feeding to satiety (Freeman, 1960a).

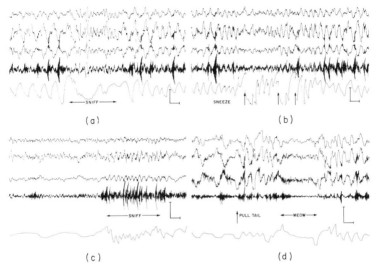

FIG. 7.2. EEG from prepyriform cortex of four different cats: (a) sniff, (b) sneeze, (c) sniff, (d) vocalize. Upper three traces in each frame with low-pass filter. Fourth trace with high-pass filter. Fifth trace from pneumograph, inspiration upward. Lines 1–3: 200 μV. Line 4: 500 μV. Time: 1 sec (Freeman, 1960a).

1964c) for food. Each period of work takes 10 sec, in which the rate of work is measured. The rms (root mean square) EEG amplitude is measured in a 10 sec period in anticipation of each trial, during work, and during the first 10 sec of lapping. Motivation is increased by taking sets of measurements at intervals of 24, 48, and 72 hr after feeding to satiety. The state of arousal is operationally defined as proportional to the rate of work done at a fixed level of food deprivation. The rms amplitude of the cortical EEG is positively correlated both with the level of deprivation and the rate of work at each level. □

The changes in EEG rms amplitude can be interpreted as due to changes in cortical excitability or to changes in cortical input from the bulb or to both. The changes in cortical excitability are studied separately by measuring cortical responses to electrical stimulation of the LOT.

The establishment of the behavioral correlates of the AEPs requires a different approach. At the outset, the state of the animal must be specified with respect to orienting to the electrical stimulus. If the LOT is stimulated intermittently at intensities less than about 5× threshold, there is no irreversible change in the AEP over a period of months.[†] If the LOT is

[†] If stimulation is given continuously at 40 pulses/sec for 3 days, a major change takes place, but this is probably a pathological change (see Section 5.4.3).

stimulated at 10 to 20× threshold for from several seconds to a minute or more, there is arrest of on-going motor activity, sniffing, and turning of the head, eyes, and ears in searching movements. This is the orienting reflex (see Magoun, 1962, pp. 109–112; Sokolov, 1963; Adey, 1967; Grastyán & Vereczkei, 1974).

Prior to an orienting reflex to the stimulus the animal is naive with respect to the stimulus. After a single orienting reflex, it enters one of three states. If specific training procedures are undertaken to make the electrical stimulus a conditioned signal for a conditioned response, such as lever-pressing or ergometer work, the animal becomes attentive. If such procedures are not undertaken, it becomes inattentive and in a state of postorienting habituation. If following the initial training a further period of specific training is given to break the connection between the conditioned response and the electrical conditioned stimulus, the animal is inattentive and the conditioned response is extinguished or in a state of extinction. At any time an animal can be habituated to the stimulus, whether it is naive, attentive or inattentive (in a state of response extinction). This is a fully reversible process in which the animal is placed in an unchanging and restricted environment (see Example A), and the electrical stimulus is maintained at a steady rate and amplitude for 1 to 2 hr. Attention and inattention are reciprocally reversible, and habituation is reversible but orienting is a form of learning (Grastyan & Vereczkei, 1974) and is not reversible.

The amplitude and frequency of the dominant component of the AEPs change in relation to the same set of variables as the EEG (degree of motivation, degree of arousal, and changes in respiratory pattern) by the same qualitative tests.

Example D. A cat with implanted electrodes is first trained to press a lever for water in response to LOT stimulation as the conditioned stimulus. The conditional response is then extinguished by withholding the reward, but the conditioned stimulus is presented at intervals of 30 to 90 sec for a period of 2 hr, and an AEP is constructed on each presentation. The cat is allowed to sit undisturbed in the training box. As time passes both the EEG and behavioral activity diminish, but the cat remains awake.

The AEPs undergo the pattern of change shown in Fig. 7.3, where 0 min denotes the AEP on the first trial after the last unrewarded pressing of the lever. The amplitude of the AEP decreases, and the frequency and decay rate increase. This is habituation. The change is rapidly reversed upon delivery of any stimulus that increases both the EEG and behavioral activity.

If, however, the extinction procedure is continued for several days, while the cat is retrained to press the lever to a light or sound stimulus, the AEP pattern seen in Fig. 7.3 at 75 min persists in the presence of high

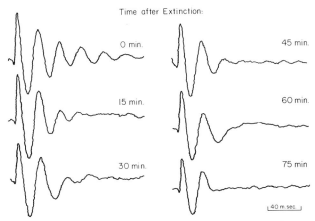

Fig. 7.3. Changes in prepyriform AEP in a cat on LOT stimulation during post-extinction habituation (Freeman, 1962b).

levels of EEG and behavioral activity. This is postextinction inattention. It is reversed only by retraining the cat to respond to the electrical stimulus.   □

Example E. AEPs are taken from a naive cat, which is working for small amounts of food in an ergometer at intervals of 24, 48, and 72 hr after feeding to satiety. The amplitudes, frequencies, and decay rates of the AEPs are averaged at each level of deprivation. The amplitudes increase with deprivation but the frequencies and decay rates are unchanged.   □

7.1.2. FACTOR ANALYSIS OF AEPs

The AEP data can be reduced by the use of digital filters for measurement (Section 2.5.3) to a set of 8 coefficients for each AEP. These 8 coefficients are constrained by the properties of KII sets and the changing state of the animal to vary in certain patterns. In a set of AEPs from a period of recording in which the behavioral variables have undergone changes, the patterns in the AEPs can be extracted by factor analysis. Specifically, each cortical AEP in a set of N AEPs is described after measurement by the parameters of two damped sine waves, which are the amplitude V_j, frequency ω_j, decay rate α_j, and phase φ_j in Eq. (203) in Chapter 2. A matrix of $N \times 8$ coefficients is factor analyzed for the principal orthogonal components of the variance.

Prior to the analysis it is convenient to transform the values for ω_j and α_j to values for K_2 and T_2 (explicit subscripts j are not needed), which are, respectively, the lumped loop gain and loop delay of the KII set described in terms of a single negative feedback loop (Section 5.4.2). The transformation restructures the variance and makes it easier to detect and measure the factor patterns (see Example C in Section 6.1.5). Then each factor is described in terms of the elements $[V_j, K_2, T_2, \varphi_j], j = 1, 2$.

The results are shown in Table 7.1 of factor analysis of the parameters from 30 cortical AEPs of each of 4 cats within each of three states (naive,

TABLE 7.1

FACTOR ANALYSIS OF AEP PARAMETERS IN DIFFERING BEHAVIORAL STATES[a]

	Naive			Attentive			Habituated		
Eigenvalues:	2.185	2.058	1.153	2.718	1.848	1.325	2.614	1.790	1.314
Proportions[b]:	.273	.530	.675	.340	.571	.736	.327	.551	.715
Factors	I	II	III	I	II	III	I	II	III
V_1	−.350	−.286	.728	−.211	.324	.699	−.360	.209	.728
T_2	.939	−.005	.038	.900	−.206	.274	.875	.018	−.054
K_2	.866	.147	−.207	.861	−.219	.181	.886	.031	−.184
φ_1	.611	−.216	.498	.864	−.287	−.000	.857	−.028	−.189
V_2	.183	−.626	.092	−.234	−.517	.455	.253	−.273	.803
T_2	−.005	.884	.118	.130	.690	.491	−.214	.753	.178
K_2	−.043	.756	.104	.405	.821	−.033	−.018	.918	.031
φ_2	.151	.405	.546	−.374	−.392	.529	−.298	−.510	−.185

[a] From Freeman (1968a).
[b] Cumulative proportions of total variance.

attentive, and postextinction habituated). In all states the largest component of the variance is called Factor I and is described by $[-V_1, +K_2, +T_2, +\varphi_1]$. That is, when K_2, T_2 and φ_1 increase together, V_1 decreases in the dominant component of the AEP. The second largest component is called Factor II and is described by $[-V_2, +K_2, +T_2, \pm\varphi_2]$ for the subsidiary component of the AEP. The third largest is Factor III and is described by $[+V_1, 0K_2, 0T_2, 0\varphi_1]$. The remaining factors have eigenvalues less than 1.0 and are not significant. When AEPs are taken during ergometer work and analyzed this way, all three factors are correlated with rate of work, mainly Factor III and to lesser extents Factor I and Factor II in that order.[†]

[†] The digital filters for measuring AEPs, which are described in Section 2.5.3, were developed and tested in this experimental situation. The hypothesis is that both the AEP and the rate of work are determined by overlapping sets of variables in the forebrain. Then some level of correlation should exist between the coefficients of the AEP and the rate of work. The digital filters are designed not merely to minimize the least squares deviation between the AEP and the fitted curve, but further to optimize the correlation between the coefficients of sets of AEPs and the concomitant rates of work (Freeman, 1964a).

Example A.   A cat with electrodes implanted in the LOT and prepyriform cortex and naive to the stimulus is trained to work in an ergometer for milk. It is fitted with a harness attached to a rope and is placed in a starting box. When the gate opens, the cat pulls on the rope against a friction device and approaches the milk. It is on a dry diet and performs 20 to 40 trials of work daily to obtain liquids. During some days' trials, the LOT is stimulated continually at 7/sec, and cortical AEPs are constructed during anticipation of work preceding opening of the gate, during work, and during lapping. On other days the rms amplitude of the EEG is measured. On the average there is an increase in the amplitude of the EEG during work in comparison to that during anticipation, and a decrease during lapping. The AEPs are measured with damped sine waves, and the values for ω and α are transformed to K_2 and T_2. On factor analysis the values for K_2 and T_2 in each behavioral state show "spontaneous" variation (Fig. 7.4). Superimposed on this variation is a larger change. Both K_2 and T_2 increase during work as compared with anticipation, and they decrease during lapping. The experimental root locus for the change with behavioral state is identical to that for "spontaneous" variation (Section 6.1.5). The theoretical root locus best approximating values for K_2 and T_2 from the dominant component is specified by KII_{AB} operation in the second mode, with $\delta_e = 0.33$, $K_o = 2.0$, and K_n ranging from 2.5 to 1.5.   □

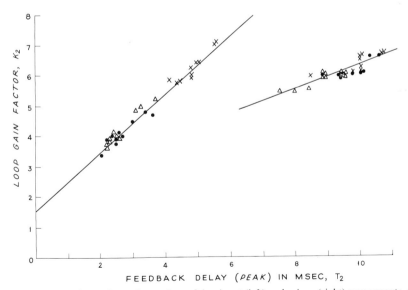

FIG. 7.4. Experimental root locus plots of dominant (left) and minor (right) components of prepyriform AEPs in $K_2 \cdot T_2$ coordinates (see Fig. 6.23) (Freeman, 1968a). △: wait; ×: work; ●: lap.

The interpretation of these patterns is as follows. Factor I is the pattern of "spontaneous" variation of AEPs. The theoretical root locus for this pattern is generated by varying K_n with fixed K_o and with $\delta_e = .33$ in the second mode (Section 6.1.5). The theoretical values for V_1 and φ_1 are found by the inverse transforms of Eqs. (27) and (33) in Section 6.1.2 for three values of K_n. Sets of values for V_1 and φ_1 are shown graphically for three values of K_n in Fig. 7.5a, c, and e, where C_{12} is the output of the KI_e or KI_A set A_{12}, and C_{34} is the output of the KI_i or KI_B set A_{34}. With

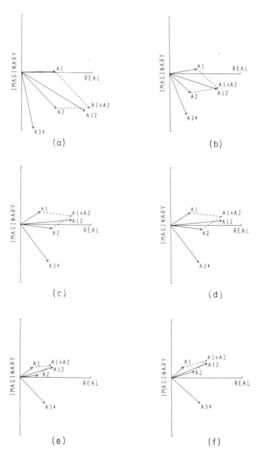

FIG. 7.5. Predicted changes in phase φ and amplitude V_1 plotted as a vector when K_n is decreased in the second mode (a, c, e) or increased in the first mode (b, d, f), by an amount sufficient to replicate the observed changes in frequency ω and decay rate α of AEPs (see Figs. 6.23a, $\delta_e = .33$, and 6.27a, $\delta_e = 1.00$). (a) Mode 2, $K_n = 2.4$; (b) mode 1, $K_n = 1.5$; (c) mode 2, $K_n = 2.0$; (d) mode 1, $K_n = 2.0$; (e) mode 2, $K_n = 1.5$; (f) mode 1, $K_n = 2.4$.

decreasing K_n, V_1 decreases and φ_1 increases, and of course both K_2 and T_2 increase. The predicted pattern is $[-V_1, +K_2, +T_2, +\varphi_1]$.

The high covariation of T_2 and φ_1 is readily explained. The phase of the AEP is determined by the duration of the initial negative peak N1 in relation to the wave period. Let the duration of N1 be T_1 and the wave period be $T_p = 2\pi/\omega$. The phase φ is given by

$$\varphi = 2\pi(\tfrac{1}{2}T_p - T_1)/T_p \tag{1}$$

in radians, where a full cycle is 2π rad. Equation (1) is reduced to

$$\varphi = \pi - \omega T_1. \tag{2}$$

If ω increases and T_1 is fixed, then φ must decrease. Experimentally, there is a very high negative correlation between ω_1 and φ_1, which is due to the fact that the duration of N1 does not change significantly during "spontaneous" variation of the AEP. The nonlinearity $G(v)$ occurs after the linear transfer function $F(s)$ in the KI_e set (Section 5.1.2), and the open loop rate constants in $F(s)$ are invariant. The sign of the correlation is reversed by the transformation of ω_1 and α_1 to K_2 and T_2.

The reason for the negative covariation of V_1 with K_2 and T_2 is not intuitively obvious. In the KII set in the second mode the decrease in K_n causes a decrease in α_1, the decay rate. In effect, the damping of the KII set is diminished. If the KII set is represented by an equivalent single negative feedback loop (Section 5.4.2), the apparent feedback gain K_2 and loop delay T_2 must increase. Due to the apparent (illusory) increase in negative feedback gain, the amplitude V_1 of the oscillatory impulse response decreases. The increase is illusory, because while K_2 increases, K_n (the postulated true negative feedback gain) decreases in mode 2. It is the global properties of the KII set that cause α to decrease in this mode.

The dynamic properties of the KII set in the second mode, when $\delta_e = .33$, are specified by K_o and K_n. At a fixed electrical stimulus input the value of K_n is determined by the EEG amplitude, which in turn (Section 6.2.3) depends on K_o. Because there are two main factors, I and III, determining the form of the dominant component, there must be at least two determinants of K_o. One is obviously the continually varying pulse input from the bulb to the cortex on the LOT which is to a large extent under motor control by the brain stem, and which partly determines the amplitude of the EEG. The other determinant must have a different source than respiration.

There is evidence that the second determinant operates by way of a centrifugal pathway from the basal forebrain into the bulb. When the bulb, anterior olfactory nucleus and prepyriform cortex are surgically undercut, so as to leave intact the receptors, PON, and LOT but sever all central neural connections, the cortical AEP retains its oscillatory form (Section

5.4.5). Factor analysis of the coefficients of the measured AEPs (Table 7.2) shows that Factor III has disappeared from sets of AEPs from the undercut cortex. The principal factor I_u has the form $[+V_j, +K_2, +T_2, +\varphi_j]$ for both the dominant and subsidiary components. This suggests that in the cortex without centrifugal control K_0 is determined solely by the peripheral input, which also controls K_n. When K_o is increased and K_n is decreased in a fixed relation, a single factor I_u emerges. In the intact cortex, K_0 is determined in part by centrifugal input and in part by peripheral input, and Factors I and III emerge for the dominant component of the AEP.

The performance of the undercut bulb and cortex shows that the KII_{MG} and KII_{AB} sets are capable of semiautonomous operation to a remarkable degree. When the animal is habituated to a monotonous environment, both the intact and undercut sides show the same abatement of burst activity in the EEG and the same pattern of change in AEP shown in Fig. 7.3. When the animal is aroused, the bursts return and the AEP reverts to its normal form on the undercut side as well as the intact side. The bursts in the second mode that manifest the limit cycle state, therefore, depend on peripheral factors, chiefly the rate of flow of air bearing odorous substances over the mucosa that is controlled by the respiratory and cranial nerve nuclei. That is, induction of the stable limit cycle state in KII sets does not require centrifugal input from the forebrain.

The most dramatic difference between the intact and undercut sides is

TABLE 7.2

FACTOR ANALYSIS OF AEP PARAMETERS FROM INTACT AND
UNDERCUT PREPYRIFORM CORTEX[a]

	Control cortex			Undercut cortex		
Eigenvalues:	2.631	1.867	1.354	4.297	1.789	.877
Proportions:	.329	.562	.731	.537	.761	.870
Factors						
	I	II	III	I	II	III
V_1	−.360	.088	.725	.879	−.288	.292
T_2	.890	−.055	−.128	.735	.545	−.214
K_2	.882	.096	−.158	.490	.740	−.374
φ_1	.638	−.158	.094	.739	.360	.157
V_1	−.429	.757	−.143	.604	.386	.630
T_2	.297	.727	.317	.840	−.493	−.089
K_2	.489	.240	.701	.803	−.528	−.059
φ_1	.108	.814	−.408	−.695	.246	.417

[a] From Freeman (1968a).

that the cortex on the undercut side fails to show the sleep pattern of the EEG, which is shown by the intact side when the animal is behaviorally asleep. This implies that in effect the centrifugal input is mainly suppressive or inhibitory and that arousal results from withdrawal of the centrifugal input. Gradations of arousal may result by graded release from inhibition of central origin. The possibility that these axons determine a minor component of the bulbar AEP on LOT stimulation (Fig. 6.5a) has been described (Section 6.1.4).

There are relatively few centrifugal afferents to the cortex, but there are many to the bulb. The most likely site of action of centrifugal input is on the granule cells (the KI_G set) in the bulb. This set receives afferents from the nucleus of the diagonal band (Price & Powell, 1970c), which is thought to receive input from the midbrain reticular formation, and from the anterior olfactory nucleus, for which the centrifugal afferents are undetermined. Sustained excitation of the KI_G set either directly through the nucleus of the diagonal band or indirectly through the anterior olfactory nucleus (Callens, 1967) can be expected to reduce K_o in the KII_{MG} set and therefore K_o in the KII_{AB} set as well. That is, the two nuclei can be viewed as control points for nonspecific centrifugal input to the bulbocortical system. There is also, of course, centrifugal input to the KI_P set (Section 5.2.3), about which little is known (Section 5.2.1).

The critical control parameters in the bulb and cortex are K_o in the KII_{MG} set and K_o in the KII_{AB} set. Both parameters depend internally on the mean pulse rates p_o and mean levels of depolarization $\bar{v}_i$ in the component KI_e and KI_i sets (Section 6.1.4) and in the KI_P set as well (Section 5.2.3). The external nonspecific determinants of the several mean pulse rates are the level of pulse input from the receptors KO_R and the centrifugal input from one or all of several sources. The patterns of operation of the KII sets can be manipulated by changing the peripheral input or the central state of the animal or both, and the resulting factor patterns display some of the general properties of the KII sets.

Now the question is considered: What are the relations between Factor I and Factor III and the levels of motivation and arousal? A clear answer cannot be given. The factors reflect some of the constraints on the KII set, as it responds to variations in central control variables and peripheral inputs. The nonspecific behavioral states are abstractions used by the experimentalist to classify a variety of loosely related manipulatory procedures available to him. The pattern of Factor I resembles the pattern of change in AEPs identified with habituation and its reversal by arousal $[+V_1, +K_2, +T_2, +\varphi_1]$ (Example D, Section 7.1.1), and that of Factor III resembles the pattern of change associated with food deprivation, $[+V_1, 0K_2, 0T_2, 0\varphi_1]$ (Example E, Section 7.1.1), and other forms of motivation.

We cannot say, however, that the factors represent changes in motivation and arousal, because the factors reflect constraints on the KII sets and not on the central state of the animal. The factors are present because motivation and arousal must operate to give the AEPs within the same constraints as other determinants of KII operation, so that the same or similar patterns arise in differing experimental conditions. The factors, then, tell us how to construct explanatory equations (Chapter 6), and the qualitative behavioral correlates tell us how to vary the peripheral and central states of the animal, which is required, because without variance there are no discernible factors.

It is reasonable and perhaps necessary to describe the manipulations of the central state with concepts that are both generalized and familiar from common experience, but there is not and cannot be an a priori relation between those concepts and the dynamics of the central neural mechanisms. The concepts are no more than heuristic tools, though we can hope that, when the operations at control points of KII sets have been defined and analyzed experimentally with their help, we may find ways to describe the dynamic processes underlying motivation and arousal in neurophysiological terms.

7.1.3. PATTERNS OF CHANGE IN AEPs WITH ATTENTION

The mechanism for selective awareness or attention is investigated by training cats with implanted electrodes to press a lever for a reward, whenever the LOT stimulus train used to evoke potentials for the AEP is turned on. Comparison is made between AEPs from the same cat in the naive state, the attentive state, and the state of extinction (Section 7.1.1).

A cat with stimulating electrodes in the LOT and recording electrodes in the prepyriform cortex is first trained in a conventional way to press the lever in response to a light stimulus. In order to establish the designated attentive state, an orienting reflex to the LOT electrical stimulus must be obtained (Section 7.1.1). This can only be done by very strong stimulation of the LOT, in which the stimulus is 8–20 times greater than that used to elicit AEPs for measurement. It is just below an intensity, which causes epileptiform seizure in the prepyriform cortex manifested in the EEG and behavioral activity in the cat. The presence of the orienting reflex is manifested behaviorally by the searching movements of the cat. After orienting to the electrical stimulus, up to 90 pairings of the light and the strong electrical stimulus on each of 3 to 5 successive days suffice for transfer of the lever-press response to the electrical stimulus alone. Thereafter, additional training is required for generalization to progressively lower intensities, until the intensity is low enough for KII operation to occur in the second mode. The state of attentiveness to the evoking stimulus is then defined as the condition in which a cat presses the lever within 15 sec on >90% of presentations of the stimulus and presses the lever no more than once between any 10 stimulus presentations. In well-trained cats, the behavioral threshold for a short train of single-shock evoked potentials is the same as the threshold for the detection by an observer of the evoked potentials on an oscilloscope screen in the presence of the normal EEG (see also Figs. 6.31).

The state of extinction is established by making three changes. First, the conditioned response is extinguished by giving the electrical stimulus and not giving the reward when the cat presses the lever. This usually requires 10–30 trials in any one day. Second, the conditioned response of pressing the lever in response to the light stimulus is reestablished by further training. Third, the LOT electrical stimulus is given either repeatedly or continually in order to habituate the cat to the stimulus. The state of extinction must be reestablished on each of 4 to 6 successive days, because the cat tends to press the lever on electrical stimulation at the start of each day, but with the passage of days even this residual disappears. Subsequently, if one or more weeks pass without habituation, the state of attention to the electrical stimulus can be again established by appropriate training.

The cortical AEPs in attentive cats are similar in many respects to those in naive cats. The operation in the first mode in respect to stimulus intensity is identical, with values for $\delta_e = \delta_i$ ranging from $-.60$ to -1.00. "Spontaneous" variation in K_2 and T_2 and the changes associated with working and lapping are indistinguishable in the two states. There are two sustained differences. First, during the first several weeks following the period of training and generalization, a new characteristic frequency emerges in the AEP that has a value slightly greater than half the value in the naive and early post training state (Fig. 7.6b). Correspondingly, the decay rate of the low frequency component of the AEP diminishes about twofold. Oscillation persists at the original frequency, but it often becomes the subsidiary component, and oscillation at the near half-frequency becomes the dominant component.

The near half-frequency component is occasionally observed in AEPs from naive cats, when the recording electrodes are in the temporal but not in the frontal prepyriform cortex. It does not enlarge or freshly appear, if the same amount of daily stimulation is given after orienting but without establishing the lever-pressing as a response to the stimulus (Fig. 7.6a).[†]

Second, the values for phase are lower in the attentive state than in the

---

[†] The values for $Q = \omega/2\alpha$ denote the sharpness of tuning of frequency response curves that are obtained by measuring the rms amplitude of cortical activity induced by trains of LOT pulses at rates varying from 10/sec to 100/sec (Freeman, 1962b). The values for Q are increased by low values for α, which are found in cats attentive to the electrical stimulus.

naive state (Table 7.3). Over the transition from the attentive state to the states of inattention and extinction, the values for phase increase with decreasing values of K_2 and T_2, and provided the level of motivation is not changed, the amplitude does not change significantly. During retraining the parameters are restored to their original values. The pattern for selective attention is specified by $[-V_1, +T_2, +K_2, -\varphi_1]$.

The negative correlation between T_2 and φ_1 is highly significant. It means that there is a positive correlation between phase and frequency in the AEP, and that the duration of N1 of the AEP is not constant. In fact, the duration of N1 must increase when the frequency decreases in order to give a lower value for the phase by Eq. (2). This pattern is not consistent with KII operation in the second mode (Section 6.1.5), because in the second mode K_2, T_2, and φ_1 are all positively correlated.

TABLE 7.3

MEAN AEP PARAMETER VALUES FROM FOUR CATS IN DIFFERING BEHAVIORAL STATES[a]

Subject	N	V_1		T_2		K_2		φ_1	
Naive									
1	33	121.0	±15.4	3.23	± .19	3.73	±.27	1.21	±.15
2	25	94.3	± 6.5	7.20	± .39	5.90	±.17	1.62	±.11
3	32	101.7	± 5.9	6.15	± .44	5.70	±.32	1.69	±.11
4	30	114.5	± 7.1	5.25	± .36	4.68	±.31	1.08	±.20
Average:		107.9		5.46		5.00		1.40	
Attentive									
1	47	128.6	±20.6	3.72	± .33	4.73	±.24	0.49	±.08
2	21	89.3	± 6.1	16.13	±1.43	8.06	±.77	0.92	±.20
3	37	103.8	±11.9	8.77	± .42	6.71	±.26	1.59	±.08
4	25	102.6	± 7.9	10.13	± .54	6.72	±.34	1.08	±.04
Average:		106.1		9.69		6.56		1.02	
Habituated									
1	54	137.7	±22.7	3.44	± .34	4.38	±.30	.54	±.10
2	34	95.3	±13.1	12.48	±1.58	7.53	±.56	1.30	±.32
3	48	126.0	±12.8	8.52	± .53	6.02	±.26	2.37	±.08
4	24	105.3	±17.2	9.65	±1.11	6.33	±.34	1.14	±.09
Average:		116.1		8.52		6.07		1.33	

[a] From Freeman (1968a). See Fig. 7.8.

Example A. A cat with electrodes implanted in the LOT and prepyriform cortex is trained to press a lever for milk in response to the onset of a light stimulus. The cat is oriented to LOT input by high-intensity single shocks. The high-intensity pulse trains are then paired with the light stimulus, in order to transfer the lever-press response to the LOT input. On every tenth

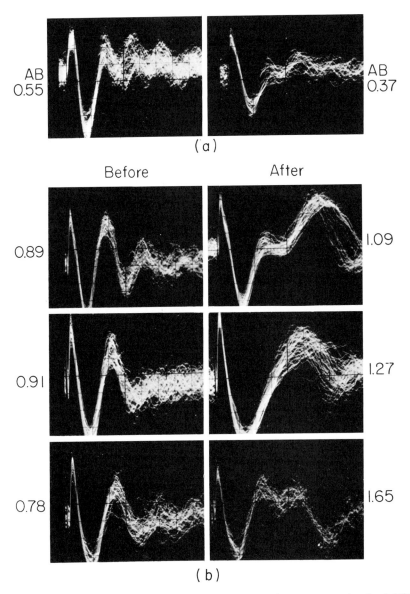

FIG. 7.6. After cats learn to press a lever for a reward in response to low-level LOT stimulation, the AEP develops a prominent low-frequency component after several weeks of daily trials. This does not occur if the cats receive stimulation without learning (see Freeman, 1962b). (a) Habituation; (b) learning.

trial, the LOT stimulus intensity is reduced to the near-threshold level used to measure the AEP, and an AEP is constructed. The procedure is repeated for a total of 270 trials (90 on each of 3 successive days). The means of the AEPs (AAEPs) are shown as dotted curves in Fig. 7.7 for three conditions: lever pressing on less than 10% of the high-intensity trials; more than 10% but less than 90% of the trials; and more than 90% of the

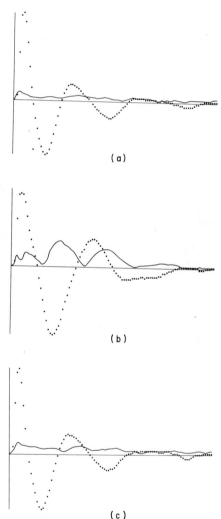

FIG. 7.7. Changes in AEP from a cat during learning to respond to the electrical stimulus as a conditioned signal. Dotted curves: ensemble mean of 9 AEPs; solid curves: standard deviations (Freeman, 1968a). (a) <10; (b) >50; (c) >90.

trials. There are 8–10 AEPs averaged to give each AAEP. The standard deviations are shown as solid curves.

In the stage of familiarization (Fig. 7.7a), the standard deviation is independent of the digitized amplitudes of the AAEP, which shows that the form of the averaged cortical responses is stable. The variation in the AEPs is due to superimposed EEG activity, which is not completely averaged out of the AEPs. During the stage of acquisition of the conditioned response (Fig. 7.7b), the AAEP frequency decay rate, and phase are reduced. This corresponds to 'he pattern $[0V_1, +T_2, +K_2, -\varphi_1]$. The pattern of the AAEP standard deviation shows that the frequency of the AEPs is varying during the stage of acquisition. In the stage of consolidation (Fig. 7.7c), the AAEP mean and standard deviation return to their forms during the naive state. This is prior to additional training for generalization of the response to the low-intensity stimulation used to collect the AEPs. Following generalization (Fig. 7.8h), the phase, frequency, and decay rate again decrease.

When attentiveness to the LOT stimulus is reduced by giving the pulse train continuously and retraining the cats to press the lever in response to the light stimulus, the phase, frequency, and decay rate again increase (Fig. 7.8i–l). The cortical change associated with attention is reversible in respect to phase but not frequency. □

Example B. A cat already trained to press a lever for milk in response to near-threshold LOT electrical stimulation is trained to work for milk

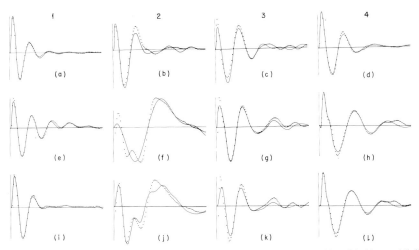

Fig. 7.8. Prepyriform AEPs from 4 cats in the naive (a–d), attentive (e–h) and habituated (i–l) states (Freeman, 1968a). See Table 7.3 for AEP parameter values.

in an ergometer. It is then trained to wait in the starting box after the gate is opened, until the LOT stimulus train is turned on. This is done in order to average the single-shock evoked potentials for each AEP across uniform states of behavior, each lasting 10 sec or more (waiting in the box for the gate to open, working, and lapping milk). The procedure is then repeated, after the response to LOT stimulation is extinguished, and the cat responds instead to the sound of a buzzer.

Examples are shown in Fig. 7.9 of the pattern of "spontaneous" variation of AEPs from two states: working for milk while attentive to the LOT stimulus, and working for milk while attentive to the buzzer. The symbols on the left side of the graph show K_2 and T_2 for the dominant component. Those on the right side show K_2 and T_2 for the minor component and are not of interest here. The solid dots show the values from AEPs when the cat is attentive to the electrical stimulus. The open triangles show the values when the cat is attentive to a buzzer. Each set of symbols reveals a pattern of "spontaneous" variation. Factor analysis of each set shows that the principle component of the variance, Factor I, has the pattern $[-V_1, +K_2,$

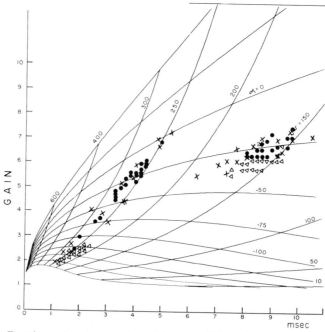

FIG. 7.9. Experimental root locus plots of dominant (left) and minor (right) components of prepyriform AEPs in $K_2 \cdot T_2$ coordinates (see Fig. 6.23). (Freeman, 1968a). ● : Attentive; △: inattentive; × : habituated.

$+ T_2, + \varphi_1]$ (see Table 7.1). The cross symbols show the values of K_2 and T_2 obtained during habituation of the cat from the attentive state. The pattern of factor I_u is $[+ V_1, + K_2, + T_2, + \varphi_1]$.

In these three patterns the change in φ_1 is positively correlated with the changes in K_2 and T_2, so the patterns reflect the changing levels of arousal. The significant pattern for attention is given by the differences between the mean values for V_1, K_2, T_2, and φ_1 in the two states (Table 7.1). This pattern is $[0V_1, + K_2, + T_2, - \varphi_1]$ in the direction of increased attentiveness.   ☐

Example C.   Electrodes are implanted in the LOT for stimulation and in the prepyriform cortex for recording in 5 cats. After recovery from the operation they are oriented to the LOT stimulus and trained to press a lever for water in response to low-level LOT stimulation at 7/sec. The criterion for attentiveness is operationally defined as the 1-sec time interval preceding each response. AEPs are constructed from the average of 8 single-shock evoked potentials on each trial summed over 12 trials to give $N = 96$ for each cat. It is assumed that following the lever press, the cat's attention is transferred from the LOT input to the water dish. AEPs are constructed in the same manner in the 1-sec time interval following the lever pressing response. The pattern for increased attentiveness, which is the reverse of the change in AEPs from before to after lever pressing, is $[0V_1, + T_2, + K_2, - \varphi_1]$ (Fig. 7.10). The entire procedure is then repeated after extinction of the lever-pressing response to LOT stimulation and retraining to press the lever in response to a light stimulus. The pattern of change in the AEP from pre- to postlever pressing is again measured. The reverse of the change is $[0V_1, + T_2, + K_2, 0\varphi_1]$ (Fig. 7.10). A two-way analysis of variance shows that the changes in T_2, K_2, and φ and the interaction for φ across the states

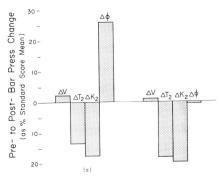

FIG. 7.10. Patterns of change from pre- to postbar press in cats attentive (a) to the electrical stimulus or (b) to a light stimulus (Emery & Freeman, 1969).

of attention and extinction, are significant at the $p = .001$ level (Emery & Freeman, 1969).

The interpretation is that in both cases there is a reduction in arousal from before to after the lever pressing, and that in one case a reduction in attentiveness to the LOT input is superimposed on the general change in the arousal state. □

7.1.4. A PROPOSED CORTICAL MECHANISM OF ATTENTION

From this evidence we conclude that the pattern of change in the AEP with increased attentiveness is $[\pm V_1, +K_2, +T_2, -\varphi_1]$. In agreement with the combined change, $-\omega$, $-\varphi$, there is an increase in the duration of N1, and often the appearance of a secondary peak on the declining part of N1 (for example, Fig. 7.8h and 1). These properties of N1 suggest that the cortical change with increased attentiveness is an increase in the level of mutual excitation among the superficial pyramidal cells forming the KI_A set. On LOT excitation the Type A neurons have two preferential poststimulus firing periods (Fig. 7.11 and Section 5.4.3). The first period begins [part (a)] less than 1 msec after the LOT compound action potential and ends before the first crest of N1. The second period begins 3 to 5 msec

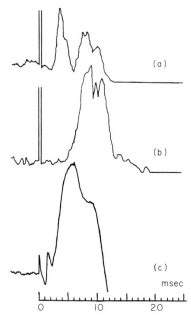

FIG. 7.11. (a) PSTH of Type A unit with $N = 408$. (b) PSTH of Type B unit with $N = 800$. (c) AEP recorded from surface of prepyriform cortex with $N = 90$ (Freeman, 1968b).

after the start of the first period and lasts several msec. It coincides with the onset of a single period of high pulse probability of Type B neurons [part (b)], and with the second crest of N1 [part (c)]. That is, Type A neurons are excited by LOT input and then excite each other in the same time period that they excite the Type B (inhibitory) neurons. Thereafter, the effects of inhibition supervene. The enhancement of the second peak of N1 and the prolongation of N1 suggest that reexcitation among Type A neurons is increased with attentiveness.

The increase in reexcitation can be represented by an increase in the feedback gain K_e of the KI_A set. As shown in Section 6.2.2, the effects on the AEP of a selective increase in K_e can be represented by increasing K_n in the KII set in the first mode with $\delta_e = \delta_i = 1$. With increasing K_n and therefore K_e (but fixed K_i) the theoretical root locus replicates the changes in ω and α, and in K_2 and T_2, which are observed experimentally with increased attentiveness (compare Figs. 6.27d and 7.9, for example). The theoretical root loci are similar to those of the KII set in the second mode,[†] but differ in that they cross the $j\omega$ axis with increasing (not decreasing) values of K_n. That is, the crossing points represent stable limit cycles according to the rule given in Section 6.2.1. By extrapolation of values of K_n from 2.0 to 2.8 (for K_o from 1.5 to 2.5), the range of frequencies of the stable limit cycles is from 235 to 268 rad/sec (37.4 to 42.6 Hz). This range is virtually identical to the observed range of frequencies in the cortical EEG, and to the convergence range for KII_{MG} limit cycle output in the second mode (Fig. 6.23a, Section 6.1.5).

This interpretation, however, is not supported by calculation of the phase of the impulse response of the KII set, which is obtained from the inverse transforms of Eq. (27) and (33) in Chapter 6. There K_n is varied from a low value (1.4) to a high value (2.4) with $K_o = 2.0$ and $\delta_e = \delta_i = 1$. The amplitude V_1 for the impulse response of the KI_A set, $c_{12}(t)$ at first increases and then decreases with increased K_n (and K_e). The predicted phase increases,

[†] The KII theoretical root loci in $K_2 \cdot T_2$ coordinates for $\delta_e = \delta_i = 1$ in the first mode and for $\delta_e = 0.33$ in the second mode are similar to each other (compare Figs. 6.23d and 6.27b) and also to yet another theoretical root locus mode (Freeman, 1967). This is generated by fixing K_e, K_i, and K_n at appropriate values and varying the passive membrane rate constant a which is fixed at $a = 220/\text{sec}$ in the calculations in the first and second modes. With decreasing values of a both K_2 and T_2 increase, as the values do in Fig. 6.27d. High values of K_2 and T_2 are associated with highly oscillatory AEPs and high amplitudes of the EEG. High levels of electrical activity imply high levels of synaptic activity, which requires that synaptic conductances for both excitation and inhibition be at high levels. If the synaptic conductance levels affect the passive membrane time constant $\tau = r_m c_m$ by changing the specific membrane resistance r_m, then τ must be decreased by increased synaptic activity, and $a = 1/\tau$ must be increased. The change in the model required to give an increase in K_2 and T_2 is a decrease in a. Therefore, this mode is excluded from consideration.

so the predicted pattern for increase in K_e is $[\pm v_1, +K_2, +T_2, +\varphi_1]$. This is shown graphically in Fig. 7.5b, d, and f. The increase in phase φ_1 is not as great as in the second mode over an equally large change (decrease) in K_n (Fig. 7.5a, c, and e), but the direction of change in φ is inconsistent with experimental data.

An explanation of the phase discrepancy can be based on closer examination of the characteristics of the input to the prepyriform cortex on electrical stimulation of the LOT. The LOT stimulus evokes an orthodromic volley that initiates cortical excitation, and an antidromic volley that excites mitral–tufted cells. These in turn excite granule cells that inhibit mitral–tufted cells and in effect deliver an inhibitory input to the cortex (Section 5.4.3). At the same time that the mitral–tufted cells excite the granule cells, they also excite each other (Green et al., 1962; Nicoll, 1971). The secondary excitation is not as prominent as it is in the cortex (see Fig. 7.11), but is readily detected at high stimulus intensity. Therefore, the input to the cortex on LOT stimulation consists of a large synchronized volley followed by a much smaller volley, which is so temporally dispersed that it is not directly recordable in the LOT. The delay between the volleys can be estimated from the separation between the two peaks of firing probability of mitral–tufted cells on antidromic excitation (3–5 msec) plus about 1-msec conduction delay in each direction (5–7 msec).

We may postulate that during increased attentiveness to the electrically induced LOT input, the increase in K_e selectively increases the sensitivity of the KI_A set to the secondary excitatory volley, and the result is prolongation of the duration of N1. The important aspect is that the secondary volley may potentiate the global effect on the KII_{AB} set of the increase in K_e, such that the characteristic frequency of the set is more sharply tuned. This is conjecture, because the mechanism has not been described mathematically.

There is some evidence that the cortical mechanism for attentiveness is under central control. The pattern of change, $[\pm V_1, +K_2, +T_2, -\varphi_1]$, can be induced in prepyriform AEPs on LOT stimulation in waking cats in the naive state by concomitant tetanization of the nonspecific nuclei of the thalamus.

Example A. Electrodes are implanted in the LOT prepyriform cortex and in the nucleus centralis lateralis of the thalamus. After a recovery period of two weeks, a control AEP is taken with LOT stimulation at near-threshold intensity. Another AEP is taken while a tetanizing pulse train is given to the thalamic nucleus at 20 V, .1-msec pulse duration, and 250 pulses/sec for 10 sec. The AEP changes (Fig. 7.12) in the pattern $[0V_1, +K_2, +T_2, -\varphi_1]$. The change is reversed on cessation of the tetanizing pulse train.

The attempt to transfer a lever-pressing response from a light stimulus to near-threshold LOT stimulation combined with tetanizing stimulation of thalamic nuclei has been unsuccessful, which implies that the cortical change induced by the tetanizing pulse train does not produce the cortical change that an orienting reflex does, when induced by high intensity LOT input.   □

Example B. A direct effect of thalamic tetanization on the level of interaction of superficial pyramidal cells is shown in deeply anesthetized cats. The prepyriform single-shock response consists of a double or dicrotic peak of N1 followed by P1 (Fig. 7.13). The first peak in N1 is due to the response of superficial pyramidal cells in the KI_A set to the LOT volley, and the second peak is due to reexcitation within the KI_A set during excitation of the KI_B set, prior to the onset of inhibition from the KI_B set.

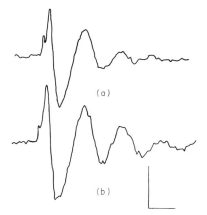

FIG. 7.12. Pattern of change in prepyriform AEP on LOT stimulation from (a) before to (b) during tetanization of the nucleus centralis lateralis, a part of the thalamic reticular system. Calibration: 100 μV, 20 msec.

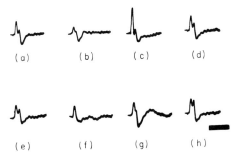

FIG. 7.13. (a)–(d) Posttetanic potentiation of the prepyriform evoked potential on LOT stimulation following tetanization of the test stimulus site. (e)–(h). Heterosynaptic facilitation of the prepyriform evoked potential after tetanization of the nucleus medialis dorsalis. Calibration: 20 msec.

Tetanic stimulation is given to the LOT by the same electrode used for testing for a period of 10 sec. Subsequently there is posttetanic potentiation of the first peak of N1 but not of the second peak of N1 or of P1. The potentiation is maximal after 1 min and abates after 3 to 4 min (Fig. 7.13a–d). Tetanic stimulation is then given to the nucleus medialis dorsalis of the thalamus. The test stimulus is subsequently given to the LOT. The second peak of N1 undergoes suppression for nearly a minute after the tetanization. Subsequently there is facilitation of the second peak of N1 and of P1 but not of the first peak of N1 (Fig. 7.13e–h). It is apparent that thalamic input can influence the level of interaction in the KI_A set by heterosynaptic defacilitation and facilitation. The pathway by which the thalamic input is carried to the cortex is undetermined. □

The most attractive feature of the proposed mechanism for attentiveness is that the selective tuning of the KII_{AB} set in the cortex is at a frequency in the same narrow range as the convergence range of the KII_{MG} set in the bulb in its stable limit cycle state in the second mode. The KII_{AB} set need not enter a stable limit cycle, and it probably should not in order to oscillate in the manner observed in the EEG, because the bulbar KII_{MG} set provides an oscillatory input. That is, during attention the active states of selected cortical subsets of neurons may oscillate because the subsets are tuned to their input frequencies. Measurements on the EEGs concomitantly recorded from the bulb and prepyriform cortex with implanted electrodes in waking cats (Boudreau, 1964) in food-seeking behavior show that there is a peak in the spectra near 40 Hz of the EEG from both structures, and that cortical EEG activity is often highly correlated with bulbar activity. These frequencies and high levels of correlation do not occur in anesthetized cats, and they occur to a lesser degree during consummatory behavior (eating or lapping), which again suggests that the basis for attention may be tuning of selected KII_{AB} subsets to the carrier frequency of their input from the KII_{MG} set.

The contrary of attention may be on the one hand nonspecific and due to lack of a pre-existing orienting response establishing a neural template as the specific basis for attentiveness, to lack of general arousal, or to direction of attentiveness elsewhere. On the other hand, the state of being inattentive may be hightly specific as in postorienting or postextinctive habituation to a stimulus. There is some evidence tentatively suggesting that specific forms of habituation involve not merely the absence of tuning or resonance but a specific form of antiresonance. Whereas attentiveness is postulated to occur as a complex pair of poles in the dynamic system of the KII set approaches the $j\omega$ axis near $\pm 250\,\mathrm{rad/sec}$ (40 Hz), during habituation a complex pair of zeros may approach these two points in the s plane.

This may happen when one or more of the neural subsets in the KII_{AB} set have characteristic frequencies that differ by 10 to 20% from the dominant frequency at 40 Hz. The result of summing the output of two subsets having characteristic frequencies, one at, say, 30 Hz and another at 50 Hz, might be the occurrence of antiresonance at or near 40 Hz. The mechanism by which the complex zeros would take a frequency near that value is described in Section 2.5.3. The existence of multimodal spectra from AEPs having the requisite form is shown in Figs. 2.25, 2.27, and 6.31b, and in Fig. 3.15a and Table 3.3 for the EEG. We have as yet no specific postulate concerning the nature of the changes in KII_{AB} feedback gains to explain these spectral patterns, but it appears that the mechanism for habituating to a stimulus is not the simple converse of the mechanism for attention.

7.2. Transformations of Neural Signals by KII Sets

The main purpose in exploring the properties of KII sets is to learn more about brain function in relation to vertebrate adaptive behavior. Even the simplest forms of such behavior depend on the activities of immense numbers of neurons, and the hierarchy of K-sets is merely a first step in understanding beyond the level of single neurons. The characteristics of teleological behavior are well known. It consists in a circular set of processes: perception, which includes sensory reception, central coding,[†] orienting, selective attending, storage (memory), recognition, and recall; and responding, which includes localization of events in external space–time, prediction, motivation, choice among a repertoire of actions, and execution; and reception of sensory input resulting from the action. It is an adaptive process. In perhaps the simplest unequivocal example it is elaborated by the forebrain of a fish, which is homing on an olfactory cue prior to mating. Conversely, it is not elaborated by the midbrain of a frog responding to visual cues (Lettvin et al., 1959).

The essential feature of the perceptual process is the elaboration by the forebrain of a coded or symbolic representation or expectation, which is a model of some aspect of the external world (Craik, 1952; Sokolov, 1963; Bongard, 1970; Grossberg, 1973). During attentiveness a continual sequence of comparisons is made between the representation or "neuronal model" (Sokolov, 1963), and the sequence of coded neural signals in an afferent system. In neurophysiological terms the coded signals consist in

---

[†] For a review of neural coding see Perkel & Bullock (1968). In common use the existence of a coding operation is taken to imply the existence of an inverse operation to retrieve the coded signal in its original form. Such an inverse operation need not exist, and there is no reason to expect that the central nervous system reconstructs its input by inverse operations.

patterns of action potentials on afferent tracts, and the symbolic representation is a pattern of excitability or sensitivity in subsets of neurons receiving
the action potentials. The nature of the response of the receiving subsets
of neurons depends on whether the patterns of excitation and excitability
are similar or dissimilar. Therefore, a description of neural signals in
perception and adaptive behavior must deal explicitly with the complementary facets of patterned excitation and patterned excitability.

A comparison between the elementary visual and olfactory mechanisms
for tracking prey or mating, respectively, in the frog and the fish may help
to clarify what is meant by the word *adaptive* in this chapter. Both
mechanisms consist of a receptor layer transmitting its signals through
a series of layers of interconnected neurons ultimately to the motorneurons.
Both systems mediate orientation of the body in space, directed locomotion,
and aimed movements of capture that involve other senses as well. The
principal site of elaboration for the fish olfactory system is in the forebrain
which has prominent EEG activity, whereas the principal site for the
frog's visual system is in the midbrain, which has been found to have less
significant EEG activity. The sensory data on the nature and location of
a stimulus to the frog's visual system are apparently represented in the
size and location of a focus of neural activity in the optic tectum of the
midbrain that provides a surface onto which the retina is mapped. The
pattern of neural connections is genetically determined (Jacobson, 1970).
The sensory data on the nature and location of an olfactory source appear
to be represented in the olfactory bulbs by a time varying amplitude of
activity that can be inferred to depend on the sequence of movements
made by the fish in swimming upstream through water containing varying
concentrations of particular chemical substances. We may presume that the
neural connectivity patterns determining a particular sensitive state for each
fish are based on learning shortly before the young fish emigrates to the
sea from its spawning waters (Hara, Ueda & Gorbman, 1965), and that
they are not genetically determined.

The most crucial difference between these systems is that visual stimuli
in the frog can be represented by a dynamic variable on a neural surface
that conforms to visual space in the external world of the frog, whereas
olfactory stimuli in the fish are represented by neural dynamic patterns that
cannot be dynamic analogs and must serve as symbols (Pattee, 1972). Each
fish must have in its forebrain a *cognitive map* (Tolman, 1948) of the external
world as the basis for its ability to plot and execute trajectories of
movement in space, but the nature of the cognitive map and the way in
which a symbolic olfactory dynamic pattern is translated into position
and direction on the map cannot be given in terms of conformal mapping
into Euclidean space. In this respect the midbrain of the frog can be

viewed as one of the most elaborate and complex developments of the deterministic neural machinery of the brainstem and spinal cord, whereas the paleocortex of the fish provides one of the most primitive identifiable examples of the non-Euclidean adaptive neural machinery of the forebrain.

The primary olfactory system can reasonably be held responsible for the earlier stages of the perceptual process in relation to odors. The main feature of reception is the chemical transduction of the incidence of active substances on the cilia of olfactory receptors to pulse trains on PON axons. The mechanism of transduction and the numbers and distributions of receptor types are not adequately known, but there are several good working hypotheses (see reviews by Moulton & Tucker, 1964; Ottoson, 1963; Wenzel & Sieck, 1967). Basically, the receptors comprise a KO set, and their function can be readily comprehended in terms of the performance of single archetypal neurons (Le Gros Clark, 1957).

About the process of central coding there is almost complete ignorance. The numerous attempts made (e.g., Beidler, 1971) to establish the existence of selective sensitivity of single bulbar and cortical neurons to differing chemical substances have not given consistent results, and it appears that olfactory equivalents (Lettvin & Gesteland, 1965) to feature detectors in the visual system (e.g. Hubel & Wiesel, 1962) do not exist in relation to known chemical substances. In the absence of a verified theory of olfactory coding, it is virtually impossible to proceed with further analysis of the perceptual process at the neural level, because the neural transformations cannot be described until the nature is known of what is being transformed.

The main thesis of this book is that olfactory central coding is a cooperative neural process, and that it can only be understood in terms of interactive neural sets. A substantiated hypothesis for coding cannot be put forward yet, but the known properties of the olfactory KII sets can be used to construct working hypotheses for experimental elaboration. Concrete examples of working hypotheses for coding and selective attention are given in the next three sections. They are based on three postulates, which can be explored and tested by experimental and mathematical techniques.

7.2.1. NEURAL CODING IN THE OLFACTORY BULB

An olfactory stimulus consists in a substance or mixture of substances, which is delivered in an air or water stream to the olfactory mucosa, which acts on varying numbers of receptors in a spatial distribution over the mucosa, and which hyperpolarizes or depolarizes their membranes. The process of reception or transduction is the conversion of a time-varying spatial distribution of the effective concentration of the substance, which depends on the air or water flow and the physiochemical properties of the substance and the receptors, to a time-varying spatial distribution of action potentials at the trigger zones of the bipolar receptors. The afferent neural signal is the distribution of action potentials at the trigger zones, which is both the effect and the specific correlate of the olfactory stimulus.

The process of central coding is the transformation of the afferent neural signal to another form, which is suitable for further transformations involved in the higher perceptual processes of orienting, attending, storage, recognition and recall.

Postulate 1.   A specific olfactory stimulus activates (excites or inhibits) a spatial distribution of receptors, which is not unique to the stimulus, but which has some general but as yet unspecified constraints.   □

The constraints mean that (a) the spatial distribution can be different on successive applications of the same stimulus, but that (b) in one or more respects it is unlike the spatial distribution of the signal for any other specific stimulus, and that (c) in some respects it is indistinguishable from the signals on previous presentations of the same stimulus.

The forms of the constraints are unknown, but that is unimportant for present purposes. The postulate requires only that a spatially nonuniform pattern of receptor activity exist during a time period equivalent to a sniff (100–200 msec). The time-dependent patterns of pulse trains from receptors are assumed to be insignificant.[†] The only important variable is the total number of pulses carried by each axon in the PON over the duration of an afferent surge of impulses induced by the stimulus flow. To express this in symbolic form, let the activity density function (Section 1.3.2) of the KO_R set in the pulse mode by designated $o_{Rp}(t, x_r, y_r, u)$, where x_r, y_r, is distance over the olfactory mucosa, t is time, and u designates the amplitude dependent nonlinearities. Further, let distance over the olfactory bulb be designated by x_b, y_b.

Transmission of the afferent signal by the PON to the glomeruli in the bulb includes the transformations of translation to a new set of surface coordinates; constriction to a smaller surface area; interspersive divergence in both surface coordinates (Section 4.5.1), which can be expressed by a

<hr/>

[†] Roitbak & Khechinashvili (1952) have shown that oscillations at frequencies near 50 Hz occur in the field potential of the olfactory mucosa, which cannot be attributed to spread of the field potential of the bulb into the mucosa. These oscillatory potentials raise the possibility that the timing of pulses in the LOT may be correlated, either with each other or with induced bulbar activity or both. These possible relations should be explored by recording of PON units. If some temporal structure is found in $p_R(x_r, t)$ at a characteristic frequency of the KII_{MG} set, its significance can be explored by introducing an appropriate input function $f_f(t) G_f(i)$ into Eqs. (5) in Chapter 6.

convergence function to each point on the bulb surface; conduction delay; and temporal dispersion (Section 2.3.3). The input to the bulb from the receptors is $o_{Rp}(t, x_b, y_b, u)$. Under Postulate 1 we may designate a time $t = 0$ at which the activity density function attains an effective summed value over a preceding time interval. This function we call $\bar{o}_{Rp}(0, x_b, y_b, u)$ and treat it as the input to the KI_M set.

In the apical dendrites of the mitral–tufted cells there is pulse to wave conversion and summation of input in accordance with the linear properties of the dendrites. Each mitral–tufted cell performs an integration over a portion of the neural signal in the mucosa. The form of the integral is determined by the interspersive convergence function for that part of the PON (Section 4.5.4). This integral transformation results in a new signal, which consists in a nonuniform spatial distribution of activity in the KI_M set of mitral–tufted cells, $o_M(t, x_b, y_b, u)$.

The PON input also excites a spatial distribution of periglomerular neurons in the KI_P set. The neurons interact with each other by axodendritic synapses and with mitral–tufted cells by apical dendrodendritic synapses (Section 5.2.1). The KI_P set generates sustained excitatory activity, which is delivered to the cell bodies and basal dendrites of mitral–tufted cells as an excitatory input bias. The bias is further transmitted to the KI_G set, which retransmits an inhibitory input bias to the KI_M set. The resulting operating bias of the KII_{MG} set is excitatory (Section 6.1.4).

The leading edge of the afferent signal in the PON induces oscillation in the KII_{MG} set in the first mode. The operating bias gives a positive value to $\delta_e = \delta_i$, so for comparable local values of $K_o(X)$ the frequency is constant near 50 Hz (the intrinsic rhythm of Adrian), and the decay rate is most rapid for higher excitatory response amplitudes. The input to the KII_{MG} set from the PON is sustained and smoothed by temporal dispersion, and the input from the KI_P set is sustained by excitatory feedback. The combination of sustained excitatory inputs raises the firing rates of the KI_M set $o_{Mp}(t, x_b, y_b, u)$ to a higher level which is easily observed (Section 3.3.2) during each inspiration in bulbar unit records. The sustained excitatory activity of the KI_M set is transmitted to the KI_G set. Excitation of the KI_G set is manifested as a surface-negative wave of potential. These sustained increases in active states cause an increase in $K_o(X)$ of the KII_{MG} set. If the increase is large enough, the KII_{MG} set enters a limit cycle state in the KII first mode (Section 6.2.2).

If the value for $K_o(X)$ is sufficiently high, and if there is also sufficient residual intrinsic wave activity in subsets of the KII_{MG} set, those subsets enter a limit cycle state in the KII second mode. Oscillatory activity increases in amplitude and converges in frequency to a narrow range near 40 Hz. We assume that the state rapidly spreads to include all subsets having sufficiently high $K_o(X)$, so a limit cycle domain is formed in the KII_{MG} set. If the distribution of frequencies over the domain is sufficiently narrow and the onset of oscillation is sufficiently well synchronized, then the dendritic potential fields of local subsets sum to give a sinusoidal wave of potential in the EEG at the mean frequency of the distribution. This, the induced wave of Adrian, is not an impulse response. It manifests a limit cycle of activity arising from the effects of the sustained PON and KI_P excitatory inputs on the KII_{MG} set (Section 6.2.3).

The range of frequency convergence is too narrow for coding of olfactory signals by frequency modulation (Hughes *et al.*, 1969). Moreover, the amplitude of oscillation of activity as well as the frequency is determined more by the characteristics of the KII_{MG} set than by the PON input. The mean rates of mitral–tufted cell firing are dependent as much on the balance between KI_M interaction, KI_G interaction, and KI_P input as on PON input. The only remaining variable is the phase of the oscillation in local subsets with respect to the mean phase of the entire limit cycle domain.

Postulate 2. The phase of oscillatory activity $\varphi_M(X)$ of local subsets in a limit cycle domain in the KII second mode varies with respect to the mean phase $\bar{\varphi}_M$ of the domain depending on the initial conditions in the local subsets. □

Just prior to the onset of the limit cycle state there are by Postulate 1 spatially nonuniform distributions of nonoscillatory activity over the KI_P, KI_M and KI_G sets. The subsets of KI_P and KI_M neurons are richly inter-connected synaptically within glomeruli and more sparsely between glomeruli (Section 4.3.1). The active states of the subset of mitral–tufted cells with apical dendrites in the same glomerulus should tend to be the same over the entire subset. The variation in active state between these subsets of the KI_M set should vary over the set at a spatial frequency, which may depend on the effective transmission distances of bulbar neurons (Section 4.5.3) and on the mean diameter of the glomeruli ($135 \pm 27\ \mu$m), for which the maximal spatial frequency is the reciprocal of twice the diameter or 3.7 ± 0.7 mm. The spatial variation in $o_M(t, x_b, y_b, u)$, $t = 0$, determines the spatial variation of $K_o(X)$. When the limit cycle state ensues, the local value of $K_o(X)$ should have negligible effect on the frequency of the oscillation (Section 6.2.3 and Fig. 6.23a), but $o_M(0, x_b, y_b, u)$ at the time of onset of the limit cycle state may critically determine the local values of the phase $\varphi_M(X)$ of the oscillation.

If this occurs, the neural signal is transformed from a surface distribution of nonoscillatory pulse densities to a surface distribution of oscillating pulse densities. The local values for the steady mean pulse densities are mapped into local values for the phase φ_M and modulation amplitude $\tilde{p}_M$ of the oscillatory activities. The phase and modulation amplitude of each local subset are the values of a vector $[\tilde{p}_M(X), \varphi_M(X)]$ for that subset. The process of central coding in the bulb is proposed to be the transformation of a steady state nonuniform surface distribution of pulse densities to the surface function of a vector, which describes the phase and amplitude modulation of the common carrier frequency of oscillatory pulse densities in the KII limit cycle domain (see also Schneider, 1974).

Phase modulation can occur because there is not sufficient strength of interaction in the KII set to cause entrainment and phase-locking (Section 6.2.3). This condition also implies that the useful duration of a burst of KII limit cycle activity is limited by the width of the frequency convergence range. If, for example, the width is 254 ± 9 rad/sec (Fig. 6.18b) and the first zero crossing is synchronous, after 8 cycles of the mean oscillation (205 msec) the zero crossings of the activities of subsets at the highest and lowest frequencies must lead and lag the mean by ± 7 msec, which is equivalent at the mean period of the oscillation (24.7 msec) to a phase lag of ± 1.77 rad, or more than a quarter cycle. Burst durations in the EEG range from 0.1 sec to over 1 sec, and the median duration is probably not far from 200 msec, particularly during sniffing (Fig. 7.2).

Some degree of synchronization, or rather a minimum of phase dispersion, is a necessary condition for the appearance of a sinusoidal burst in the EEG, but it is not a condition for the transformation of an olfactory signal. A burst need not occur in the EEG during the maintenance of a signal by the KII_{MG} set in the limit cycle second mode, and instances occur in which the EEG amplitude diminishes during a sniff (Fig. 7.2a), though they are less common than the occurrences of an increase (Fig. 7.2c).

The KII limit cycle state and the EEG burst may outlast the useful duration over which phase relations can be defined in the presence of a frequency distribution. Both may outlast the withdrawal of PON input at the end of inspiration. Termination of the wave and reimposition of a KII equilibrium stable state is required before a new signal can be coded. This is apparently done by the act of expiration.

According to Postulate 1 the afferent neural signal consists in a surface distribution of pulse densities, which are averaged by neurons in the KI_M set over a time period long enough to establish a KII limit cycle state in the second mode and to impose modulation on that state. The afferent signal can be described as a spatiotemporally patterned volley of impulses. According to Postulate 2 the coded neural signal consists in oscillatory cooperative activity. This can be thought of as a *wave packet* occupying a location in some fraction X_M of the KII_{MG} surface area (176 mm^2) for a limited time on the order of 100 to 200 msec, ΔT_M, beginning at some time T. It has a characteristic carrier frequency ω_t of about 250 rad/sec

(40 Hz) which undergoes amplitude $\tilde{p}_M$, and phase modulation φ_M at a spatial frequency ω_x on the order of 4/mm. The main function of the bulb may be to generate a sequence of wave packets which represent olfactory stimuli, and to transmit them to the prepyriform cortex over the LOT. The wave packet consists of pulses p in a certain kind of order. We may represent the variables $(t, \tilde{p}_M, \varphi_M, \omega_x, \omega_t, X_M, \Delta T_M)$ by Ω and define the wave packet as an active state having the form specified by

$$o_M(\Omega) \triangleq o_{Mp}(t, \tilde{p}_M, \varphi_M, \omega_x, \omega_t, X_M, \Delta T_M). \tag{3}$$

7.2.2. BULBAR MECHANISMS FOR PHASE MODULATION

The mechanism for phase modulation can be described mathematically in a simple way. At the onset of stable limit cycle activity in the second mode the KII set as a dynamic system has 12 poles and 10 zeros (Section 6.1.2). One of the pairs of complex conjugate poles lies on the $j\omega$ axis in the s plane. The remaining 10 poles and 10 zeros lie far to the left of the $j\omega$ axis, and their total contribution to the transfer function is negligible. When the phase of the impulse response is computed for the KII set in the second mode at the required low value for K_n, the phase of the output of the KI_e set is very near zero (see Fig. 7.5e). That is, the higher-order poles and zeros can be said to cancel. Then the differential equation required to represent the KII set in the stable limit cycle state of the second mode is linear and second order. The observable output of each subset in the KI_M set, $p_M(X, t)$ in the pulse mode is governed by

$$\partial^2 p_M(X, t)/\partial t^2 = -\omega^2 p_M(X, t), \tag{4}$$

where ω is the limit cycle frequency in radians per second. When $p_M(X, 0)$ is the initial condition at each local subset, and p_o is the mean pulse rate of the entire KII_{MG} set as previously defined (Section 6.1.1), the solution is

$$p_M(X, t) = p_M(X, o) \sin[\omega t + \varphi_M(X)], \tag{5}$$

where

$$\varphi_M(X) = 0, \qquad p_M(X, 0) = p_o, \tag{6}$$

$$\varphi_M(X) > 0, \qquad p_M(X, 0) > p_o, \tag{7}$$

$$\varphi_M(X) < 0, \qquad p_M(X, 0) < p_o. \tag{8}$$

That is, the phase for each subset in KI_M depends on the initial conditions in that subset.

Physiological evidence bearing on this hypothesis is from the EEG and AEP. The existence of wave packets $o_M(\Omega)$ is manifested in pulse probability waves from mitral–tufted cells, both singly and in local subsets recorded from the same microelectrode (Section 3.3.3 and Fig. 3.18). In the bulb the frequency of each wave is always the same as the dominant frequency of the EEG, and the modulation amplitude of the wave is closely related to the amplitude of the EEG bursts. The phase difference expected intuitively (Section 5.3.3) between the outputs of the KI_M set in the pulse mode and of the KI_G set in the wave mode is 1.57 rad (one-quarter of the period of the oscillation). The phase difference calculated between the outputs of the KI_e and KI_i sets in the KII set by Eq. (28) in Chapter 6 is predicted to be 1.00 rad (the difference in Fig. 7.5 between output A_{12} and A_{34}) in Sections 7.1.2 and 7.1.4 (Table 7.4). This range (1.00–1.57 rad) includes the observed means (Section 3.3.4).

TABLE 7.4

VARIATION IN PHASE OF PULSE PROBABILITY WAVE

| | Phase | | Delay |
	(rad)	(deg)	(msec)[a]
Predicted			
Section 5.3.3	1.57	90	6.25
Section 7.1.2	1.01	58	4.00
Observed mean	1.40	80	5.55
Range	2.29	134	9.30
Standard deviation	±.71	±41	±2.85
Mean absolute deviation	±.57	±33	±2.25

[a] Computed on the basis of frequency of 250 rad/sec giving a period of 25 msec.

When pulse trains from two, three, or multiple units are recorded simultaneously from the same electrode, the phase values of the several pulse probability waves are almost always equal within the limits of experimental error (.1 rad), though they vary on sequential trials (Fig. 7.14). When single or multiple unit trains are recorded simultaneously from multiple microelectrodes at different locations in the same cooperative focus in the bulb, the phase values vary significantly between sites and at the same sites over successive recording periods. The first result shows that the similarity exists in active state of neurons in local subsets, which is required by Postulate 2 (but see the footnote in Section 4.5.1). The second result shows that the possibility exists of variation in phase and modulation amplitude with time and distance, which is required for neural coding in wave packets $o_\mu(\Omega_v)$.

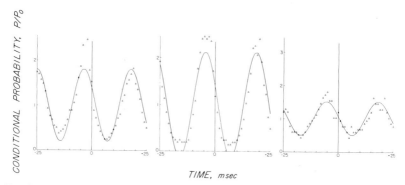

FIG. 7.14. Successive measurements of the pulse probability wave of a mitral–tufted pulse train from an anesthetized cat. The wave is characterized by a frequency equal to the frequency of the EEG, an amplitude expressed as a fraction of the mean pulse probability, and a phase measured with respect to the phase of the EEG (see Section 3.3.4).

Example A. A multiple microelectrode is made by cementing 10 insulated stainless steel wires, each 25 μm in diameter into a ribbon, which is cut at an angle, so that the tips are 150 μm apart center to center over a distance of 1350 μm. The array is inserted into an active focus in the olfactory bulb of a waking minimally restrained rabbit and into the external plexiform layer in a direction parallel to the bulbar surface. Multiple unit trains are recorded from each electrode and amplified on separate channels, and the EEG is sampled on number 5 electrode from the tip. The unit trains are filtered to remove the EEG and passed through a threshold device, which is set to deliver a standard 5-V 1.0-msec pulse for each neural pulse above the threshold. Multiple units are recorded at average rates of 20/sec. The EEG is filtered to remove units and the respiratory wave (3 dB falloff at 10 and 130 Hz). Each of the 11 channels is sampled 1000 times in 1 sec, and the data are read onto magnetic tape in a block in the next 1.5 sec. A pulse probability table is constructed for each channel from 20 blocks of 1000 measurements extending over 20 sec of recording time and 50 sec of real time. The phase and modulation amplitude are determined by fitting a sine wave to the two experimental pulse probability waves from each channel (Section 3.3.3). The means and differences between the two estimates for phase and amplitude for each channel are shown in Fig. 7.15.

The procedure is repeated 5 times during rest and 5 times during eating. The successive sets of values for phase and amplitude at each site varying with time are shown in Fig. 7.16, in the form of perspective drawings of the three-dimensional figures. The results show that the parameters specified for signal representation in wave packets can vary concomitantly with distance and sequentially with time, as they are required to by Postulate 2.

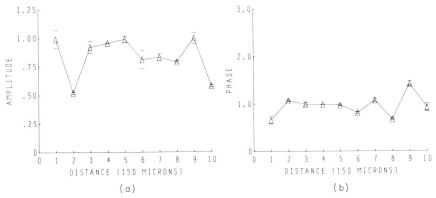

(a)   (b)

FIG. 7.15. Simultaneous measurement of the amplitude and phase of pulse probability waves of mitral–tufted unit clusters at 10 points on a line parallel to the bulbar surface in a waking rabbit. Upper and lower bars: values derived from $\hat{P}_+(T)$ and $\hat{P}_-(T)$; triangle: means (see Section 3.3.4).

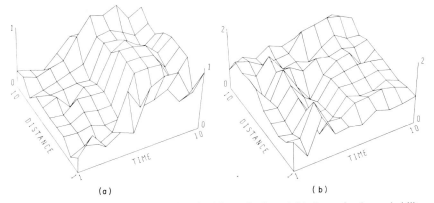

(a)   (b)

FIG. 7.16. Ten sequential sets of values for (a) amplitude and (b) phase of pulse probability waves at 10 points $150\,\mu$m apart in the olfactory bulb of a waking rabbit. The first five sets precede eating, and the second five sets accompany eating.

However, neither the spatial nor the temporal resolution is adequate as yet to support correlations between values of the parameters and particular olfactory stimuli. □

Variations are also observed in the phase difference between AEPs and PSTHs simultaneously collected in the bulb on LOT or PON stimulation (Sections 5.3.3 and 5.3.4). The variations significantly exceed the limits of experimental error (Section 6.2.4). The mean phase difference is $1.49 \pm .25$ rad with a range in variation of .77 rad. The distribution of values is flatter than expected for random variation.

Examination of AEPs and PSTHs in relation to changes in stimulus intensity gives a clue to a mechanism by which an excitatory or inhibitory bias can contribute to the determination of phase. Figure 6.15 shows pairs of AEPs and PSTHs on LOT and PON stimulation at three levels of intensity. For near threshold input there is minimal saturation displayed in the PSTH (a and d). With increasing stimulus intensity saturation is augmented, which causes the decrease in both AEP and PSTH frequency (b and e). Above the range of piecewise linear approximation (c and f) there is marked prolongation both in the period of complete block of firing and in the duration of P1. However, the burst of pulses at the end of saturation precedes the crest of N2 of the AEP by a fixed interval.

These relations hold in the lower range of input intensity, though it is less obvious. With increasing input intensity the AEP and PSTH frequency decreases, but the interval between the second crest of the PSTH and N2 is fixed. The phase lead of the PSTH oscillation decreases with respect to the phase of the AEP oscillation. The effect of increasing the input intensity in this respect is to increase the effect of saturation by threshold, which is equivalent to an inhibitory operating bias. More generally, an inhibitory bias should decrease the phase difference between the AEP and PSTH, and an excitatory operating bias should increase it.

The phase of pulse probability waves is measured with respect to the phase of the bulbar EEG, which is taken as the mean over the cooperative domain. The expected mean phase is about a quarter cycle of lead. If the phase lead of the pulse probability wave at a site is more than 1.57 rad, that site can be inferred to have more excitatory bias than the average over the domain. If it is less than 1.57 rad, the site has more inhibitory bias by this inference.

Local variations in bias may have four sources, namely the PON and the KI_P, and KI_M, and KI_G sets. Doubtless the most important is the input signal from the PON, which by Postulate 1 is nonuniformly distributed to the KI_M set. The subsets of mitral–tufted cells receiving the highest density of PON input should have the strongest phase lead in their pulse probability waves with respect to the EEG [Eq. (5)].

The KI_P set also provides excitatory bias to the KI_M subsets receiving PON input (Section 6.1.3). This input bias, however, appears to be neutralized by the inhibitory bias, which is generated by the KI_G set and directed onto the same KI_M subsets (Section 6.1.4). Tertiary effects may occur in several forms. The most prominent form derives from the fact that the inhibitory focus following focal excitation of the KI_M set has a larger diameter than the excitatory focus (Section 4.5.3). This pattern consists in synaptic divergence of inhibition. It is not surround inhibition, which only occurs concomitantly around a focus of excitation.

Synaptic divergence of excitation occurs in the glomerular layer. Divergence of activity in the KI_P set in the glomerular layer by successive excitation is not detectable in responses to PON electrical stimulation, because the surface distribution of the input is too wide. The axons of periglomerular neurons, however, extend across 3 or 4 glomerular diameters, which implies that when neighboring glomeruli receive significantly different amplitudes of PON input, some divergence of excitation must occur in the glomerular layer (Section 4.5.4).

Another source of divergent excitation is the interaction of mitral–tufted cells of the KI_M set through axon collaterals in the external and internal plexiform layers. The extent to which divergence occurs in the KI_G set, possibly by way of the axons of stellate cells (Section 4.3.1), is not known. Each KI_G subset, which is excited by a KI_M subset, must inhibit other KI_G subsets, which lie in a focus of larger diameter. The inhibited KI_G subsets disinhibit (excite) neighboring mitral–tufted KI_M subsets as well as other KI_G subsets. This constitutes a third form of excitatory divergence.

These several forms of excitatory divergence are in opposition to the main tertiary effect of inhibitory divergence. They are probably negligible. It is possible that the average length of mitral–tufted basal dendrites which determines the radius of inhibitory divergence (Section 4.5.3) is adapted to a distance sufficient to prevent excitatory divergence by the three mechanisms described. A similar cancellation of the effects of stimulus dispersion (by light scattering) by mutually inhibitory neural interactions has been described in the eye of Limulus (Kirschfeld & Reichardt, 1964).

If these inferences are correct, the transformation of a signal from an afferent volley to a wave packet is by the conversion of each local value of pulse density entering the glomeruli to a locally determined value for phase of the induced pulse probability wave of the corresponding subset of mitral-tufted cells. That is, the pulse density function is mapped one-to-one into a phase function over the same surface

$$o_M(t, x_b, y_b, u), z_b = H_b[o_{Rp}(0, x_b, y_b, u), z_b]. \tag{9}$$

Some of the other subsidiary properties of the KI_P and KI_G sets can now be explained in terms of the basic role of the KII_{MG} set. The KI_P set, in addition to providing sustained and transient excitatory bias, provides automatic volume control of PON input (Section 5.2.3), because glomerular transmission attenuation occurs as a side effect of periglomerular activity. Each glomerulus in the cat receives on the order of 5×10^4 PON axons. The number of excited axons sufficient to evoke oscillatory bulbar activity in response to odors may vary over 3 orders of magnitude, depending on the concentration of the olfactory stimulus and on other factors. The reduction in effectiveness of PON input in proportion to its amplitude in the glomeruli is essential to adapt the wide dynamic range of the input KO set to the relatively narrow near-linear range of optimal function of the KII_{MG} set.

The KI_G set, through the mechanism of inhibitory feedback, provides for signal normalization (Grossberg, 1973). In addition the KI_G subsets provide an entry into the KII_{MG} system for axons coming from the ipsilateral and contralateral anterior olfactory nuclei and from the nucleus of the diagonal band (Price & Powell, 1970c). These inputs as well as the centrifugal input to the KI_P set provide a basis for regulation of the output of the KI_M set, particularly in relation to the states of sleep and arousal (Section 5.4.5).

7.2.3. ATTENTION AND THE CORTICAL EXPECTATION FUNCTION

The wave packet established at the trigger zones of mitral–tufted cells in the KI_M set is transmitted by pulses on the LOT, first to the lateral part of the anterior olfactory nucleus by collaterals and synapses en passant, and then to the prepyriform and periamygdaloid cortex. There is an orderly topographic arrangement in the nucleus (Section 5.4.3), such that each part receives from KI_M subsets in one segment of the bulb and transmits its output to KI_G subsets in the same part of the bulb. The topology suggests that the nucleus serves to monitor the output of the bulb and to provide for feedback regulation of the amplitude or frequency or both of every part of the wave packet. The mechanism needs further study, but its topology and geometry are relatively simple, so that quantitative analysis and lumped circuit mathematical description appear feasible without extensive further development of theory.

The transmission channel to the cortex presents more difficult problems. In addition to translation $(x_b, y_b) \rightarrow (x_c, y_c)$, on reaching the cortex the activity in LOT undergoes extensive interspersion, and there is a high degree of collateral divergence (Section 4.4.2). Each local subset of the KI_A set receives axons from up to three-fourths of the KI_M set, and each KI_M neuron transmits to an undefined number and distribution of neurons in the KI_A set. At the simplest level it is reasonable to conclude that the LOT and KI_A set perform an integral transformation on the wave packet, $o_M(\Omega_c)$, which consists of convolution of the LOT input with the LOT convergence function to each point on the prepyriform cortex. Neither is known quantitatively.

This transformation can be regarded as a key step in the process of pattern recognition in the olfactory system. Every pattern of spatially distributed activity consists in the relation of the parameter values in each part to all other parts. Because each part of the KII_{AB} set receives input from virtually every part of the KII_{MG} set (excluding the dorsomedial bulb), the anatomical basis is provided for pattern analysis. If the activities of every subset of mitral–tufted cells are not uniformly and simultaneously distributed to the KI_A set, then the divergence function is not uniform, and spatially distributed information coded in the bulbar wave packet is not destroyed by the integration. The wave packet $o_M(\Omega_b)$ has a single frequency, bounded amplitude, and a maximal and possibly characteristic spatial frequency, so the integration can probably be described in a relatively simple linear form.

Before this can be done, however, some crucial data are needed on the characteristic length, width and periodicity of single LOT axon terminal distributions, including the spatial frequency of axon collaterals and en passant synapses, and on the characteristic spatial frequencies of the KII_{AB} set. These must depend on the effective transmission distances and lengths of fibers of the Type A and B neurons, as in the case of mitral–tufted and granule cells in the bulb (Sections 4.5.3 and 4.5.4).

Each Type A neuron receives axons from an unspecified number of mitral–tufted cells, as well as from other Type A neurons and Type B neurons. It performs two kinds of running integration over the inputs from these axons. The first is a scalar summation of the steady levels of p_o on the axons. The second is a vector summation of the pulse probability waves. For each input frequency the resultant is a sine wave at the same frequency. The phase and amplitude of output of each Type A neuron are given by the vector sum of the phases and amplitudes of the pulse probability waves at that frequency. Corresponding to each output frequency there is an input frequency, if the KII_{AB} set is operating in a linear range.

Each Type A neuron is embedded in the KII_{AB} set, and if it generates a detectable pulse probability wave, the frequency is usually though not invariably at the dominant frequency of the EEG. Exceptions occur when there are two peaks in the spectrum of the EEG in the vicinity of 40 Hz, and the pulse probability wave frequency then has a value between the EEG frequency values (Table 3.3 in Section 3.5.5).

The pulse probability wave of a Type A neuron or of a subset of the KI_A set can have maximal modulation amplitude only when the frequencies of the pulse probability waves on both LOT and intracortical axons converge to a narrow range. This is postulated to depend on the conjunction of two conditions. First, the bulbar KII_{MG} set must enter the stable limit cycle state in the second mode, in which a substantial fraction of the KII_{MG} set transmits pulse probability waves at a frequency near 40 Hz (Section 6.2.3). Second, the value for K_e for the subset in the KI_A set must increase to a value, which is sufficiently large to cause the KII_{AB} subset to approach the KII limit cycle state in the first mode (Section 7.1.4). That is, the characteristic frequency of the KII_{AB} set must be tuned to the output frequency of the KII_{MG} set (Fig. 7.17).

On the one hand, if the bulb is in an equilibrium state in either mode or

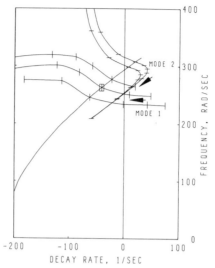

FIG. 7.17. It is suggested that bursts of EEG activity at 40 Hz occur in the prepyriform cortex upon the conjunction of two conditions: stable limit cycle activity in the bulbar KII_{MG} set in the second mode, and tuning of the characteristic frequency of the cortical KII_{AB} set to a value near 40 Hz by an increase in K_e in the first mode. $\square$: $K_o = K_n = 2.00$.

in a limit cycle state in the first mode, such that there is a distribution of intrinsic frequencies, the vector sum by each KI_A subset over a collection of KI_M subsets continually averages near zero. It is only when the KI_M subsets transmit at frequencies in the narrow convergence range, as when a wave packet is transmitted, that a nonzero vector sum results from the integral transformation performed by the LOT and the KI_A set.

On the other hand, the KII_{MG} set can be regarded as transmitting a signal at a certain carrier frequency, and the KII_{AB} set can be considered as a receiver with a variable tuned frequency. The optimal condition for transmitting and receiving occurs when the two frequencies coincide. Studies of AEPs in attentive cats suggest that K_e in the KII_{AB} set is increased during attentiveness to the stimulus evoking the responses, which are averaged to give the AEP (Section 7.1.3). Therefore, attentiveness may involve the selective increase in forward gain $K_e^{.5}$ of certain subsets within the KI_A set, such that the characteristic frequencies of the corresponding KII_{AB} sets are sharply tuned to a range near 40 Hz.

The difficulty with this hypothesis as stated in Section 7.1.4 is that the predicted phase does not decrease with increased $K_e^{.5}$, whereas the observed phase of AEPs does decrease with attentiveness. This difficulty can be resolved if attentiveness is conceived not merely as a state of excitability, but as the relation between an excitable state (an expectation function) and that which is expected (an excitation function). Specifically we are concerned with a possible relation between the input function on the LOT, $\varphi_M(X_c)$, which is determined by $\varphi_M(X_b)$ in the bulb and the divergence property of the LOT, and an expectation function which we postulate to have the form of a spatially varying forward gain, $K_e^{.5}(X_c)$ of the KI_A set.

The critical parameter of the input signal is the phase of the pulse probability wave, because KI_M subsets from strongly activated glomeruli are postulated to transmit with relative phase lead and those from weakly or nonactivated glomeruli with relative phase lag. During the rising part of an impulse response of the KI_A set there is a sequence of two time periods at which the pulse probability is highest with an intervening interval of from 3 to 6 msec (Fig. 7.11). The mean absolute deviation in phase of pulse probability waves from KI_M subsets is .57 rad or 33° (Table 7.4 in Section 7.2.2). The average phase difference between leading and lagging pulse probability waves is 1.14 rad or 66°. At a carrier frequency of 40 Hz this is equivalent to a delay in arrival time between leading and lagging waves of 4.5 msec. The KI_A subsets which synapse with axons of mitral-tufted cells from strongly activated glomeruli, as well as with other KI_M cells, receive LOT pulses in pairs with an average time separation of 4.5 msec. The KI_A subsets which synapse only with a mitral–tufted cells from nonactivated glomeruli receive LOT pulses singly at a time corresponding only to the second peak of KI_A excitation. It is postulated that the effect of the pulse pairs is to potentiate the effect of any preexisting increase in $K_e^{.5}(X_c)$ for the KI_A subsets receiving them.

Postulate 3.   The maximal activation of subsets in a receiving KII set depends on the critical tuning of the characteristic frequency to the carrier input frequency of the KII subsets, first by a local increase in $K_e^{.5}(X_c)$, and second by receipt of pulse probability waves having relative phase lead.   □

According to this postulate attention results in a maximal oscillatory response of selected cortical KI_A subsets, if there is correspondence between two spatial patterns. One is the pattern of cortical excitability invested in the spatial function of $K_e^{.5}(X_c)$ over the KI_A set, which constitutes an expectation of a sensory input. The other is the pattern of excitation, $\varphi_M(X_c)$, invested in the spatial function of phase in the transformed wave packet $o_M(\Omega_c)$ arriving at the surface of the KI_A set, which constitutes a present event. If the functions are similar (Fig. 7.18a), the corresponding KII_{AB} sets become tuned to the carrier frequency of the wave packet $o_M(\Omega_c)$. A signal is entered in the cortex. The corresponding subsets of KI_A and KI_B sets undergo prolonged oscillation in the cortex. If the patterns are dissimilar (Fig. 7.18b), the KII_{AB} subsets are not tuned to the carrier frequency, and

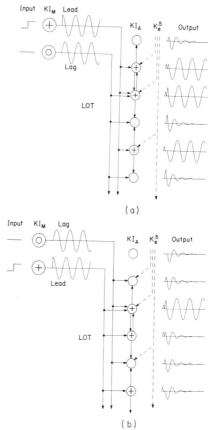

(a)

(b)

FIG. 7.18. A suggested model for the cortical mechanism of attention. (a) Conformance and (b) nonconformance of excitation and excitability functions.

the wave packet is rejected. The evoked KII_{AB} activity decays more or less rapidly to an equilibrium state in the first mode.

The result of similarity is the formation in the KII_{AB} set of a new wave packet $o_A(\Omega_c)$, which is manifested by a sinusoidal burst in the EEG. The precise value of the carrier frequency of the KII_{AB} receiving set is not important, provided it is sufficiently close to the transmitting frequency of the KII_{MG} set, so that phase distortion does not occur over the useful lifetime of the wave packet. The cortical wave packet is not merely a decision function, which signifies the level of correspondence and which is the output of an ordinary correlation filter. Rather the wave packet $o_A(\Omega_c)$ contains a signal based on the sensory input, which has been filtered by attentiveness, and which is in a form suitable for further filtering or for combination with other signals in the same form.

The value of this proposed mechanism for filtering appears to lie first in the recovery of a facsimile of the original signal after selective filtering, and second in the reliance on locally determined time or phase relations among pulses. There is relative insensitivity to local variations in mean pulse rates or to variations in carrier frequency from one wave packet to the next. The peculiarity of the mechanism is that the cortical signal is presumed to be based as much on the expectation function as on the excitation function. We may postulate that the animal perceives the stimulus it models or expects to receive rather than the stimulus it receives (see Section 1.1.1), unless the received input differs slightly to moderately from expectation so that the input is rejected or it triggers an orienting reflex (Section 7.1.1) or differs greatly so that it is rejected.

The proposed requirement for the structure of a signal in the LOT to be receivable by the cortex, consisting of an ordered set of delays between pulses on the order of 3 to 7 msec, may be the reason why cats can be trained to LOT stimulation only with high stimulus intensity and with prolonged training (Section 7.1.3). The use of pairs of electrical pulses separated by 4–5 msec might be more effective for orienting and training, provided other unknown constraints on LOT input are not violated, particularly in the spatial domain.

The increase in K_e associated with attentiveness is the result of a dynamic process, and the level in respect to an electrical stimulus can change within the time interval of two successive stimuli (140 msec) in a pulse train used to test for it (Emery & Freeman, 1969). During normal behavior there may be continual variation in the spatial functions for phase and for K_e, which underlies the continually varying sequence of bursts in the prepyriform EEG. According to this hypothesis, for each matching pair of functions, there must have been earlier an orienting response (Section 7.1.1), in which the stimulus wave packet provided a template during learning (Grastyán & Vereczkei, 1974) for the development of an excitability pattern or "neural model of the stimulus" (Sokolov, 1963). The neural mechanism for the orienting response and the nature and location of the permanent change in excitability (memory) are unknown, but they must be at least as broadly distributed as the wave packet is.[†]

[†] We conceive the process of template formation during orienting to involve the prepyriform cortex as the subsequent site of reversible elaboration and dissolution of an excitability function, but we have not localized the site of template formation, which may take place in the cortex or in the bulb and other parts of the forebrain and involve the cortex secondarily. The mechanism of template formation may be related to the mechanism of imprinting as described for immature salmon, which is subsequently demonstrated in the behavior of the adult fish homing on olfactory stimuli (Hara et al., 1965). Imprinting, however, occurs only at a critical state of maturation, whereas orienting occurs at times throughout the lifespan of an animal.

7.2.4. POSSIBLE MECHANISMS OF CORTICAL OUTPUT

The disposition of the wave packet following filtering by selective attention is not known. Anatomical and electrophysiological studies show that cortical output is transmitted to several structures in the forebrain, including the olfactory tubercle, the nuclei gemini in the thalamus, the ventral striatum, the hypothalamus, amygdaloid nucleus and entorhinal cortex (Heimer, 1969, Price, 1973). According to Postulates 2 and 3, signals can be transmitted by wave packet only if the characteristic frequencies of the transmitting and receiving KII sets are tuned to the same value. EEG activity in the amygdala and hypothalamus is commonly found in the 40-Hz range, but activity at lower frequencies is more common in the thalamus and entorhinal cortex.

This suggests two mechanisms for further study. The oscillatory activity in the wave packet may undergo rectification and smoothing by high-threshold or directionally sensitive neurons in the cortex. Evidence has been found in the visual system by stimulation with sine wave modulated light (Lopes da Silva, 1970; Spekreijse, 1969) for the existence there of an essential nonlinearity which is characterized as rectification. The process has not yet been looked for in the prepyriform cortex. If it exists, its effect might be to convert a function for modulation amplitude of pulse probability waves over the KI_A set or KI_B set to a pulse density function, which is the same type as that delivered by the PON to the glomeruli. This function might then be reconverted at a lower frequency by the interaction of KII_{AB} and KI_C sets to a phase function at a lower frequency (Section 6.2.4), that is transmitted as a wave packet to other structures tuned to that frequency. Alternatively, there may be a direct transformation of the wave packets at 40 Hz in the KII_{AB} set to a wave packet at 22 Hz in the KI_C set that is manifested by the occurrence of bursts of sinusoidal activity at the lower frequency (see Fig. 7.19, lower EEG traces, and Fig. 6.31 in Section 6.2.4).

In either case the prepyriform output is a wave packet that may be transmitted simultaneously to multiple KII or KIII sets. Reception should be detectable in the form of transient increases in the covariance of the EEGs and pulse probability waves of subsets of neurons in the transmitting and receiving subsets at the common carrier frequency.

Direct feedback from a receiving subset to a transmitting subset is not required to establish communality of frequency. However, a physiological basis for feedback to the prepyriform cortex does exist, which is manifested in the nonspecific centrifugal influences on cortical function. It is likely that feedback has the effects of optimization of the carrier frequency and amplitude of the wave packets. More generally, there may be changes in the expectation function $K_e^{.5}(X_c)$ over the KI_A set that maximize the spatial

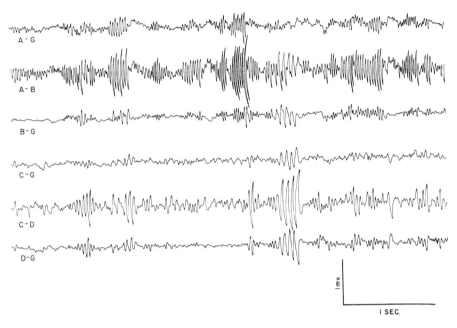

FIG. 7.19. Simultaneous bipolar and monopolar records of prepyriform EEG from prepyriform (A − B) and periamygdaloid (C − D) cortex (Freeman, 1959).

correlation between the phase function in the LOT wave packet $\varphi_M(X_c)$ and
the expectation function of the KI_A set. Such a mechanism must exist
to account for the adaptiveness of teleological behavior, though it cannot be
described yet at the neural level.

These three postulates raise many unanswered questions. How, for
example, might changes in the levels of nonspecific arousal inputs result in
an increase in the level of correspondence between specific spatial patterns
of excitation and excitability? How can some odors induce the state of
selective attention, as when attention is drawn by the unexpected odor of
smoke? The purpose of the postulates is to show how an understanding
of the properties of KI and KII sets can be used to predict the mechanisms
by which neural signals are encoded, transformed and filtered by mass actions,
so that these and other questions can be refined and answered. The key
point is the following. If a signal is represented by the active state of a KI
set, the identity of the signal must be established by taking ensemble time
averages over the subsets in each local part of the set. If the active
state were in the nature of impulse responses to the input signal, the averages
could be made with respect to the time of the onset of the sensory
stimulus. But the time of onset of the stable limit cycle states in KII sets

is not precisely locked to the time of onset of the sensory stimulus, and the ensemble averages must be taken with respect to the carrier frequency of the limit cycle domain and not the stimulus. Therefore the signal cannot be detected in the neural mass without resort to the ensemble averages over the domain, and such averages are only accessible through a theory of mass actions.

7.3. Comments concerning Neocortical Mass Actions

All neural masses in the vertebrate central nervous system generate extra-cellular fields of potential though not all the fields are detectable. With respect to the patterns of time variation in potential there are two types of neural mass. Those in the forebrain comprising the bulb, paleocortex, neocortex, striatum, and thalamus generate oscillatory potentials with frequencies in the range of 1 to 100 Hz. Those in the brainstem, cerebellum, and spinal cord generate irregular slow and spiky potentials that are seldom rhythmic. The theory of neural masses can be applied to both types of mass but in different forms. The masses in the forebrain display limit cycle activity, and their dynamics are best described by networks of KII sets. Those outside the forebrain seldom show limit cycle activity and may best be described by networks of KO and KI sets. Their most interesting properties will probably be found in the dynamic changes which accompany shifts from one set of nonzero equilibrium states to another and in the spatial frequencies of steady state activity that occur in KI_i sets (Section 1.3.4; Eccles et al., 1967; Wilson & Cowan, 1973).

The experimental data described here do not provide a basis for extensive commentary on networks of KI sets. Some progress has been achieved in developing a KO network modelling the electrophysiological properties (as distinct from the behaviorally determined input–output properties) of the cerebellum (Bantli, 1974a–c), but the model does not yet incorporate KI sets.

The forebrain masses particularly in the neocortex display EEG activity over a wide range of frequencies, including the alpha (8–12 Hz), low beta (12–30 Hz), theta (4–7 Hz), delta (<4 Hz), and high beta (30–100 Hz) ranges. Again the experimental data given here provide little basis for comment for two reasons. First, the KII model can be used only to explain activity in the high beta range. An extensive development of models at the KIII or higher levels may be required to explain activity in the lower and more commonly observed frequency ranges. Second, the development of a testable K model for a nucleus or an area of cortex requires such an array of anatomical, electrophysiological, pharmacological, mathematical, and be-havioral data as to require a monograph for each mass.

The key test of a K model is the successful prediction of electrophysiological measurements. Certain general principles and postulates have arisen in the study of KII sets in the olfactory system that may be useful in electro-physiological testing of other parts of the forebrain. There are five methods in present use. These are the measurements of internally regulated rhythmic potentials (Petsche, 1972; Ajmone Marsan, 1973); of the effects of rhythmic stimulation; of steady or so-called dc (direct current) potentials (Caspers, 1974); of the effects of dc polarization; and of the behavioral and EEG correlates of unit activity.[†] Brief comments are made on each method.

7.3.1. RHYTHMIC POTENTIALS AND RHYTHMIC STIMULATION

The direct applicability of K models to the mechanisms of the EEGs in other parts of the brain is undetermined. It is quite clear that the neocortical EEG is not the sum of extracellular cortical action potentials, and that it is chiefly the sum of potentials of extracellular dendritic loop currents as in the bulb (Section 4.3.2) and prepyriform cortex (Section 4.4.2). Comparisons of simultaneous extracellular recordings from cortex and intracellular recordings from neocortical neurons have shown the existence of fluctuations in potential in both recordings with similar spectral properties (Creutzfeldt, Watanabe & Lux, 1966a, b; Elul, 1967), as for evoked potentials in the prepyriform cortex (Biedenbach and Stevens, 1969a, b). Elul (1972) has emphasized the finding that the level of correlation between simultaneous intracellular and extracellular recordings is usually quite low but occasionally rises to high levels. He suggests that the EEG is the manifestation of synchrony among a small subset (for example, 10%) of cortical neurons in each area, and that membership in the subset changes by a scanning mechanism under thalamic control at intervals no longer than a few hundred milliseconds.

The mechanism of synchronization postulated by Elul (1972) and by most other physiologists[‡] is rhythmic stimulation from other parts of the brain,

---

[†] A sixth method is notable for its nonuse. This is study of the behavioral effects of stimulation of single units. When a microelectrode is driven through the cortex, there is a succession of high frequency pulse trains from injured neurons, which sound like buzzes and squeals on an audiomonitor. If as Barlow (1972) proposes each percept and memory, what McCulloch (1965) has called a "psychon," is stored in a single neuron or "cardinal cell," then driving an electrode through at least some parts of the human cortex in waking patients should cause a cascade of vivid memories to be reported. The fact that this phenomenon has not been reported is evidence against the psychon and cardinal cell hypotheses.

[‡] One form of the evidence for believing that neocortical EEG waves are driven by an extracortical pacemaker and are not emergent is that the oscillations disappear when the cortex is undercut (Burns, 1958). The prepyriform cortex behaves the same way when it is undercut, but its capacity for oscillatory activity reappears when it is subjected to tetanization (Section 5.4.3) or anodal dc polarization (Section 7.3.2). The isolated neocortical slab should be reexamined with these techniques, with particular attention paid to observation on a range of frequencies. For example, beta activity may be emergent whereas alpha or theta activity may be driven, or vice versa.

such as from the thalamus for neocortical bursts under pentobarbital that resemble alpha waves (Andersen and Andersson, 1968) and from the septum for the hippocampal theta waves (Stumpf, 1965). Some theorists postulate the existence of limit cycle activity as the basis for waves in neocortex (Dewan, 1964) and thalamus (Wilson & Cowan, 1973). The degree of interaction required among cortical neurons for the appearance of limit cycle behavior is usually predicated on the existence of synaptic connections between neurons, as proposed here. Additionally Adey (1967) has evidence for the sensitivity of cortical neurons to changes in the ionic constitution of the extracellular medium and to transcortical potential gradients, which raises the question whether the potential gradients of the EEG might serve to couple neocortical neurons into cooperative domains (see Section 7.3.2 for an appraisal).

The major unsolved problem in the analysis of the EEG of the neocortex and basal ganglia (including the thalamus) is that the precise neurons of origin are unknown. Each nucleus and area of cortex consists of a certain number of KO and KI sets (Section 1.3.1), some of which may contribute to the local field potential and others of which may not. The fields of those that do are overlapping (Section 4.2.3) and in turn are overlapped by fields of externally situated KI sets. To use the EEG for K-set analysis we must know which of a network of KI sets it is coming from.

The most obvious frequencies in the EEG are at the lower end of the spectrum, but they may not be the most informative. Activity at high spatial and temporal frequencies is more strongly degraded by divergence (Section 4.5.1) and dispersion (Section 2.3.3). It is likely that more information could be obtained from the neocortical EEG by greater use of corrective filters to restore the higher frequencies (e.g., Sheer, 1970). Narrow band-pass filters may be most effective, particularly if combined with prior use of auto-correlation and power spectrum analysis (Section 3.3.1) and with measurement of pulse probability waves (Section 3.3.3). The conditional pulse probability is a much more powerful way of determining the characteristic frequency of subsets in a KII set than autocorrelation is, and more useful information about a K set may be extracted by use of narrow band filtering across its range of characteristic frequency, prior to calculation of conditional pulse probabilities.

According to Postulate 3 in Section 7.2.3, transmission of signals in wave packets $o_\mu(\Omega_v)$ between KII sets occurs only when they are tuned to a common carrier frequency. The period of tuning may be for periods of 100 to 200 msec or for an irregular series of short periods. Trush & Efremova (1972) and Efremova & Trush (1971, 1973) in recording the EEGs of the visual and motor cortices of dogs report a low correlation between them prior to conditioning. When the dogs are conditioned to make a response to a visual stimulus, the correlation increases, and it is highest at the time of conditioned stimulation and response. Dumenko (1968, 1970) similarly reports that dogs, which are trained to perform a conditioned response to a visual stimulus and to an auditory stimulus given on separate unrelated trials, have relatively high correlations between the EEGs of the motor cortex and the EEGs respectively of the visual and auditory cortices, but not between the EEGs of the two sensory cortices even if the stimuli are given on the same trial. When the dogs are further trained in a "dynamic stereotype," so that the order of presentation of the visual and auditory stimuli is the cue, there is a high correlation between the EEGs of the visual and auditory cortices. The maximal correlations in both sets of experiments are found in the upper theta range (5–7 Hz). This frequency is too low to be the carrier for KII transmission. It may represent the frequency at which a series of wave packets $o_\mu(\Omega_v)$ is transmitted between the designated areas of cortex. These remarkable studies should therefore be extended to include examination of EEG activity in the upper beta range.

John (1967, 1972) has studied closely related phenomena in cats by giving rhythmic stimuli, either clicks, light flashes, or electrical pulses with implanted electrodes as conditioned signals and measuring the AEPs from the same stimuli in conjunction with conditioned response formation. Depending on the nature of the preceding conditioning of the animals to these stimuli, the AEPs recorded in numerous parts of the forebrain have shared frequencies and common patterns on factor analysis of the digitized values of potential. His interpretation is that the neural signals representing the stimulus events are encoded in the shared frequencies of oscillation (factor components) observed in sets of the AEPs. This is based on the hypothesis that the relevant neural activity is carried in the statistical averages of the active states of sets of neurons in coherent (not necessarily cooperative) domains, and that the ensemble average in each domain has the same time function as the AEP. This differs from the KII hypothesis of coding, which treats the ensemble average over a domain as the manifestation of a carrier frequency. The signal is conceived to be carried in the spatial patterns of phase differences from the average. These phase differences in John's interpretation must be considered as random and essentially meaningless deviations from the average.

According to the KII hypothesis the observable output from active states of KI sets in the pulse mode can be in phase with the output in the wave mode only if both outputs are from the same KI set in a KII set, and only if certain constraints are found to hold on the KI set geometry (Sections 4.3.3 and 4.4.3). If a KI set generates a dipole field in the wave mode, the activity in the pulse and wave modes may appear in phase or

$180°$ out of phase (Fig. 4.44), depending on which side of the zero isopotential surface the wave activity is recorded in. For the olfactory bulb an example is shown of an AEP generated by one set (KI_G) with two components, each related to activity in the pulse mode in two other sets (KI_P in Fig. 6.12 and KI_M in Fig. 5.20) but not in the same set. From these data we should expect to find some PSTHs with the same time function as concomitantly recorded AEPs, but such occurrences should be occasional and not universal.

However, John's deeper-lying hypothesis that neural signals are carried in time-dependent mass activity rather than in space-dependent mass activity at selected frequencies constitutes an alternative to the form of coding proposed here (Sections 7.2.1 and 7.2.2). The theory of mass actions may provide a basis for postulating how neural coding, transmission, and selective filtering take place according to his model.

7.3.2. DC POLARIZATION AND STEADY POTENTIALS

A classical rule in electrophysiology is that when current is passed through an axon by a pair of external electrodes, excitation occurs at the cathode. This is because the current outflow from the axon at the cathode depolarizes the adjacent part of the axon membrane, while the membrane at the anode is hyperpolarized by inward current. But when current is passed through two electrodes on the surface of cortex, excitation occurs beneath the anode. This is because the anodal current flowing from the surface to the base of the cortex passes into the cortical pyramidal cells across their apical dendritic membranes and outwardly across their axonal membranes in the deeper layers of the cortex. The depolarization takes place at the axonal membranes.

Rusinov (1973) uses anodal dc to create what he calls a "dominant focus." His technique is to expose the motor cortex and search with brief anodal pulses for the point on the cortex at which pulse stimulation causes a motor response such as leg flexion. He then passes a weak anodal dc (less than $100\,\mu A/mm^2$) through the cortex at that point, and gives a series of sensory stimuli, such as a repeated light flash. After a number of stimulus repetitions, the leg flexes with each stimulus presentation. His interpretation is based on the Pavlovian hypothesis of the corticocortical temporary connection and the Wedensky theory of inhibition, which states that a weak steady excitatory stimulus can bring a nerve or a neural tissue to an optimal state of activity, whereas a stronger excitatory stimulus causes paradoxical or "transmarginal" inhibition. Thus strong anodal currents do not establish a dominant focus. At present he is exploring the possible role of the cortical neuroglia in establishing dominant foci in normal conditioning without resort to anodal polarization.

The interpretation according to the KII hypothesis is that steady trans-cortical anodal current increases the pulse probability p_o of pyramidal neurons formed into KI_e sets. This increases K_e in the KI_e set. If the KI_e set is part of a KII set, the result is an increase in K_o in the first mode with $\delta_e = \delta_i = 1$ (Fig. 6.27c). With sufficient increase in K_o the KII set approaches and may enter a stable limit cycle state. Evidence that this may occur is shown in Fig. 7.20. Anodal polarizing current across the

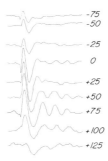

-75
-50
-25
0
$+25$
$+50$
$+75$
$+100$
$+125$

FIG. 7.20. Effect on the prepyriform AEP of direct current polarization ($\mu A/mm^2$) of the cortex through the exposed surface, both anodal ($+$) and cathodal ($-$). Time base: 125 msec.

prepyriform cortex in densities of 25 to $75\,\mu A/mm^2$ causes decreases in both the frequency and the decay rate of AEPs from LOT stimulation. Cathodal polarizing current causes the reverse pattern of change. That is, weak anodal polarization can cause critical tuning of a KII set to its characteristic frequency.

We may postulate on the basis of evoked potential studies (John, 1967) that a novel external stimulus is broadly transmitted from the primary sensory cortex or thalamus to other parts of the cortex including the motor cortex. On the basis of Postulate 3 (Section 7.2.3) we can hypothesize that KII transmission occurs at some characteristic frequency, and that reception occurs in KII sets tuned to that frequency. If this is correct, then activities in the sensory and motor cortices in the high beta range should be highly correlated during the operation of a dominant focus.

Also according to the KII hypothesis, the natural occurrence of a sensitive cortical domain equivalent to a dominant focus requires a steady source of excitation. One plausible source is a KI_e set, such as the periglomerular KI_p set in the olfactory bulb, which provides depolarizing bias for the KII_{MG} set in the bulb. That is, in addition to a search for KII sets in neocortex as the basis for limit cycle activity, the existence of KO, KI_e, and KI_i sets should be sought, because these are required to maintain KII sets in nonzero equilibrium states and to switch them into stable limit cycle states or sharply tuned nonzero equilibrium states.

The operations of KI sets may be manifested directly or indirectly in the form of transcortical steady potentials. These so-called dc potentials have numerous and complex origins (Plonsey, 1969), some of which are neural and others not. Some sudden changes in steady potential might be traced to changes in the equilibrium states of one or more KI sets within or transmitting to a KII set. An example is the baseline shift in the bulbar AEP on PON stimulation, which is generated as a field potential by the granule cells in the KI_G set, but which is the response of the KI_G set to the impulse response of the KI_P set transmitted through the KI_M set (Sections 6.1.3 and 6.1.4).

One of the better known shifts in steady cortical potential is called the contingent negative variation (CNV). It is a negative-going slow potential detected over the sensory and motor cortices accompanying expectation (see Hillyard, 1974). By the KII set hypothesis the CNV can be interpreted as the manifestation of an excitatory bias from a KI_e set, which acts to increase the tuning of a motor cortical KII set, so that it can receive sensory input prior to or during the execution of output.

The remarkable sensitivity of areas of cortex to weak polarizing currents raises the question, whether the currents of the EEG are sufficient to influence neural activity significantly and thereby to contribute to the formation of cooperative domains (Terzuolo & Bullock, 1956; Adey, 1969). The answer for the prepyriform cortex is "no," for two reasons. First, the minimal anodal current required to change the AEP is about $25 \, \mu A/mm^2$ (Fig. 7.20). The typical transcortical EEG current, which is estimated from the specific resistance of the cortical tissue (about $250 \, ohm \, cm^2/cm$) and the transcortical potential difference (about $1 \, mV$ over a distance of $1.5 \, mm$, see Fig. 7.19) is about $0.25 \, \mu A/mm^2$, or 2 orders of magnitude too small.

Second, cats trained to press a lever for milk on electrical stimulation of the LOT can perceive the input, when the evoked potential amplitude is no greater than that of the on-going EEG. When thirsty, they are very sensitive. The potential field of the EEG is then simulated by using arrays of transcortical electrodes to set up a dipole field and passing an oscillatory current across the cortex in bursts at $40 \, Hz$. The recorded amplitude of exogenous transcortical potential must be increased more than 100-fold above the amplitude of the EEG before the cats respond to the current bursts as a conditioned signal. At this level the current densities at the generating electrodes are great enough to excite LOT axons directly (Freeman, 1962e).

Though the brain appears to be sensitive to weak global electrical fields (Adey, 1969), we may postulate, conversely, that the cortex is structurally designed to minimize the effects of the extracellular currents of the EEG, because the glia provide a low resistance path for the currents to shunt the neurons. The question is not trivial, because if EEG currents were to cause entrainment of neural activity in cooperative domains, neural signals represented by phase functions in wave packets (Section 7.2.1) would be subjected to phase locking and signal degradation.

7.3.3. UNIT ACTIVITY CORRELATED WITH SENSORY AND MOTOR EVENTS

The cortex (from the Greek word for tree bark) forms the outer shell of the forebrain in all vertebrates. There are two main types. Paleocortex comprises the olfactory bulb, the primary olfactory cortex (including the prepyriform cortex), the septum, and the hippocampus and is found in all vertebrates. Neocortex (Chow & Leiman, 1970) is present only in mammals, where it comprises the greater part of the surface of the forebrain.

Both types of cortex consist of sheets of intermingled and densely interconnected excitatory and inhibitory neurons. They receive arrays of afferent axons over the entire surface and extend efferent axons in arrays over the entire surface. Within the cortex the afferent and efferent axons and the main dendritic and axonal fibers of the cortical neurons tend to an orientation perpendicular to the surface, and side branches providing the basis for interconnection extend parallel to the surface. The neurons beneath each local area of the surface tend to form functional groupings by virtue of their interconnections and common afferent connections. These are called columns (Mountcastle, 1974). They are dynamic entities without anatomical boundaries (with some exceptions such as the glomerular layer in the bulb). Their size depends on the effective radii of interactions (Section 4.5.3) and may vary from $25 \mu m$ to over $250 \mu m$. The continuum of intermingling of interconnecting fibers suggests that the locations and sizes of columns may vary from moment to moment, depending on the characteristics of the on-going afferent activity (Sholl, 1956).

The two types of cortex differ mainly in respect to the degree of laminar complexity, paleocortex being traditionally described as three-layered and neocortex as six-layered. The terms refer to cellular architectural appearance, not to functional organization. The pyramidal cells of paleocortex are characteristically bipolar with dendritic trunks extending both toward and away from the surface and tend to generate dipole fields of potential, whereas the neocortical pyramidal cells tend to have large *apical dendrites* extending toward the surface and several *basal dendrites* radiating parallel to the surface, which lead to closed fields of potentials (Section 4.2.2). Both features can account in large part for the fact that paleocortical potential fields have higher amplitudes than neocortical fields. Additionally, paleocortex has the peculiarity that its main afferent tract enters on the surface side, and its efferent tract leaves on the deep side of the surface, which gives an experimental advantage. The afferent and efferent tracts of neocortex are mixed on the deep side.

Each area of paleocortex and neocortex has its peculiarities of neuron structure and laminar architecture, which invite functional exploration. The primary sensory cortex for both vision and somatic sensation and the motor cortex are traditionally classified as neocortex, but they are as different from general neocortex as the paleocortex is, each in its own way. They share a common attribute, however, which has made them the most carefully studied of all areas of cortex. This is the high degree of topographic specificity in their connections respectively with the retinal surface, the body surface, and the array of skeletal musculature. Focal electrical stimulation at points on the motor cortex causes contraction of small groups of muscles, though the precise relation between each point and the pattern of movement is plastic and depends on the recent history of stimulation. The motor cortex is not tuned like a piano keyboard. Focal excitation of the skin or deep tissue activates a local region in the somatosensory cortex, and illumination of a point in the retina activates a local region in primary visual cortex. In each case if the stimulus is moved by an appropriate step over the input surface, the response moves by an equivalent step over the cortical surface and in the skeletal musculature. The functional and anatomical relations between these areas of cortex and the receptor or motor "surfaces" with which they are connected can be described in terms approaching one-to-one mapping.

The degree of refinement in topographic specificity is astonishing, as it is revealed by recording pulse trains of single cortical neurons during focal stimulation of the body or of the retina. (For examples, see Mountcastle, 1974, Chapters 10 and 16.) Two lines of interpretation are laid on these data. First, by mechanisms of divergent excitation and lateral inhibition the activity of a single receptor, for example in a joint or attached to a hair, may excite the cortical neurons in an entire column. By this means the activity level may be multiplied from that of one cell to that of thousands but with preservation of the precise location of the input in time and the surface coordinates. Second, by mechanisms of convergent excitation and inhibition the input from the receptor array may be preprocessed, so that certain features of a stimulus are extracted and transmitted and others are suppressed. For example, a set of retinal ganglion cells, which is optimally sensitive to a spot of light with a dark surrounding ring, may transmit convergently to one neuron in the visual cortex, which responds optimally either to a fixed bar of light at a certain angle on the retina (Hubel & Wiesel, 1962), or to a spot of light moving across the retina in a certain direction (Barlow, 1969), independently of the level of illumination.

The further disposition of topographically specific activity patterns from primary sensory cortex to the general neocortex is now unclear. Barlow

(1972) and others believe that the same or similar mechanisms of feature extraction continue to operate on afferent activity patterns successively in different parts of the forebrain, so that the pulse trains of single neurons in the general neocortex signify sensory events of ever greater complexity, culminating in what Barlow calls "cardinal cells," which encode percepts, memories, complex actions, etc.

Barlow's hypothesis is formulated in five "dogmas." (a) The operations of the brain relating to behavior exist and are to be understood in the form of interactions at the level of neurons in networks, rather than at molecular or microscopic levels. (b) The sensory neural networks are designed to represent signals in the activity of a "minimum number of active neurons". (c) The "trigger features" of single neurons are matched to stimulus patterns by the genetic and experiential processes. (d) Perception consists in the activity of a small number among the cardinal cells in the cortex, each corresponding to the level of complexity of a word in a sentence. (e) The pulse rate of each cardinal cell corresponds to the degree of subjective certainty of the percept.

Difficulties are encountered at several levels in testing this hypothesis. The first three dogmas are generalized restatements of the observed phenomena at the level of single neurons. They contain no explicit reference to the topological properties and dynamics of neurons, which are to be assembled in order to explain network behavior and do not comprise a model as defined in Section 1.1.2. They provide no anatomical or physiological basis for predicting forms of trigger features beyond those already known. In the fourth dogma, the appeal to the concept of "word" as an atomic element of the percept invokes the unresolved problems raised by Russell, Whitehead, Wittgenstein, Carnap, and others in the attempt to define and structure logical discourse in terms of "atomic propositions." Barlow's hypothesis can be interpreted as the neurophysiological aspect of logical positivism, to which the search for the percepts of cardinal cells must eventually lead. Historically, this seems to have been a philosophical cul de sac, and it is unlikely to provide a basis for identification and classification of cardinal cells.

The main difficulty with Barlow's hypothesis and with similar pulse logic hypotheses applied to the brain is that testing cannot be carried out within the framework established by the dogmas. The fifth dogma assigns a probability measure to a unit pulse train but without defining the physiological set of neurons and their states on which the probability measure is based. We may suppose that in a contiguous distribution of cortical neurons each testable neuron responds maximally to a particular sensory pattern such as a bar of light at a certain angle on the retina, but it responds to a lesser degree to other related stimuli such as a bar of light at a different angle. The neural event occurring in the visual cortex for a bar of light at each angle or position on the retina is by inference a distribution of increased and decreased activity of many neurons. The neuron under observation whose output has been maximized may or may not be the most rapidly firing neuron in the distribution, and the output from the distribution may or may not be focussed by convergence mechanisms into a smaller distribution. Experimental testing of these implicit assertions will require use of techniques for studying mass actions.

Further, the neural mechanisms for convergence of activity by surround inhibition in the visual cortex are unknown. It is unlikely that the model of mutual inhibition derived from studies of the Limulus eye (Hartline & Ratliff, 1958) is applicable, because it is likely that the visual cortex contains both excitatory and inhibitory neurons. Before a quantitative study of the spatial and temporal dynamics can be undertaken, the topological problem should be resolved whether there is forward inhibition as in the cerebellum (Section 1.3.1) or feedback inhibition as in the olfactory bulb (Section 5.3.1) or both as in the prepyriform cortex (Section 5.4.1). It appears feasible to construct mass action models of the visual cortex (e.g. Wilson & Cowan, 1973) and to test them physiologically as the means for solving this problem, because the interactions giving rise to the simple and complex response configurations of visual cortical neurons (Hubel & Wiesel, 1962) are local properties based on local connection densities within the visual system. These neural mechanisms should be clearly understood, before extrapolations are made to their operations on global retinal patterns or on sensory patterns involving multiple modalities. Some of the difficulties of handling global transformations are discussed in Section 7.2.1. Briefly, it is likely that feature extraction in relation to contours and to motion is based on local topologies, which are described with partial differential equations, but that feature extraction in relation to complex patterns depends also on interspersive divergence in tracts (Section 4.5.1) between KII sets and is global.

The relevant unit studies on sensory neocortex are mostly done in paralyzed and anesthetized animals. From evoked potential studies comparing the responses of waking, freely moving animals with those in anesthetized animals, it is obvious that, for this form of measurement, focal sensory stimulation evokes widespread activity in waking animals and topographically restricted activity only under deep anesthesia. That is, the convergence mechanisms seem to be enhanced by anesthesia, and the divergence mechanisms seem to be dominant in normal behavior. The pulse logic hypothesis is not easily adapted to description of the divergence property.

From the viewpoint of a theory of mass action, the primary somatosensory and visual cortices may be regarded as specialized systems, that are inappropriate to serve as models for the general neocortex. Their function is to extract information about the local organization of a sensory event, such as a moving spot on the retina or an insect crawling on the skin or the sequence of receptors excited by a moving joint, and to amplify the activity of a very few receptors to the activity of the number of neurons in a cortical column, before the signal is entered through an integral transformation into a distributed KI or KII set with its inherent background noise.

The necessity for these two types of preprocessing seems not to exist in the olfactory system, though the presence of other forms of preprocessing (automatic volume control and input normalization, Sections 5.2.3, 6.2.5, and 7.2.2) have been noted, which are equivalent to operations performed in the retina and spinal cord in the visual and somesthetic systems. Because of the absence of a high degree of topographic specificity, the olfactory system is inherently different from the neocortical parts of the visual and somesthetic systems, and it may serve as a more appropriate model for the study of visual and somesthetic information processing after the level of the primary sensory cortices. It would be interesting to learn, for example, whether the neurons in the primary sensory areas are formed into KII sets, whether the cortical sets have stable limit cycles, and whether some of the neurons there generate pulse probability waves, suggesting coding of output in wave packets.

Similar considerations hold regarding the unit correlates of conditioned reflex behavior in the sensory and motor cortices (e.g., Evarts, 1967, 1971; Phillips, 1973), in which the search is made for "command" neurons, whose output is uniquely identifiable with particular movements or aspects of movements. It is already apparent that each movement is preceded and followed by a constellation of cortical neural pulse trains. From the viewpoint of mass action the motor cortex can be conceived as consisting of a network of KI or KII sets. Prior to a movement some subsets of the network must be "switched on," meaning that the levels of p_o in the subsets must be increased, as the network changes from zero or near-zero resting equilibrium to a nonzero equilibrium state or a limit cycle state. Then increased unit activity for periods of a few hundred milliseconds should readily be observed in many neurons. The specifics of the signals for particular movements should be sought in the measurement of pulse density functions $p(t, X)$ if an equilibrium state prevails (Section 7.2.1) or a phase function $\varphi(X)$ if a stable limit cycle state prevails (Section 7.2.2). That is, if the neural signal correlated with a movement is conceived as the property of a KI set, the signal is a function of the active state of the entire set, and the observed activity of selected units is treated as a sample of local activity densities over the activity density function. The problems, then, are how to define the KI set and how to predict an activity density function, which can be tested experimentally by recording units at selected points in the KI set. The spatial extent of a KI set can be limited by restricting the movement to a small set of muscles in an extremity, but the prediction of an activity density function is much more difficult and may depend on the development of a general theory of coding in KII sets.

Considering that cortex has important properties at microscopic and macroscopic levels, the most fruitful approach appears to be to treat definable areas of cortex as specialized elements supporting mass action, which are embedded in discrete networks of neurons. There is no doubt that the input and output of the central nervous system is based on collections of individual receptors and motor units that can and often do function in particulate ways. Local operations concerning input and output such as signal normalization, feature extraction of lines or moving spots, localization of proprioceptive feedback to relevant motorneurons, etc., may best be treated by means of models based on discrete networks. The assembly of the sensory signals from numerous receptors into symbolic representations in the vehicle of dynamic patterns and the subsequent operations on those patterns leading eventually to the patterned firing of motorneurons may best be treated by use of mass action models. The convergence points between the network and mass action paradigms (Section 1.1.3), then, are the neural interfaces between networks and K sets, which may be the primary sensory and motor cortices. The areas of association cortex would appear to have only macroscopic functions or "mass actions" (Lashley, 1929) and therein might more closely resemble the olfactory cortex than the primary sensory neocortex.

There are two additional reasons for suggesting the olfactory system as a model for distributed or parallel processing in the neocortex. One is the requirement for cross-modality signal compatibility. At some level in the central nervous system there must be a common code, so that signals from several sensory systems can be combined and can then be delivered to the motor system generally (including the basal ganglia as well as the sensori-motor cortex). KII sets appear to have only the requirement of a common carrier frequency for mixing input from different sources, and even this restriction may be relaxed for KIII sets to admit simultaneous operations on wave packets $o_\mu(\Omega_v)$ at two or more carrier frequencies (Section 7.2.4).

The other reason is that KII sets provide a form of encoding, in which the timing of the signals is an independent variable, both internally and externally with respect to the time of onset of the initiating stimulus or stimuli. Whereas the neural events observed in the brainstem, cerebellum, and spinal cord are locked tightly to the external timing of sensory and motor events, as in the forms of locomotion, the timing of neural events in the cerebrum during adaptive behavior is less precisely predictable. A well-trained cat, for example, when given a conditioned signal may sit motionless interminably before performing its conditioned response. This degree of freedom from the immediacy of external events is a crucial aspect of all higher neural activity, such as abstraction, prediction, and creation, and a valid neural theory of behavior must explain it. Perhaps this indeterminacy can be traced ultimately to the fact that when the background state of a KII set is raised sufficiently by a steady input, the time that the set requires to switch from an equilibrium stable state to a limit cycle stable state is uncertain and only partly under peripheral and central control.

References

Adey, W. R.   Intrinsic organization of cerebral tissue in alerting, orienting, and discriminative responses. In G. C. Quarton, T. Melnechuk, & F. O. Schmitt (Eds.), *Neurosciences— A study program*, pp. 615–633. New York: Rockefeller Univ. Press, 1967.

Adey, W. R.   Slow electrical phenomena in the central nervous system. *Neurosciences Research Program Bulletin*, 1969, **7**, 75–180.

Adrian, E. D.   The electrical activity of the mammalian olfactory bulb. *Electroencephalography and clinical Neurophysiology*, 1950, **2**, 377–388.

Adrian, R. H.   The effect of internal and external potassium concentration on the membrane potential of frog muscle. *Journal of Physiology*, 1956, **133**, 631–658.

Ahn, S. M., & Freeman, W. J.   Steady-state and limit cycle activity of mass of neurons forming simple feedback loops (I): Lumped circuit model. *Kybernetik*, 1974, **16**, 87–91. (a).

Ahn, S. M., & Freeman, W. J.   Steady-state and limit cycle activity of mass of neurons forming simple feedback loops (II): Distributed parameter model. *Kybernetik*, 1974, in **16**, 127–132. (b).

Ajmone Marsan, C.   Electrocorticography. In A. Rémond (Ed.), *Handbook of electroencephalography and clinical neurophysiology*, Vol. 10C. Amsterdam: Elsevier, 1973.

Andersen, P., & Andersson, S. A. *Physiological basis for the alpha rhythm*. New York: Appleton, 1968.

Anderson, T. W. *Introduction to multivariate statistical analysis*. New York: Wiley, 1958.

Anninos, P. A., Beck, B., Csermely, T. J., Harth, E. M., & Pertile, G.   Dynamics of neural structures. *Journal of Theoretical Biology*, 1970, **26**, 121–148.

Bantli, H.   Analysis of difference between potentials evoked by climbing fibers in cerebellum of cat and turtle. *Journal of Neurophysiology*, 1974, **37**, 573–593. (a).

Bantli, H.   Analysis of the dynamic behavior of neuron populations in the turtle cerebellum: I. General topological model. II. Lumped circuit model. *Kybernetic*, 1974, **15**, 203–212, 213–225. (b).

Barlow, H. B.   Summation and inhibition in the frog's retina. *Journal of Physiology*, 1953, **119**, 69–88.

Barlow, H. B.   Trigger features, adaptation and economy of impulses. In K. N. Leibovic (Ed.), *Information processing in the nervous system*, pp. 209–226. Berlin and New York: Springer-Verlag, 1969.

462

Barlow, H. B. Single units and sensation: A neuron doctrine for perceptual psychology? *Perception*, 1972, **1**, 371–394.

Becker, C. J., & Freeman, W. J. Prepyriform electrical activity after loss of peripheral or central input or both. *Physiology and Behavior*, 1968, 597–599.

Beidler, L. M. Olfaction. In *Handbook of sensory physiology*, Vol. IV. Berlin and New York: Springer-Verlag, 1971.

Beurle, R. L. Properties of a mass of cells capable of regenerating pulses. *Transactions of Royal Society (London), Ser. B*, 1956, **240**, 55–94.

Biedenbach, M. A. Effects of anesthetics and cholinergic drugs on prepyriform electrical activity in cats. *Experimental Neurology*, 1966, **16**, 464–479.

Biedenbach, M. A., & Freeman, W. J. Click-evoked potential map from the superior olivary nucleus of cats. *American Journal of Physiology*, 1964, **206**, 1408–1414.

Biedenbach, M. A., & Freeman, W. J. Linear domain of potential from the prepyriform cortex with respect to stimulus parameters. *Experimental Neurology*, 1965, **11**, 400–417.

Biedenbach, M. A., & Stevens, C. F. Electrical activity in cat olfactory cortex produced by synchronous orthodromic volleys. *Journal of Neurophysiology*, 1969, **32**, 193–203. (a).

Biedenbach, M. A., & Stevens, C. F. Synaptic organization of cat olfactory cortex as revealed by intracellular recording. *Journal of Neurophysiology*, 1969, **32**, 201–214. (b).

Bongard, M. *Pattern recognition* (T. Cheron, Transl.). New York: Spartan, 1970.

Boudreau, J. C. Computer analysis of electrical activity in the olfactory system of the cat. *Nature*, 1964, **201**, 155–158.

Boudreau, J. C., & Freeman, W. J. Spectral analysis of electrical activity in the prepyriform of the cat. *Experimental Neurology*, **8**, 1963, 423–439.

Brazier, M. A. B., Walter, D. O., & Schneider, D. (Eds.) *Neural modeling*. Los Angeles: University of California Press, 1973.

Bullock, T. H. The neuron doctrine and electrophysiology. *Science*, 1959, **129**, 997–1002.

Burns, B. D. *The mammalian cerebral cortex*. Baltimore, Maryland: Williams & Wilkins, 1958.

Byzov, A. L., Polyshchuk, N. A., & Zenkin, G. M. On the transmission of signals in vertebrate retina by means of spike generating mechanism and without it. *Neurofyziologia*, 1970, **2**, 536–543.

Caianiello, E. R. (Ed.) *Neural networks*. Berlin and New York: Springer-Verlag, 1967.

Callens, M. *Peripheral and central regulatory mechanisms of the excitability in the olfactory system*. Brussels: Presses Academiques Européennes, 1967.

Caspers, H. DC potentials recorded directly from the cortex. In A. Rémond (Ed.), *Handbook of electroencephalography and clinical neurophysiology*, Vol. 10A. Amsterdam: Elsevier, 1974.

Chow, K. L., & Leiman, A. L. The structural and functional organization of the neocortex, *Neurosciences Research Program Bulletin*, 1970, **8**, 153–220.

Cole, K. S., & Curtis, H. J. Electric impedance of the giant squid axon during activity. *Journal of general Physiology*, 1939, **22**, 649–670.

Coombs, J. S., Eccles, J. C., & Fatt, P. The electrical properties of the motoneurone membrane. *Journal of Physiology*, 1955, **130**, 291–325.

Cragg, B. G., & Temperley, H. N. V. The organisation of neurones: A co-operative analogy. *Electroencephalography and clinical Neurophysiology*, 1954, **6**, 85–92.

Craik, K. J. W. *The nature of explanation*. London and New York: Cambridge Univ. Press, 1952.

Creutzfeldt, O. D., Watanabe, S., & Lux, H. D. Relations between EEG phenomena and potentials of single cortical cells. I. Evoked responses after thalamic and epicortical stimulation. *Electroencephalography and clinical Neurophysiology*, 1966, **20**, 1–18. (a).

Creutzfeldt, O. D., Watanabe, S., & Lux, H. D.   Relations between EEG phenomena and potentials of single cortical cells. II. Spontaneous and convulsoid activity. *Electroencephalography and clinical Neurophysiology*, 1966, **20**, 19–37. (b).

Dennis, B. I., & Kerr, D. I. B.   An evoked potential study of centripetal and centrifugal connections of the olfactory bulb in the cat. *Brain Research*, 1968, **11**, 373–396.

Dewan, E. M.   Nonlinear oscillations and electroencephalography. *Journal of Theoretical Biology*, 1964, **7**, 141–159.

DiStefano, J. J., Stubberud, A. R., & Williams, I. J.   *Control systems*. New York: McGraw-Hill, 1967.

Dodge, F. A. Jr.   On the transduction of visual, mechanical, and chemical stimuli. *International Journal of Neuroscience*, 1972, **3**, 5–14.

Dumenko, V. N.   Electrophysiological characteristics of the dynamic stereotype (in Russian, English summary). *Zhurnal Vysshei Nervnoi Deyatel nosti*, 1968, **18**, 187–195.

Dumenko, V. N.   Electroencephalographic investigation of cortical relationships in dogs during formation of a conditioned reflex stereotype. In V. S. Rusinov (ed.), *Electrophysiology of the Central Nervous System* (B. Haigh, transl.; R. W. Doty, transl. ed.), pp. 107–118. New York: Plenum Press, 1970.

Eccles, J. C.   *The physiology of nerve cells*. Baltimore, Maryland: Johns Hopkins Press, 1957.

Eccles, J. C.   *The physiology of synapses*. New York: Academic Press, 1964.

Eccles, J. C., Ito, M., & Szentagothai, J.   *The cerebellum as neuronal machine*. Berlin and New York: Springer-Verlag, 1967.

Efremova, T. M., & Trush, V. D.   Dynamics of frequency characteristics of cortical biopotentials in rabbits during formation of a defensive conditioned reflex. *Zhurnal Vysshei Nervnoi Deyatel'nosti*, 1971, **21**, 963–970.

Efremova, T. M., & Trush, V. D.   Power spectra of cortical electrical activity in the rabbit in relation to conditioned reflexes. *Acta Neurobiol. Exp.*, 1973, **33**, 743–755.

Elul, R.   Statistical mechanisms in generation of the EEG. In L. Fogel & F. George (Eds.), *Progress in biomedical engineering*, pp. 131–151. Washington, D.C.: Spartan, 1967.

Elul, R.   The genesis of the EEG. *International Review of Neurobiology*, 1972, **15**, 227–272.

Emery, J. D., & Freeman, W. J.   Pattern analysis of cortical evoked potential parameters during attention changes. *Physiology and Behavior*, 1969, **4**, 69–77.

Evarts, E. V.   Representation of movements and muscles by pyramidal tract neurons of the precentral motor cortex. In M. D. Yahr & D. P. Purpura (Eds.), *Neurophysiological basis of normal and abnormal motor activities*, pp. 215–254. New York: Raven Press, 1967.

Evarts, E. V.   Central control of movement, *Neurosciences Research Program Bulletin*, 1971, **9**, 1–170.

Freeman, W. J.   Distribution in time and space of prepyriform electrical activity. *Journal of Neurophysiology*, 1959, **22**, 644–666.

Freeman, W. J.   Correlation of electrical activity of prepyriform cortex and behavior in cat. *Journal of Neurophysiology*, 1960, **23**, 111–131. (a).

Freeman, W. J.   Repetitive electrical stimulation of prepyriform cortex in cat. *Journal of Neurophysiology*, 1960, **23**, 383–396. (b).

Freeman, W. J.   Linear approximation of prepyriform evoked potential in cats. *Experimental Neurology*, 1962, **5**, 477–499. (a).

Freeman, W. J.   Phasic and long-term excitability changes in prepyriform cortex of cats. *Experimental Neurology*, 1962, **5**, 500–518. (b).

Freeman, W. J.   Changes in prepyriform evoked potential with food deprivation and consumption. *Experimental Neurology*, 1962, **6**, 12–29. (c).

Freeman, W. J.   Alterations in prepyriform evoked potential in relation to stimulus intensity. *Experimental Neurology*, 1962, **6**, 70–84. (d).

Freeman, W. J.   Comparison of thresholds for behavioral and electrical responses to cortical electrical stimulation in cats. *Experimental Neurology*, 1962, **6**, 315–331. (e).

Freeman, W. J.   The electrical activity of a primary sensory cortex: Analysis of EEG waves. *International Review of Neurobiology*, 1963, **5**, 53–119.

Freeman, W. J.   Use of digital adaptive filters for measuring prepyriform evoked potentials from cats. *Experimental Neurology*, 1964, **10**, 475–492. (a).

Freeman, W. J.   A linear distributed feedback model for prepyriform cortex. *Experimental Neurology*, 1964, **10**, 525–547. (b).

Freeman, W. J.   Correlation of goal-directed work with sensory cortical excitability. *Recent Advances in Biological Psychiatry*, 1964, **7**, 243–250. (c).

Freeman, W. J.   Analysis of function of cerebral cortex by use of control systems theory. *Logistics Review*, 1967, **3**, 5–40.

Freeman, W. J.   Patterns of variation in waveform of averaged evoked potentials from prepyriform cortex of cats. *Journal of Neurophysiology*, 1968, **31**, 1–13. (a).

Freeman, W. J.   Relations between unit activity and evoked potentials in prepyriform cortex of cats. *Journal of Neurophysiology*, 1968, **31**, 337–348. (b).

Freeman, W. J.   Effects of surgical isolation and tetanization on prepyriform cortex in cats. *Journal of Neurophysiology*, 1968, **31**, 349–357. (c).

Freeman, W. J.   Spectral analysis of prepyriform averaged evoked potentials in cats. *Journal of Biomedical Systems*, 1970, **1**, 3–22.

Freeman, W. J.   Spatial divergence and temporal dispersion in primary olfactory nerve of cat. *Journal of Neurophysiology*, 1972, **35**, 733–744. (a).

Freeman, W. J.   Measurement of open-loop responses to electrical stimulation in olfactory bulb of cat. *Journal of Neurophysiology*, 1972, **35**, 745–761. (b).

Freeman, W. J.   Measurement of oscillatory responses to electrical stimulation in olfactory bulb of cat. *Journal of Neurophysiology*, 1972, **35**, 762–779. (c).

Freeman, W. J.   Depth recording of averaged evoked potential of olfactory bulb. *Journal of Neurophysiology*, 1972, **35**, 780–796. (d).

Freeman, W. J.   Linear analysis of the dynamics of neural masses. *Annual Review of Biophysics and Bioengineering*, 1972, **1**, 225–256. (e).

Freeman, W. J.   Waves, pulses and the theory of neural masses. *Progress in Theoretical Biology*, 1972, **2**, 87–165. (f).

Freeman, W. J.   A model of the olfactory system. In M. A. B. Brazier, D. O. Walter, & D. Schneider (Eds.), *Neural modeling*, pp. 41–62. Los Angeles: Univ. of California, 1973.

Freeman, W. J.   Topographic organization of primary olfactory nerve in cat and rabbit as shown by evoked potentials. *Electroencephalography and clinical Neurophysiology*, 1974, **36**, 33–45. (a).

Freeman, W. J.   Average transmission distance from mitral tufted to granule cells in olfactory bulb. *Electroencephalography and clinical Neurophysiology*, 1974, **36**, 609–618. (b).

Freeman, W. J.   Attenuation of transmission through glomeruli of olfactory bulb on paired shock stimulation. *Brain Research*, 1974, **65**, 77–90. (c).

Freeman, W. J.   Relation of glomerular neuronal activity to glomerular transmission attenuation. *Brain Research*, 1974, **65**, 91–107. (d).

Freeman, W. J.   A model for mutual excitation in a neuron population in olfactory bulb. *IEEE Transactions on Biomedical Engineering*, 1974, **BME-21**, 350–358. (e).

Freeman, W. J.   Stability characteristics of positive feedback in a neural population. *IEEE Transactions on Biomedical Engineering*, 1974, **BME-21**, 358–364. (f).

Freeman, W. J., & Patel, H. H.   Extraneuronal potential fields evoked in septal region of cat by stimulation of fornix. *Electroencephalography and clinical Neurophysiology*, 1968, **24**, 444–457.

Gardner, E.   *Fundamentals of neurology* (5th ed.). Philadelphia, Pennsylvania: Saunders, 1968.

Gasser, H. S., & Grundfest, H.   Axon diameters in relation to the spike dimensions and the conduction velocity in mammalian A fibers. *American Journal of Physiology*, 1939, **127**, 393–414.

Gault, F. P., & Leaton, R. N.   Electrical activity of the olfactory system. *Electroencephalography and clinical Neurophysiology*, 1963, **15**, 299–304.

Gerard, R. W.   Neurophysiology: an integration. In J. Field, H. W. Magoun, & V. E. Hall (Eds.), *Handbook of physiology*. Vol. III. pp. 1919–1965. Washington, D.C.: Amer. Physiol. Soc., 1960.

Gerstein, G. L., & Kiang, N. Y.-S.   An approach to the quantitative analysis of electrophysiological data from single neurons. *Biophysics Journal*, 1960, **1**, 15–28.

Glansdorff, P., & Prigogine, I.   *Thermodynamic theory of structure, stability and fluctuations*, New York: Wiley, 1971.

Goldman, D. E.   Potential, impedance and rectification in membranes. *Journal of general Physiology*, 1943, **27**, 37–60.

Goodman, L. S., Gilman, A.   *Pharmacological basis of therapeutics* (4th ed.). New York: Macmillan, 1970.

Goodwin, B. C.   *Temporal organization of cells*. New York: Academic Press, 1963.

Granit, R.   Recurrent inhibition as a mechanism of control. *Progress in Brain Research*, 1963, **1**, 23–37.

Granit, R., Kellerth, J.-O., & Williams, T. D.   "Adjacent" and "remote" post-synaptic inhibition in motoneurons stimulated by muscle stretch. *Journal of Physiology*, 1964, **174**, 453–472.

Granit, R., Kernell, D., & Shortess, G. K.   Quantitative aspects of repetitive firing of mammalian motoneurones caused by injected currents. *Journal of Physiology*, 1963, **168**, 911–931.

Granit, R., & Renkin, B.   Net depolarization and discharge rate of motorneurons, as measured by recurrent inhibition. *Journal of Physiology*, 1961, **158**, 461–475.

Grastyán, E., & Vereczkei, L.   Effects of spatial separation of the conditioned signal from the reinforcement: A demonstration of the conditioned character of the orienting response or the orientational character of conditioning. *Behavioral Biology*, 1974, **10**, 121–146.

Green, J. D., Mancia, M., & von Baumgarten, R.   Recurrent inhibition in the olfactory bulb. I. Effects of antidromic stimulation of the lateral olfactory tract. *Journal of Neurophysiology*, 1962, **25**, 467–488.

Griffith, J. S.   On the stability of brain-like structures. *Biophysical Journal*, 1963, **3**, 299–308.

Griffith, J. S.   *Mathematical neurobiology*. New York: Academic Press, 1971.

Grossberg, S.   Embedding fields: Underlying philosophy, mathematics, and applications to psychology, physiology, and anatomy. *Journal of Cybernetics*, 1971, **1**, 28–50.

Grossberg, S.   Contour enhancement, short term memory, and constancies in reverberating neural networks, *Studies in Applied Mathematics*, 1973, **52**, 213–257. (a).

Grossberg, S.   Classical and instrumental learning by neural networks. *Progress in Theoretical Biology*, 1974, **3**, 51–141.

Gusel'nikova, K. G., Gusel'nikov, V. I., Tsytolovskii, L. E., Engovatov, V. V., & Voronkov, G. S.   Some properties of olfactory bulb dendrites in frogs. *Neuroscience Translations*, 1970. **13**, 88–92.

Haberly, L. B.   Summed potentials evoked in opossum prepyriform cortex. *Journal of Neurophysiology*, 1973, **36**, 775–788.

Haberly, L. B., & Shepherd, G. M.   Current-density analysis of summed evoked potentials in opossum prepyriform cortex. *Journal of Neurophysiology*, 1973, **36**, 789–802.

Hagiwara, S., & Tasaki, S.   A study on the mechanism of impulse transmission across the giant synapse of the squid. *Journal of Physiology*, 1958, **143**, 114–137.

Hara, T. J., Ueda, K., & Gorbman, A.   Electroencephalographic studies of homing salmon. *Science*, 1965, **149**, 884–885.

Harth, E. M., Csermely, T. J., Beek, B., & Lindsay, R. D.   Brain functions and neural dynamics, *Journal of Theoretical Biology*, 1970, **26**, 93–120.

Hartline, H. K., & Ratliff, F.   Spatial summation of inhibitory influences in the eye of Limulus and the mutual interaction of receptor units. *Journal of general Physiology*, 1958, **41**, 1049–1066.

Hebb, D. O.   *The organization of behavior: A neuropsychological theory.* New York: Wiley, 1949.

Hebb, D. O.   *A textbook of psychology.* Philadelphia, Pennsylvania: Saunders, 1958.

Heimer, L.   Synaptic distribution of centripetal and centrifugal nerve fibres in the olfactory system of the rat. An experimental anatomical study. *Journal of Anatomy*, 1968, **103**, 413–432.

Heimer, L.   The secondary olfactory connections in mammals, reptiles, and sharks. *Annals of the New York Academy of Science*, 1969, **167**, 129–146.

Highstone, H. H.   Anterior olfactory nucleus and forebrain evoked potentials. M.A. Thesis in Physiology. Berkeley: Univ. of California, 1970.

Hillyard, S. A.   Methodological issues in CNV research. In R. F. Thompson & M. M. Patterson (Eds.), *Bioelectric recording techniques*, Part B, Chap. 8. New York: Academic Press, 1974.

Hodgkin, A. L.   *The conduction of the nervous impulse.* Liverpool, England: Univ. of Liverpool Press, 1964.

Hodgkin, A. L., & Huxley, A. F.   A quantitative description of membrane current and its application to conduction and excitation in nerve. *Journal of Physiology*, 1952, **117**, 500–544.

Hodgkin, A. L., & Rushton, W. A. H.   Electrical constants of a crustacean nerve fiber. *Proceedings of the Royal Society (London)*, 1946, **133B**, 444–479.

Horowitz, J. M.   Evoked activity of single units and neural populations in the hippocampus of the cat. *Electroencephalography and clinical Neurophysiology*, 1972, **32**, 227–240.

Horowitz, J. M., & Freeman, W. J.   Evoked potentials arising from neural population elements at different times on a warped surface. *Bulletin of Mathematical Biophysics*, 1966, **28**, 519–536.

Horowitz, J. M., Freeman, W. J., & Stoll, P. J.   A neural network with a background level of excitation in the cat hippocampus. *International Journal of Neuroscience*, 1973, **5**, 113–123.

Howland, B., Lettvin, J. Y., McCulloch, W. S., Pitts, W. H., & Wall, P. D.   Reflex inhibition by dorsal root interaction. *Journal of Neurophysiology*, 1955, **18**, 1–17.

Hubel, D. H., & Wiesel, T. N.   Receptive fields, binocular interaction and functional architecture in the cat's visual cortex. *Journal of Physiology*, 1962, **160**, 106–154.

Hughes, J. R., Hendrix, D. E., Wetzel, N. S., Johnston, J. W., Jr. Correlations between electrophysiological activity from the human olfactory bulb and the subjective response to odoriferous stimuli. In C. Pfaffman (Ed.), *Olfaction and Taste III*. New York, Rockefeller Press, 1969.

Huxley, A. F., & Stämpfli, R.   Evidence for saltatory conduction in peripheral myelinated nerve fibers. *Journal of Physiology*, 1949, **108**, 315–339.

Jacobson, M.   *Developmental neurobiology.* New York: Holt, 1970.

John, E. R.   *Mechanisms of memory.* New York: Academic Press, 1967.

John, E. R.   Switchboard versus statistical theories of learning and memory. *Science*, 1972, **177**, 850–864.

Kandel, E. R., Frazier, W. T., & Coggeshall, R. E.   Opposite synaptic actions mediated by different branches of an identifiable interneuron in Aplysia. *Science*, 1967, **155**, 346–348.

468   REFERENCES

Kandel, E. R., & Spencer, W. A. Electrophysiological properties of an archicortical neuron. *Annals of the New York Academy of Sciences*, 1961, **94**, 570–603.

Katchalsky, A. Biological flow structures and their relation to chemodiffusional coupling. *Neurosciences Research Program Bulletin*, 1971, **9**, 397–413.

Katchalsky, A., Rowland, V., & Blumenthal, R. (Eds.) Dynamic patterns of brain cell assemblies. *Neurosciences Research Program Bulletin*, 1974, **12**, 3–187.

Katz, B. *Electric excitation of nerve*. London and New York: Oxford Univ. Press, 1939.

Katz, B. *Nerve muscle, and synapse*. New York: McGraw-Hill, 1966.

Kirschfeld, K., & Reichardt, W. Die Verarbeitung stationärer optischer Nachrichten im Komplexauge von Limulus. *Kybernetik*, 1964, **2**, 43–64.

Knight, B. W., Toyoda, J., & Dodge, F. A. A quantitative description of the dynamics of excitation and inhibition in the eye of Limulus. *Journal of general Physiology*, 1970, **56**, 421–437.

Köhler, W. *Dynamics in psychology*. New York: Grove Press, 1940.

Kuhn, T. S. *The structure of scientific revolutions* (2nd ed.) Chicago: Univ. of Chicago Press, 1970.

Lashley, K. S. *Brain mechanisms and intelligence*. Chicago: Univ. of Chicago Press, 1929.

LeGros Clark, W. E. Inquiries into the anatomical basis of olfactory discrimination. *Proceedings of the Royal Society (London)*, 1957, **146B**, 299–319.

Lettvin, J. Y. & Gesteland, R. C. Speculations on smell. *Cold Spring Harbor Symposia on Quantitative Biology*, 1965, **30**, 217–225.

Lettvin, J. Y., Maturana, H. R., McCulloch, W. S., & Pitts, W. H. What the frog's eye tells the frog's brain. *Proceedings of the IRE*, 1959, **47**, 1940–1951.

Libet, B., & Gerard, R. W. Control of the potential rhythm of the isolated frog brain. *Journal of Neurophysiology*, 1939, **2**, 153–169.

Liebovic, K. N. (Ed.) *Information processing in the nervous system*. Berlin and New York: Springer-Verlag, 1969.

Lilly, J. C., & Cherry, R. B. Surface movements of click responses from acoustic cerebral cortex of cat: leading and trailing edges of a response figure. *Journal of Neurophysiology*, 1954, **17**, 521–532.

Lindsley, D. B. Attention, consciousness, sleep and wakefulness. In J. Field, H. W. Magoun & V. E. Hall (Eds.), *Handbook of physiology*, Vol. III, Section 1. Washington, D.C.: Amer. Physiol. Soc., 1960.

Llinás, R., & Nicholson, C. Electrophysiological properties of dendrites and somata in alligator Purkinje cells, *Journal of Neurophysiology*, 1971, **34**, 532–551.

Lloyd, D. P. L. Synaptic transmission. In J. F. Fulton (Ed.), *Textbook of physiology* (17th ed.). Philadelphia, Pennsylvania: Saunders, 1955.

Loewenstein, W. R. Mechano-electric transduction in the pacinian corpuscle, initiation of sensory impulses in mechanoreceptors. In W. R. Loewenstein (Ed.), *Handbook of sensory physiology*, Vol. 1, pp. 269–290. Berlin and New York: Springer-Verlag, 1971.

Lopes da Silva, F. H. *Dynamic characteristics of visual evoked potentials* (Report 1.5.63-3). Utrecht, Netherlands: Inst. Med. Phys., T.N.O., 1970.

Lopes da Silva, F. H., van Rotterdam, A., Storm van Leeuwen, W., & Thielen, A. M. Dynamic characteristics of visual evoked potentials in the dog. II. Beta frequency selectivity in evoked potentials and background activity. *Electroencephalography and clinical Neurophysiology*, 1970, **29**, 260–268.

Lorente de Nó, R. Action potentials of the motoneurons of the hypoglossus nucleus, *Journal of cellular and comparative Physiology*, 1947, **29**, 207–287. (a).

Lorente de Nó, R. *A Study of Nerve Physiology*, Part 2, Vol. 132. New York: Rockefeller Inst. Med. Res., 1947. (b).

Magoun, H. W. *The waking brain* (2nd ed.). Springfield, Illinois: Thomas, 1962.

Matoušek, M.   Frequency and correlation analysis. In A. Rémond (Ed.), *Handbook of electro-encephalography and clinical neurophysiology*, Vol. 5A. Amsterdam: Elsevier, 1973.

McCulloch, W. S.   *Embodiments of mind*. Cambridge, Massachusetts: MIT Press, 1965.

McCulloch, W. S., & Pitts, W. H.   A logical calculus of the ideas immanent in nervous activity. *Bulletin of Mathematical Biophysics*, 1943, **5**, 115–133.

Minor, A. V., Flerova, G. I., & Byzov, A. L.   Integral evoked potentials and activity of single neurons in the frog olfactory bulb (in Russian).*Neurophysiologica*, 1969, **1**, 269–278.

Moulton, D. G., & Tucker, D.   Electrophysiology of the olfactory system, *Annals of the New York Academy of Sciences*, 1964, **116**, 380–428.

Mountcastle, V. B.   Modality and topographic properties of single neurons of cat's somatic cortex. *Journal of Neurophysiology*, 1957, **20**, 408–434.

Mountcastle, V. B.   The neural replication of sensory events in the somatic afferent system. In J. C. Eccles (Ed.), *Brain and conscious experience*, pp. 85–115. Berlin and New York: Springer-Verlag, 1966.

Mountcastle, V. B. (Ed.) *Medical physiology*, 13th ed., Vol. I. St. Louis, Missouri: Mosby, 1974.

Nastuk, W. L., & Hodgkin, A. L.   The electrical activity of single muscle fibers. *Journal of Cellular and comparative Physiology*, 1950, **35**, 39–75.

Nicholson, C.   Theoretical analysis of field potentials in anisotropic ensembles of neuronal elements, *IEEE Transactions on Biomedical Engineering*, 1973, **BME-20**, 278–288.

Nicholson, C., & Llinás, R.   Field potentials in the alligator cerebellum and theory of their relationship to Purkinje cell dendrite spikes, *Journal of Neurophysiology*, 1971, **34**, 509–531.

Nicoll, R. A.   Recurrent excitation of secondary olfactory neurons: a possible mechanism for signal amplification, *Science*, 1971, **171**, 824–825.

O'Leary, J.   Structure of the primary olfactory cortex of the mouse. *Journal of Comparative Neurology*, 1937, **67**, 1–31, 1937.

Ottoson, D.   Some aspects of the function of the olfactory system. *Pharmacological Review*, 1963, **15**, 1–42.

Pappas, G. D., & Purpura, D. P. (Eds.)   *Structure and function of synapses*. New York: Raven Press, 1972.

Parzen, E.   *Modern probability theory and its applications*. New York: Wiley, 1960.

Pattee, H. H.   Laws and constraints, symbols and languages. In C. H. Waddington (Ed.), *Towards a theoretical biology*, Vol. 4, pp. 248–258. Edinburgh: Edinburgh Univ. Press, 1972.

Perkel, D. H., & Bullock, T. H.   Neural coding. *Neurosciences Research Program Bulletin*, 1968, **6** (3), 221–348.

Petsche, H.   EEG topography. In A. Rémond (Ed.), *Handbook of electroencephalography and clinical neurophysiology*, Vol. 5B. Amsterdam: Elsevier, 1972.

Phillips, I. I. (Ed.)   *Brain unit activity during behavior*. Springfield, Illinois: Thomas, 1973.

Pickering, S., & Freeman, W. J.   Variations of the superior colliculus evoked response in cats. *Experimental Neurology*, 1967, **19**, 127–139.

Pigache, R. M.   The anatomy of "paleocortex," A critical review. *Advances in Anatomy, Embryology, and Cell Biology*, 1970, **43** (6).

Pinching, A. J., & Powell, T. P. S.   Ultrastructural features of transneuronal cell degeneration in the olfactory system, *Journal of Cell Science*, 1971, **8**, 253–287. (a).

Pinching, A. J., & Powell, T. P. S.   The neuron types of the glomerular layer of the olfactory bulb. *Journal of Cell Science*, 1971, **9**, 305–345. (b).

Pinching, A. J., J., & Powell, T. P. S.   The neuropil of the glomeruli of the olfactory bulb. *Journal of Cell Science*, 1971, **9**, 347–377. (c).

Pinching, A. J., & Powell, T. P.S.   The neuropil of the periglomerular region of the olfactory bulb. *Journal of Cell Science*, 1971, **9**, 379–409. (d).

Pinching, A. J., & Powell, T. P. S.   The termination of centrifugal fibres in the glomerular layer of the olfactory bulb. *Journal of Cell Science*, 1972, **10**, 621–635. (a).

Pinching, A. J., & Powell, T. P. S. Experimental studies on the axons intrinsic to the glomerular layer of the olfactory bulb. *Journal of Cell Science*, 1972, **10**, 637–655. (b).

Plonsey, R. *Bioelectric phenomena*. New York: McGraw-Hill, 1969.

Pradhan, S. N., & Dutta, S. N. Central cholinergic mechanism and behavior. *International Review of Neurobiology*, 1971, **14**, 173–231.

Pribram, K. H. *Languages of the brain*. Englewood Cliffs, New Jersey: Prentice-Hall, 1971.

Price, J. L. An autoradiographic study of complementary laminar patterns of termination of afferent fibers to the olfactory cortex. *Journal of Comparative Neurology*, 1973, **150**, 87–108.

Price, J. L., & Powell, T. P. S. The synaptology of the granule cells of the olfactory bulb. *Journal of Cell Science*, 1970, **7**, 125–155. (a).

Price, J. L., & Powell, T. P. S. An electron microscopic study of the termination of the afferent fibers to the olfactory bulb from the cerebral hemisphere. *Journal of Cell Science*, 1970, **7**, 157–180. (b).

Price, J. L., & Powell, T. P. S. An experimental study of the origin and the course of the centrifugal fibres to the olfactory bulb in the rat. *Journal of Anatomy (London)*, 1970, **107**, 215–237. (c).

Price, J. L., & Powell, T. P. S. The mitral and short-axon cells of the olfactory bulb. *Journal of Cell Science*, 1970, **7**, 631–651. (d).

Prigogine, I. Structure, dissipation and life. Paper presented at the First International Conference on Theoretical Physics and Biology, Versailles, 1967, pp. 23–52. Amsterdam, North-Holland Publ., 1969.

Prigogine, I., & Nicolis, G. Fluctuations and the mechanism of instabilities. Proceeding of the Third International Conference on Theoretical Physics and Biology, Versailles, 1971, pp. 89–109. Basel, Karger, 1973.

Rall, W. A statistical theory of monosynaptic input–output relations. *Journal of cellular and comparative Physiology*, 1955, **46**, 373–411.

Rall, W. Branching dendritic trees and motoneuron membrane resistivity. *Experimental Neurology*, 1959, **1**, 491–527.

Rall, W. Membrane potential transients and membrane time constant of motoneurons, *Experimental Neurology*, 1960, **2**, 503–532.

Rall, W. Electrophysiology of a dendritic neuron model. *Biophysics Journal*, 1962, **2**, 145–167.

Rall, W. Synaptic activity of dendritic locations: theory and experiment. In E. R. Caianiello (Ed.), *Neural networks*, 1–5 pp. Berlin and New York: Springer-Verlag, 1968.

Rall, W., & Hunt, C. C. Analysis of reflex variability in terms of partially correlated excitability fluctuation in a population of motoneurons. *Journal of general Physiology*, 1956, **39**, 397–422.

Rall, W., & Shepherd, G. M. Theoretical reconstruction of field potentials and dendrodendritic synaptic interactions in olfactory bulb. *Journal of Neurophysiology*, 1968, **31**, 884–915.

Rall, W., Shepherd, G. M., Reese, T. S., & Brightman, M. W. Dendrodendritic synaptic pathway for inhibition in the olfactory bulb. *Experimental Neurology*, 1966, **14**, 44–56.

Ramón y Cajal, S. *Studies on the cerebral cortex (limbic structures)*. (L. M. Kraft, transl.). Chicago, Illinois: Yearbook Publ., 1955.

Reese, T. S., & Shepherd, G. M. Dendrodendritic synapses in the central nervous system. In G. D. Pappas & D. P. Purpura (Eds.), *Structure and function of synapses*, pp. 121–136. New York: Raven Press, 1972.

Rodieck, R. W., & Stone, J. Analysis of receptive fields of cat retinal ganglion cells. *Journal of Neurophysiology*, 1965, **28**, 883–849.

Rogers, W. E. *Introduction to electric fields*. New York: McGraw-Hill, 1954.

Roitbak, A. I., & Khechinashvili, S. N. On the mechanisms of E. D. Adrian's electrical activity of mammalian olfactory bulb (in Russian). *Journal of Physiology USSR*, 1952, **38**, 350–365.

Rushton, W. A.   Visual adaptation. The Ferrier lecture, 1962. *Proceedings of the Royal Society* (*London*), 1965, **162b**, 20–46.

Rusinov, V. S.   *The dominant focus, electrophysiological investigations* (B. Haigh, transl.; R. W. Doty, transl. ed.). New York: Consultants Bureau, 1973.

Schneider, W.   Phase-shift theory of neural information processing in the cortex: theoretical consideration and physiological evidence. 4th Annual Meeting, Society for Neuroscience, October 1974. p. 414. (Abstract.)

Sheer, D. E.   Electrophysiological correlates of memory consolidation. In G. Ungar (Ed.), *Molecular mechanisms in memory and learning*, pp. 177–211. New York: Plenum Press, 1970.

Shepherd, G. M.   Synaptic organization of the mammalian olfactory bulb. *Physiological Review*, 1972, **52**, 864–917.

Shepherd, G. M., & Haberly, L. B.   Partial activation of olfactory bulb: analysis of field potentials and topographic relation between bulb and lateral olfactory tract. *Journal of Neurophysiology*, 1970, **33**, 643–653.

Sherrington, C. S.   *The integrative action of the nervous system*. New Haven, Connecticut: Yale Univ. Press, 1906.

Sherrington, C. S.   Some functional problems attaching to convergence. *Proceedings of the Royal Society* (*London*), 1929, **105B**, 332–362.

Sholl, D. A.   *The organization of the cerebral cortex*. New York: Wiley, 1956.

Simon, W.   *Mathematical techniques for physiology and medicine*. New York: Academic Press, 1972.

Smith, O. J. M.   *Feedback control systems*. New York: McGraw-Hill, 1958.

Sokolov, Ye. N.   *Perception and the conditioned reflex* (S. W. Waydenfeld, transl.). Oxford: Pergamon Press, 1963.

Spekreijse, H.   Rectification in the goldfish retina: analysis by sinusoidal and auxiliary stimulations. *Vision Research*, 1969, **9**, 1461–1472.

Sperry, R. W.   Mechanisms of neural maturation. In S. S. Stevens (Ed.), *Handbook of experimental psychology*, pp. 236–280. New York: Wiley, 1951.

Stellar, E., & Corbit, J. D. (Eds)   Neural control of motivated behavior. *Neurosciences Research Program Bulletin*, 1973, **11**, 296–410.

Stevens, C. F.   Structure of cat frontal olfactory cortex. *Journal of Neurophysiology*, 1969, **32**, 184–192.

Stumpf, C.   Drug action on the electrical activity of the hippocampus. *International Review of Neurobiology*, 1965, **8**, 77–138.

Ten Hoopen, M., & Verveen, A. A.   Nerve-model experiments on fluctuation in excitability. *Progress in Brain Research*, 1963, **2**, 8–21.

Terzuolo, C. A., & Bullock, T. H.   Measurement of imposed voltage gradient adequate to modulate neuronal firing. *Proceedings of the National Academy of Sciences, Washington, D.D.*, 1956, **42**, 687–694.

Tolman, E. C.   Cognitive maps in rats and men. *Psychological Reviews*, 1948, **55**, 189–208.

Trush, V. D., & Efremova, T. M.   Orienting reflex and spectral characteristics of cortical biopotentials in rabbits, *Neuroscience and Behavioral Physiology*, 1972, **5**, 347–354.

Turing, A. M.   The chemical basis of morphogenesis. *Philosophical Transactions of the Royal Society*, 1952, **237B**, 37–72.

Valverde, F.   *Studies on the pyriform lobe*. Cambridge, Massachusetts: Harvard Univ. Press, 1965.

von Neumann, J.   *The computer and the brain*. New Haven, Connecticut: Yale Univ. Press, 1958.

Voronkov, G. S., & Gusel'nikova, K. G.   Presynaptic inhibition in the frog olfactory bulb. *Neuroscience Translation*, 1969, **7**, 775–777.

Wall, P. D.   The origin of a spinal-cord slow potential, *Journal of Physiology*, 1962, **164**, 508–526.

Wall, P. D.   Presynaptic control of impulses at the first central synapse in the cutaneous pathway. *Progress in Brain Research*, 1964, **12**, 92–118.

Walter, W. G.   *The living brain*. New York: Norton, 1953.

Wenzel, B. M., & Sieck, M. H.   Olfaction. *Annual Review of Physiology*, 1966, **28**, 381–434.

Werblin, F. S., & Dowling, J. E.   Organization of the retina of the mudpuppy Necturus maculosus. II. Intracellular recording. *Journal of Neurophysiology*, 1969, **32**, 339 335.

Willey, T. J.   The ultrastructure of the cat olfactory bulb. *Journal of comparative Neurology*, 1973, **152**, 211–232.

Willey, T. J., & Freeman, W.J.   Alteration of prepyriform evoked response following prolonged electrical stimulation. *American Journal of Physiology*, 1968, **215**, 1435–1441.

Wilson, H. R., & Cowan, J. D.   Excitatory and inhibitory interactions in localized populations of model neurons. *Biophysics Journal*, 1972, **12**, 1–24.

Wilson, H. R., & Cowan, J. D.   A mathematical theory of the functional dynamics of cortical and thalamic nervous tissue. *Kybernetik*, 1973, **13**, 55–80.

Woodbury, J. W.   Potentials in a volume conductor. In H. D. Patton, J. W. Woodbury, & A. L. Towe (Eds.), *Neurophysiology*, pp. 83–91. Philadelphia, Pennsylvania: Saunders, 1961.

Yamamoto. C., & Yamamoto, T.   Oscillation potential in strychninized olfactory bulb. *Japanese Journal of Physiology*, 1962, **12**, 14–24.

Zetterberg, L. H.   *Stochastic activity in a population of neurons* (Report No. 2.3. 153/1). Utrecht, Netherlands: Med.-Fys. Inst., T.N.O., 1973.

Author Index

Numbers in italics refer to the pages on which the complete references are listed.

A

Adey, W. R., 406, 450, 454, *462*
Adrian, E. D., 386–387, 431, *462*
Adrian, R. H., 124, *462*
Ahn, S. M., 379, *462*,
Ajmone Marsan, C., 449, *462*
Andersen, P., 450, *462*
Anderson, T. W., xii, *462*
Andersson, S. A., 450, *462*
Anninos, P. A., 400, *462*

B

Bantli, H., 31, 271, 448, *462*
Barlow, H. B., 4, 252, 449, 456–457, *462*, *463*
Becker, C. J., 341, *463*
Beek, B., 400, *463*, *467*
Beidler, L. M., 429, *463*
Beurle, R. L., 5, 396, *463*
Biedenbach, M. A., 107, 204, 244, 329, 449, *463*
Blumenthal, R., 6, *463*, *468*
Bongard, M., 427, *463*
Boudreau, J. C., 150, 390, 426, *463*
Brazier, M. A. B., 24, *463*
Brightman, M. W., 19, *463*, *470*
Bullock, T. H., 12, 427, 454, *463*, *469*, *471*
Burns, B. D., 341, 449, *463*
Byzov, 18, 286, *463*, *469*

C

Caianiello, E. R., 24, *463*
Callens, M., 324, *463*
Carnap, R. P., 457,
Caspers, H., 449, *463*
Cherry, R. B., 5, *468*
Chow, K. L., 455, *463*
Coggeshall, R. E., 19, *467*
Cole, K. S., 63, 91, 137, *463*
Coombs, J. S., 97, *463*
Corbit, J. D., 403, *470*
Cowan, J. D., 5, 171, 271, 396–400, 448, 450, 458, *472*
Cragg, B. G., 5, *463*
Craik, K. J. W., 427, *463*
Creutzfeldt, O. D., 449, *463*, *464*
Csermely, T. J., 400, *462*, *467*
Curtis, H. J., 63, 91, 137, *463*

D

Dennis, B. I., 324, *464*
Dewan, E. M., 390, 450, *464*
Di Stefano, J. J., xii, 69, *464*
Dodge, F. A., 271, *464*, *468*
Dowling, J. E., 18, *472*
Dumenko, V. N., 451, *464*
Dutta, S. N., 384, *470*

473

E

Eccles, J. C., 9, 18, 97, 99–100, 304, 448, *463*, *464*
Efremova, T. M., 450, *464*, *471*
Elul, R., 271, 449, *464*
Emery, J. D., 445, *464*
Engovatov, V. V., 18, *466*
Evarts, E. V., 459, *464*

F

Fatt, P., 97, *463*
Flerova, G. I., 286, *469*
Frazier, W. T., 19, *467*
Freeman, W. J., 7, 104, 107, 173, 214, 227, 257, 271, 329, 341, 379, 383, 403–409, 445, 447, *462*, *463*, *464*, *465*, *467*, *469*, *472*

G

Gardner, E., xii, *466*
Gasser, H. S., 74, *466*
Gault, F. P., 383, *466*
Gerard, R. W., 5, 383, *466*, *468*
Gerstein, G. L., 153, *466*
Gesteland, R. C., 429, *468*
Gilman, A., xii, *466*
Glansdorff, P., 6, 8, *466*
Goldman, D. E., 128, *466*
Goodman, L. S., xii, *466*
Goodwin, B. C., 7, *466*
Gorbman, A., 428, *467*
Granit, R., 101, 102, 145, *466*
Grastyán, E., 406, 445, *466*
Green, J. D., 333, *466*
Griffith, J. S., 5, 7, *466*
Grossberg, S., 5, 171, 399–400, 427, 440, *466*
Grundfest, H., 74, *466*
Gusel'nikov, V. I., 18, *466*
Gusel'nikova, K. G., 18, 304, *466*, *471*

H

Haberly, L. B., 173, 235, 244, 266, *466*, *471*
Hagiwara, S., 144, *467*
Hara, T. J., 428, *467*
Harth, E. M., 400, *462*, *467*
Hartline, H. K., 458, *467*
Hebb, D. O., xii, 4, 9, 24, *467*
Heimer, L., 236, 238, *467*
Hendrix, D. E., 432, *467*
Highstone, H. H., 331, *467*

Hillyard, S. A., 454, *467*
Hodgkin, A. L., 3, 90, 129–132, 136, *467*, *469*
Horowitz, J. M., 173, 214, 271, *467*
Howland, B., 173, *467*
Hubel, D. H., 252, 456, 458, *467*
Hughes, J. R., 432, *467*
Hunt, C. C., 160, *470*
Huxley, A. F., 3, 129, 132, 190, *467*

I

Ito, M., 448, *464*

J

Jacobson, M., 428, *467*
John, E. R., 5, 451, *464*
Johnson, J. W., 432, *467*

K

Kandel, E. R., 18–19, 288, *467*
Katchalsky, A., 6, 7 n., 26, *468*
Katz, B., xii, 121, *468*
Kellerth, J.-O., 145, *466*
Kernell, D., 101, *466*
Kerr, D. I. B., 324, *464*
Khechinashvili, S. N., 430 n., *470*
Kiang, N. Y.-S., 153, *466*
Kirschfeld, K., 439, *468*
Knight, B. W., 271, *468*
Köhler, W., 5, *468*
Kuhn, T. S., 8, *468*

L

Lashley, K. S., 5, 460, *468*
Leaton, R. N., 383, *466*
Le Gros Clark, W. E., xi, 257, 429, *468*
Leiman, A. L., 455, *463*
Lettvin, J. Y., 4, 427, 429, *467*, *468*
Libet, B., 383, *468*
Liebovic, K. N., 24, *468*
Lilly, J. C., 5, *468*
Lindsay, R. D., 400, *467*
Lindsley, D. B., 403, *468*
Llinás, R., 18, *468*, *469*
Lloyd, D. P. L., 28, *468*
Loewenstein, W. R., 18, *468*
Lopes da Silva, F. H., 271, *468*
Lorente de Nó, R., 173, 185–186, 203, *468*
Lux, H. D., 449, *463*, *464*

M

Magoun, H. W., 406, *468*
Mancia, M., 333, *466*
Matoušek, M., 149, *468*
Maturana, H. R., 4, *468*
McCulloch, W. S., 4, 9, 24, *467, 468, 469*
Minor, A. V., 286, *469*
Moulton, D. G., xi, 429, *469*
Mountcastle, V. B., 4, 252, 455–456, *469*

N

Nastuk, W. L., 129, *469*
Nicholson, C., 18, 173, *468, 469*
Nicolis, G., 8, *470*
Nicoll, R. A., 333, 424, *469*

O

O'Leary, J., 236, *469*
Ottoson, D., xi, 429, *469*

P

Pappas, G. D., 18, *469*
Parzen, E., xii, 152, *469*
Patel, H. H., *465*
Pattee, H. H., 428, *465*
Perkel, D. H., 427, *469*
Pertile, G., 400, *462*
Petsche, H., 449, *469*
Phillips, I. I., 459, *469*
Pickering, S., 329, *469*
Pigache, R. M., 236, *469*
Pinching, A. J., 286, 288, 413, *469, 470*
Pitts, W. H., 4, 9, 24, *467, 468, 469*
Plonsey, R., 173, 454, *470*
Polyshchuk, N. A., 18, *463*
Powell, T. P. S., 286, 288, 413, *469, 470*
Pradhan, S. N., 384, *470*
Pribram, K. H., 5, *470*
Price, J. L., 236, 238, 324, 413, *470*
Prigogine, I., 6, 8, *466, 470*
Purpura, D. P., 18, *469*

R

Rall, W., 19, 90–91, 160, 173, 190, 214, 231, *470*
Ramón y Cajal, S., 236, *470*
Ratliff, F., 458, *467*
Reese, T. S., 19, *470*

Reichardt, W., 439, *468*
Renkin, B., 101, *466*
Rodieck, R. W., 252, *470*
Rogers, W. E., xii, *470*
Roitbak, A. I., 430 n., *470*
Rowland, V., 6, *468*
Rushton, W. A. H., 90, 305, *467, 471*
Rusinov, V. S., 452, *471*
Russell, B., 457

S

Schneider, D., 24, *463*
Schneider, W., 433, *471*
Sheer, D. E., 450, *471*
Shepherd, G. M., xi, 19, 173, 214, 231, 235, 244, 266, *466, 470, 471*
Sherrington, C. S., 4, 9, *471*
Sholl, D. A., 455, *471*
Shortess, G. K., 101, *466*
Sieck, M. H., xi, 429, *472*
Simon, W., 104, *471*
Sokolov, Ye. N., 406, 427, 445, *471*
Spekreijse, H., 271, 446, *471*
Spencer, W. A., 18, *467*
Sperry, R. W., 4, *471*
Stämpfli, R., 190, *467*
Stellar, E., 403, *471*
Stevens, C. F., 236, 244, 449, *463, 471*
Stoll, P. J., 271, *467*
Stone, J., 252, *470*
Storm van Leeuwen, W., 271, *468*
Stubberud, A. R., xii, 69, *464*
Stumpf, C., 450, *471*
Szentagothai, J., 448, *464*

T

Tasaki, S., 144, *467*
Temperley, H. N. V., 5, *463*
Ten Hoopen, M., 140, *471*
Terzuolo, C. A., 454, *471*
Thielen, A. M., 271, *468*
Tolman, E. C., 5, 428, *471*
Toyoda, J., 271, *468*
Trush, V. D., 450, *464, 471*
Tsytolovskii, L. E., 18, *466*
Tucker, D., xi, 429, *469*
Turing, A. M., 6, *471*

U

Ueda, V., 428, *467*

V

Valverde, F., 236, 238, *471*
Van Rotterdam, A., 271, *468*
Vereczkei, L., 406, 445, *466*
Verveen, A. A., 140, *471*
Von Baumgarten, R., 333, *466*
Von Neumann, J., 5, *471*
Voronkov, G. S., 18, 304, *466, 471*

W

Wall, P. D., 304, *467, 472*
Walter, D. O., 24, *463*
Walter, W. G., 4, 24, *472*
Watanabe, S., 449, *463, 464*
Wenzel, B. M., xi, 429, *472*
Werblin, F. S., 18, *472*
Wetzel, N., 432, *467*

Whitehead, A. N., 457
Wiesel, T. N., 252, 416, 458, *467*
Willey, T. J., 32, 333, *472*
Williams, I. J., xii, 69, *464*
Williams, T. D., 145, *466*
Wilson, H. R., 5, 171, 271, 396–400, 448, 450, 458, *472*
Wittgenstein, L., 457
Woodbury, J. W., 173, *472*

Y

Yamamoto, C., 383, *472*
Yamamoto, T., 383, *472*

Z

Zenkin, G. M., 18, *463*
Zetterberg, L. H., 400, *472*

Subject Index

A

AAEP (ensemble average of AEPs), 56, 229, 418–419

Accommodation, in wave-to-pulse conversion, 21, 145, 163

Acetylcholine chloride, AEP and, 384

Action potential
  absence of, 392
  antidromic or orthodromic propagation of, 95, 332
  average number of per second, 59
  compound, 74, 84, 333
  field of, 187–189, 256
  monopolar recording of, 84, 187, 239–240, 254

Active states
  of neural sets, 34–36
  of neuron, 14–15, 17
  in olfactory bulb, 287, 306–307
  in prepyriform cortex, 245–249
  rate of change in, 196, 205, 274
  spatial distribution of, 251–260
  specification of, 16–19
  state variables in, 17–18

Activity density, defined, 34

Activity density function, 35
  conversion of to source–sink distribution, 250
  for neural sets, 250

Activity distribution, 35, 251–260
  symbols for, 253

Adaptation, in wave-to-pulse conversion, 21, 145, 163

AEP (averaged evoked potential), 37, 39, 43
  acetylcholine chloride and, 384
  changed patterns of in attentive state, 414–422
  characteristic frequency of, 110–112, 324–325, 342–343, 407
  dominant oscillatory component of, 331
  EEG changes and, 369, 375, 406, 409
  errors of measurement, 390–391
  factor analysis of, 407–414
  fitting with basis functions, 105–106, 110–120
  Fourier transforms of, 112, 150, 394
  from KII set, 110
  LOT stimulus and, 406–407
  measurement techniques for, 110–120, 392
  in multichannel recording, 195, 221
  neural mass components of, 205–211
  open-loop, 44, 107, 309–310, 330
  pattern of change for, 117, 414–422
  in piecewise linear lumped circuit approximation, 325
  PON stimulus and, 315
  potential field of, 220
  in prepyriform cortex, 118, 246–247
  PSTH frequency and, 315, 335, 438
  root loci and, 357–359, 392
  spectrum, 112, 150, 394
  "spontaneous" variation of, 395, 390, 409–410, 420

AEP, *(continued)*
transmembrane potential and, 233, 244, 249, 269
AEP amplitude, root loci and, 357–359
AEP frequency, background activity and, 330, 366
Amplitude probability density, EEG, 146, 155
Anatomical connection, versus functional, 25–26
Anesthesia, effect of on AEP, 106, 309–310, 361, 383
Anterior olfactory nucleus (AON), 234–235, 267–268, 331, 413
Antiresonance, 117, 426
Arousal, 341, 403, 413
Attentive state
change patterns for AEPs in, 414–422
cortical expectation function and, 440–448
proposed cortical mechanism of, 422, 427
Attenuation, 41, 397
see also Glomerular transmission
Autocorrelation
of EEG, 149
of pulse trains, 153
Autoexcitation, 41, 400
Autoinhibition, 41, 397, 400
Automatic gain control, 305, 439, 459
Averaged evoked potential, *see* AEP
Axons
branching of, 11–13, 81
conduction velocity in, 137
divergence by, 12, 252
firing of, 138–139
potential fields of, 185–188
probability distribution in, 138–139
pulse train of, 12
single-shock input and, 60
threshold uncertainty in, 138–140

B

Background activity
of neural masses, 146–150
in pulse mode, 150–154
as "spontaneous," 146, 150, 381
in wave mode, 146–150
Basis function(s)
adaptive, 54
defined, 39, 52
examples of, 53–55
family of, basis, 52
fitting of AEP with, 107–108

linear family, 61
neural masses and, 39
for potential fields of neural masses, 196–202
for potential in current fields, 177–180
for potential measurement in space, 173–176
Bernstein model, for neural membrane, 124
Bias control, of characteristic frequency, 366–370
Bipolar neurons, 198
Bipolar recording, 175
Brainstem, in Sherringtonian paradigm, 9
Brain systems, new technology and, 5–6
Branched fibers, nodes of, 188–193
Bulbar mechanisms, for phase modulation, 434–440

C

Cable equation, synaptic delay and, 91–92
Capacitance, electrical, 63, 87
Carbaminoylcholine (carbachol), 384
Cardinal cells, 457
Cat
behavioral states and AEP patterns in, 408–422
forebrain of, 212–213, 234
prepyriform cortex of, 111–116, 161
Cathodal block, 145
Cell body, soma of neuron, 11
Cell layer, *see* Mitral cells; Mitral-tufted cells
Center(s)
mosaic of, 4–5
versus neurons, 4–5
Centrifugal input to bulb, 341, 412–413
Cerebellum, 9, 18, 30–31, 271, 288, 448
Cerebrospinal fluid, conductance of, 179
Characteristic frequency
antiresonance, 427
bias control of, 366–370
equilibrium states and, 342–378
tuning, 442
Cholinesterase, blocking of, 384
Chronaxie, 60
Click stimulation, in cat superior olivary complex, 204–206
Closed loop cases, differential equations for, 314–321
Closed field of potential, *see* Monopole field
Closed loop trasnfer function, 279, 281–282
Cluster, unit, 49, 146, 193
CNV (contingent negative variation), 454
Coactive versus interactive states, 26
Coded neural signals, 427–428

Coding, neural, *see* Neural coding
Cognitive map, 428
Columns, cortical, 455
Component, AEP, dominant, minor, 110–112, 324–325
Compound action potential, 74, 84, 333
Compound potential fields, 202–211
  see also Potential fields
Conduction velocity, axon diameter and, 137
Constant field equation, 127–128
Contingent negative variation (CNV), 454
Convergence, 252
Convolution, in neuron models, 72–76, 100
Convolution theorem, 76–80
Core conductor
  defined, 86
  model of, 86–91
  potential functions for, 180–185
  reduction of branches to, 191
Cortex
  see also Prepyriform cortex
  differential equations for, 326–329
  macroscopic forms of neural activity in, 7
  mass action and, 460
  negative feedback loop in, 331
  oscillatory AEP from, 327
  periamygdaloid stimulation and, 338
  pulse–wave relations in, 334–337
  two types of, 455
Cortical expectation function, attention and, 440–448
Cortical impulse response, in LOT stimulation, 330
Cortical open-loop response, 326–329
Cortical output, possible mechanisms of, 446–448
Current, force and potential relations in, 178
Current fields, 177–180
Current vector fields, 173

D

DC polarization, 452–455
Deafferentation, cortical, 330, 332, 366
Deep neuron, in prepyriform cortex, 238
Deep pyramidal cell, 238
Delta function, 60
Dendrites, 11
  apical and basal, 216–218, 455
  function of, 12
  postsynaptic potentials in, 140–143
  pulse-to-wave conversion in, 17, 163–165

Dendritic membrane, ion flow in, 140–141
Dendritic membrane conductance, excitatory and inhibitory changes in, 95, 423
Dendritic tree, 8, 95, 191
Dendrodendritic synapses, 19, 218
Depolarization, of neural membrane, 130–134
Describing functions, 101, 343, 348
Dialectic, 2, 48
Differencing technique, for source–sink distribution, 173, 180
Differential equations
  input–output pairs and, 96–98
  KII set equilibrium states and, 346–355
  for neural masses, 49–50
  for neural membrane model, 64–67
Digitizing, defined, 53
Dilative divergence, 252
Dipole field, 183, 199, 200–203, 218, 222, 232, 245, 337
Dipole generators
  in olfactory bulb, 218
  in prepyriform cortex, 244
Dipole moment, solid angle and, 173, 199
Dirac delta function, 60
Dispersion, in axon bundles, 12, 81, 93, 293, 311, 424
Dissipative structures, 6, 47
Divergence, neural, 251, 439
  at axon, 12
  collateral, 252
  dilative, 252
  interspersive, 252
  in neural sets, 37, 249–252
  synaptic, 252, 260–264
  tractile, 252, 264–269
Divergence, in potential field, 175
Dogmas, in Barlow's hypothesis, 457–458
Dominant transient, 110–112, 314, 324–325
Dorsomedial quadrant, of olfactory bulb, 235
Drugs, effects on AEPs, 381–386
Dynamic modes of KII set, 356
Dynamic pattern, in theoretical chemistry, 6, 47

E

EEG (electroencephalographic) activity, 45, 143
  AEP amplitude and, 369
  AEP changes in presence of, 375, 406, 409
  bursts of sinusoidal activity in, 386, 388, 433, 435, 442
  behavioral correlates of, 403
  characteristic frequency of, 342–343, 441

EEG activity, *(continued)*
  coded neural signals and, 428
  as collection of nonstationary processes, 393, 449
  as correlates of KO and KI active states, 403
  cortical and bulbar activity compared in, 426
  as coupling for neocortical neurons, 389, 450
  dendritic currents and, 389
  filtering of, 436
  intrinsic versus induced bulbar, 386, 432
  KII level and, 308, 348 n.
  leptokurtosis in distribution, 148
  limit cycle states and, 378–401
  as manifestation of synchrony among cortical neurons, 449
  of neural mass and pulse trains, 154
  neuron populations and, 147
  in olfactory bulb, 336, 384, 387
  in prepyriform cortex, 147, 447
  probability density function from, 148
  pulse probability wave and, 441
  sinusoidal bursts in, 386, 388, 433, 435, 442
EEG amplitude
  change in, 168–169
  odors and, 404–405
  root loci and, 356, 370–378
  variation in, 161, 369
EEG field compared with AEP field, 211–212
Electric circuit theory, 63
Electromotive forces, in membrane, 13, 122
Electrophysiology, basis of, 51–52
Ensemble average, derivation of, 56
  see also AEP
Entrainment, EEG, and, 389–390, 455
EPL (external plexiform layer), of olfactory bulb, 215, 253
EPSP (excitatory postsynaptic potential), 20–21, 97, 142
  afterpotential, 97, 109, 142
  average equilibrium potential and, 164
  in KO neural set, 106
  in motorneurons, 142
  in prepyriform cortex stimulation, 244
  in spinal motorneuron, 97
Equilibrium potential, 126–129
Equilibrium states, in multiple feedback loops, 342–378
Equivalent electrostatic field, 173
Events, neural, representation of by functions, 51–55
Excitatory changes, in dendritic membrane conductance, 95

Excitatory inputs, 19
Expectation density, pulse, 153
Expectation function, 2, 427, 443–445
Extinction, response, 406

F

Factors, I–III
  in AEP analysis, 408, 413–414
  in potential fields, 210–211
Faradic stimulator, 6
Feedback
  concept of, 271
  differential equations for, 49–50, 272
  gain, 39
  lumped, 270
  topological property of, 24, 39, 275
  types of, 40–42, 271–273, 342–349
Feedback channels, 25
Feedback equation, 41
Feedback gain
  evaluation of, 40
  excitatory, 299
  as parameter for interaction, 39–42
  root locus as function of, 278–284
  three types of, 40–42, 271–273, 342–349
Feedback inhibition, in prepyriform cortex, 458
Feedback loops
  equilibrium states and, 342–378
  multiple, 342–401
  positive, 272
  single, 270–341
Force, current and potential relations in, 122, 178
Forward connections, 24–26
Forward gain, 165–171, 302–303, 346, 392
Frog, midbrain of, 428–429
Functional connection, versus anatomical, 25–26
Functions, representation of events by, 51–55

G

Gain contour, 283
Gemmules, of neuron, 11
Glomerular layer, 214–215
  functions of, 288, 304, 331, 367–369, 438–439
  in olfactory bulb, 214
  periglomerular neurons in, 253
  spatial structure of, 216
  topological analysis of, 285–291
Glomerular PST histograms, 296
Glomerular transmission attenuation, 288–293, 304, 439

Goldman constant field equation, 128
Golgi types I and II neurons, 202
Granule cell field potential, 226, 340
Granule cell layer
  of olfactory bulb, 215, 218, 238
  wave-to-pulse nonlinearity in, 392

H

Habituation, 406
Hierarchy
  of interactive sets, 25–34
  models in, 3–5
Hippocampus, 18, 203, 271, 288, 329, 450
Hodgkin–Huxley equations and model, 14, 103, 130–134, 138–139
Horseshoe crab, see Limulus

I

Impulse function, Laplace transform of, 70
Impulse response, 60–61
Inductance, electrical, 63
Inhibition
  see also Glomerular, transmission attenuation
  forward (divergent), 258–263, 438
  presynaptic, 20, 30, 163, 304
  surround, 438, 458
  synaptic, 19, 95, 143
  transmarginal, 452
  Wedensky theory of, 452
Inhibitory inputs, 19
Inhibitory postsynaptic potentials, see IPSPs
Input–output functions, 55–57
Input–output pairs, 52
  differential equations in, 96–98
  examples of, 58–59
  ordered, 55
Input–output relations, amplitude-dependent, 144–146
Interactive sets, topological hierarchy of, 25–34
Internal plexiform layer, see IPL
Interspersive divergence, 252
Interval histogram, pulse train and, 153–154
Ionic hypothesis, 121–125
IPL (internal plexiform layer), 215, 220, 225
IPSPs (inhibitory postsynaptic potentials, 19, 95, 143
  average equilibrium potential of, 164
  grading of, 140
  in prepryiform cortex, 244
Isopotential surface, defined, 174

K

KO set, 26
  amplitude-dependent nonlinearity in, 345
  compound potential fields and, 202
  defined, 26–28
  dynamical system in, 109
  EEG in analysis of, 450
  feedback in, 270, 324
  impulse response, 107, 309, 330
  input–output function for, 70, 273
  lumped circuit approximation, 273–278
  network of, 26–29, 42, 448
  neural signal in, 402
  neuron threshold variation in, 160, 399
  observability of, 47–48
  piecewise linear approximation of dynamics in, 170
  potential fields for, 196
  state variables of, 34–36
  topology of, 26, 110
KO subsets
  feedback loop between, 40, 165, 287
  pulse-to-wave conversion in, 166
  wave-to-pulse conversion in, 166
KI level, reduction of feedback from, 285–305
KI set, 26
  activity density function and, 460
  compound potential fields and, 202
  cortical output mechanism and, 447–448
  defined, 29, 273
  differential equations for, 291
  EEG values in, 154
  examples of, 29–31
  feedback elements in, 41–42, 270
  forward gain and, 165–171
  interaction level of, 43–44
  linear output of, 43
  neural signal in, 402
  observability of, 47
  olfactory bulb potential field and, 225
  piecewise linear approximations in, 390
  potential fields for, 196
  in prepyriform cortex, 245
  pulse probabilities in, 162–163
  pulse-to-wave conversion in, 163–165
  periglomerular neurons as, 286
  reduction to lumped piecewise linear approximation, 273–278
  root locus plot for, 292
  self-stabilization of, 299–305
  stable nonzero equilibrium and, 46

KI set, *(continued)*
  stable zero equilibrium domain of, 44
  state space of, 42
  topology of, 29
  wave–pulse relations in, 154–155, 159–162
KII set, 26
  attention mechanism and, 422–423
  behavioral correlates of wave activity in,
    402–430
  in bulb and cortex, 331
  characteristic frequency of, 342–344
  coding hypothesis and, 451–452
  cortical output mechanisms and, 447–448
  differential equations for, 346–355, 394–396
  dynamic properties in second mode, 411
  encoding in, 460
  equilibrium states in, 433
  examples of, 31–33
  feedback in, 47, 305–321
  interaction level for, 43–44, 171
  limit cycle state of, 49, 388–389, 433
  linearization of, 348–349
  in lumped circuit representation, 269
  negative feedback loop in, 347
  neocortical mass actions and, 448
  neural signal transformation and, 427–448
  observability of, 47–48
  operating bias in, 381
  oscillatory responses from, 110–120
  piecewise linear approximations in, 390
  PON input to, 366
  in prepyriform cortex, 238
  primary sensory areas as, 459
  reduced, 31, 307, 324, 359
  representation of, 42
  root locus plots for, 319, 356–359, 375
  semiautonomous operation in, 412
  stable zero equilibrium domain of, 44
  stability properties of, 378–381
  state space of, 42
  state variables of, 36
  theory of, 400–401
  topology of, 31
  transfer function from KI output in, 350
KIII level, 34
  and channels for centrifugal input, 338–341
  as lowest level of behavioral analysis, 47
  and pulse–wave relations in cortex and bulb,
    334–337
  reduction of to lumped linear piecewise level,
    321–341

KIII sets, wave packets and 460
Kirchhoff's laws, 62, 64–67, 87
K model, key test of, 448–449

L

Laplace transform, 67–70
  in convolution theorem, 76–77
  defined, 76
  for neural membrane, 70–72
Lateral olfactory tract, *see* LOT
Leptokurtosis, of EEG amplitude density, 148
Limit cycle states
  comparisons with related mathematical mod-
    els, 396–401
  EEG mechanism and, 378–401
  in first mode, 381–386
  in second mode, 386–390
  neural sets, 45
  neurons, single, 23
Limulus, eye of, 29, 46, 271, 439, 458
Linear models, for neurons, 94–103
Longitudinal polarization, axon, 186
Loop current
  in membrane, 13
  for neuron, 62, 177
  postsynaptic potentials of, 140
LOT (lateral olfactory tract), 215
  mitral-tufted axon organization in, 266
  prepyriform cortex and, 235–238
  primary olfactory cortex and, 234
LOT axons, convergence of, 268, 440
LOT input, transfer function for, 334
LOT input channel
  impulse response of, 311
  transfer function of, 330–334
LOT stimulation, 223–224, 231
  AEP in response to, 316, 386, 405–406, 409
  AEP decay rate and, 453
  antidromic, 288
  in attentive state, 414–415
  attenuation effect in, 290
  behavioral states and, 416–422
  cat behavior and, 394
  characteristic frequency in, 367
  closed-loop response to, 314
  cortical excitability in, 405
  cortical impulse response and, 330
  divergence and, 266
  field potential evoked by, 340
  impulse responses to, 307

inhibitory bias and, 369
long-term, 332
mitral-tufted cells in, 424
negative peak decrease and, 332
neural signal transformations in, 438–439
olfactory bulb and, 305
open-loop response and, 107, 313
orthodromic transmission and, 333
orthodromic volley following, 424
in piecewise linear lumped circuit approximation, 325
root loci and, 356
single-shock, 238, 356, 364
tractile divergence and, 266
Lumped circuit model, 41
Lumped piecewise linear approximation
derivation of, 273–278
reduction from KI level, 288–305
reduction from KII level, 305–314
reduction from KIII level, 321–341

M

Macroscopic activity, distribution in brain, 7
Macroscopic states (macrostates), 5, 36
Mass action
cortex and, 460
paradigm of, 10
theory of, 458
MCL (mitral cell layer), see Mitral cells
Membrane, 10
electromotive forces in, 13, 122
neural, see Neural membrane
Membrane capacitance, discharge of, 63–67, 137
Membrane potential
active state and, 13–15, 233, 249, 269
fluctuations in, 126
synaptic noise in, 145
Mitral-tufted cells, 215, 218, 253
in divergence and convergence, 218, 253, 258–259
interaction of, 333, 424, 439
in LOT stimulus, 422
in olfactory bulb, 331
transmission distance, 261–262
wave-to-pulse nonlinearity in, 392
Mode
of activity, wave or pulse, 13, 37
of KII set dynamics, 356
Models
of brain function, 2–3

in hierarchy, 3–5
linear, 94–103
for neuron parts, 72–94
"neuronal" (expectational), 406, 427, 445
synaptic interaction and, 5
Molecular layer, of prepyriform cortex, 236
Monopolar recording, 175, 186
Monopole field, closed, 183, 192, 200–203, 205, 215, 218, 222, 245, 337
Motivation, 403–404, 413
Motor cortex, as network of KI and KII sets, 459
see also Cortex; Prepyriform cortex
Motorneurons, spinal, 18, 29, 35, 97, 142
Multichannel recording, of potential fields, 195, 221, 437
Multiple feedback loops
limit cycle states and, 378–401
with variable gain, 342–401
Multiple stable states
interaction levels and, 42–45
neural signals and, 46–47, 402, 427
Myelin, 11, 74

N

Negative feedback, root locus plot for, 283
see also Feedback
Negative feedback loop
characteristic frequency of, 351–352
in cortex, 331
for KII set, 347
Neocortex
common neuron orientation in, 203
in mammals, 455
mass actions of, 448–461
neural structure of, 456
parallel processing in, 460
Nernst equation, 124, 127–128, 130
Nerve action potential, 81, 128, 134–138, 185–189
Network representations, 24–34
Networks, of neurons, 4–5, 9, 24–25
see also Neural sets; Neuron(s)
Neural activity
assumptions about, 7–8
defined, 17
fine structure in, 4
macroscopic forms of, 5–10
new technology and, 5–6
Neural coding, in olfactory bulb, 429–434
Neural events
macroscopic versus individual, 8

Neural events, *(continued)*
  measurement of, 51–61, 174–175
Neural masses, 25–50
  activity density function in, 250
  approach to, 1–10
  background activity of, 146–150
  basis functions in, 39, 196–202
  differential equations for, 49–50
  divergence and convergence in, 249–269
  EEG of, 154
  global description of fields for, 198
  linear models for, 103–120
  nonlinear models for, 146–171
  nonlinear regression in models of, 103–106
  observable electrical activity of, 250
  observed fields measurement for, 193–196
  optimal values of parameters for, 104
  potential fields of, 193–211
  relation to neural sets, 25
  signal processing by, 402–461
  synaptic interaction in, 5
Neural membrane
  Bernstein model of, 124
  capacitance discharge in, 137
  conductance changes in, 125
  as current generator, 134
  depolarization of, 130–134
  differential equations for model of, 64–67
  differential polarization of, 134
  equation for, 123
  Laplace transform and, 67–72
  linear models for, 61–72
  metabolic forces in, 125–126
  molecular structure of, 121–122
  nonlinear models for, 121–134
  potential fluctuations in, 126
  sodium and potassium flux of, 125–126
  topology of, 61–64
  transactional events in, 126
  transmembrane potential in, 127
Neural network, topologies for, 25
Neural pulse trains, 151–154
Neural sets, 5
  see also KO set; KI set; KII set
  averaged evoked potential in, 37
  examples of, 28–34
  feedback gain as parameter for interaction in, 39
  networks of, 26–27
  operations of, 37–38
  sigmoid nonlinear input–output curve for, 171

Neural signal
  activity density function and, 47
  coded, 427–428
  defined, 402
  multiple stabilities and, 46–47
  synchronization in, 433
  transformation of by KII sets, 427–448
Neural system, parameters of, 17–18
Neuron(s)
  active state of, 14–19, 245–260
  amplitude-dependent properties of, 121–171
  anatomical concept of, 94–95
  autoexcitatory or autoinhibitory, 25, 397–398
  axon of, *see* Axons
  behavior and, 4–5
  bipolar, 198
  cell body or soma of, 11
  cells in, 10, 218
  as columns, 455
  common orientation of, 203
  convergence among, 24–25
  coupling of by EEG, 450
  cytoplasm in, 10, 16–17
  "deep" type, in prepyriform cortex, 238
  divergence among, 25, 249–269
  dynamic versus anatomical concept of, 94–95
  excitatory or inhibitory output of, 19
  feedback channel and, 25
  function of, 16
  Golgi types I and II, 202
  granule cells, 218
  input–output relations of, 19–20
  interpretation of parameters in model of, 99–100
  in KI sets, 273–274
  linear models for, 72–103
  loop current in, 13, 62
  membrane of, *see* Neural membrane
  mitral cells, 218
  multiple stable states of, 22–24
  networks of, 4, 9
  nodes and branched fibers in, 188–193
  nonlinear models for, 134–146
  operation of, 11–13
  in parallel, 25
  periglomerular, 215, 264, 286, 288, 292–293
  potential fields of, 172–193
  single, 10–25
  space-dependent properties of, 172–269
  spines and gemmules of, 11
  stable zero equilibrium in, 23

state of, 14
state variables of, 13–15, 95
structure of, 10–11
synapses of, 5, 11–12, 91–94, 260–264
time-dependent properties of, 51–120
topological properties of, 1–50
transmembrane potential of, 127, 140–141, 288
trigger features of, 457
tufted cells, 218, 253, 258–259
type A and Type B, 441
unstable, 22
Neuron doctrine, in neurophysiology, 10
Neuron geometry
reduction to spherical soma, 192
reduction of to a cylinder, 191
Neuron networks, basic topologies of, 9, 24–25
Neuron sets, *see* Neural sets
Neurophysiology
neuron doctrine in, 10
paradigms in, 9
two traditions in, 4
Nodes
branched fibers and, 188–193
of Ranvier, 130, 137, 190, 196
Nonlinear models, for neural masses, 146–171, 342–355

O

Observed fields, measurement of for neural masses, 193–196
Odors, EEG activity and, 403–405
Ohm's law, 90, 122, 178
ionic equivalent to, 122
Olfactory bulb
artificial input to, 305
cortex and, 330
deafferentation and, 331, 366
dorsomedial quadrant of, 235
EEG in, 336–337
equilibrium state of, 441–442
external plexiform layer in, 215
geometry and topology of, 212–219
granule cell layer in, 215, 220, 225
internal plexiform layer in, 215, 220, 225
isolation of, 331, 373, 411–412
local geometry of, 215
mitral-tufted cells in, 215, 331
neural coding in, 429–434
potential fields in, 211–234, 222–223

pulse–wave relations in, 334–337
quadrants of, 235
response domain of, 233
sections through, 215
in sleep–wake cycle, 341
time-dependent activity in, 228–234
topological analysis of, 305–309
ventrolateral quadrant of, 235
Olfactory nerve, primary, *see* PON
Open-loop AEPs, differential equations for, 309–310
Open-loop responses, in PON stimulation, 310–312
Open-loop state, 44
in feedback, 278
Open-loop transfer function, 279
of neuron subsets, 400
Operations, state variables in, 17, 37
Ordered pairs, input–output, 55
Orienting response, 405–406
Orthodromic propagation, in action potential, 95
Oscillatory, AEP, from cortex, 327
Oscillatory responses, from KII set, 110–120

P

Paleocortex, 429, 455–456
Parameters, of neural system, 17–18
Parts of neurons, nonlinear models for, 134–146
see also Neuron(s)
Periglomerular neurons, 218
see also Glomerular layer
in glomerular layer, 253
as KI set, 286
PSTHs of, 288 n.
transfer function and, 293
Pharmacological techniques
study of feedback with, 329–330, 381–386
Phase
bulbar mechanisms for modulation, 434–440
coding in wave packets, 432–434
gradient, 230, 233, 245, 268, 390
locking, 389, 455
measurement in AEPs and PSTHs, 110, 316, 327
predicted for closed loop, 320, 337
of pulse probability waves, 159, 435
Poisson process, pulse train as, 151–152
Poles, in Laplace transform, 69–70, 278
PON (primary olfactory nerve), 81–82
compound action potential of, 84, 254

PON, *(continued)*
   monopolar stimulation of, 256–258
   single-shock stimulation of, 253, 362, 372
   transmission of afferent signal by, 430
   transsection of, 302
PON axons, 218–219, 265
PON conduction velocity, 82
PON input
   apical dendritic action potential response to, 341
   glomerular transmission attenuation of, 304–305
PON stimulation, 307
   AEP amplitude of, 289
   in cat olfactory bulb, 357
   characteristic frequency and, 367
   closed-loop responses to, 314
   compound action potential, 84
   feedback and, 286
   open-loop responses on, 310–312
   pentobarbital and, 383
   periglomerular neuron distribution and, 431
   root loci and, 372
   single-shock, 253, 362, 372
   width of active focus of, 258
Positive feedback
   see also Feedback
   closed-loop transfer function for, 279
   root locus plot for, 280–282
Poststimulus time histogram, *see* PSTH
Postsynaptic potential, *see* PSP
Posttetanic depression, 20, 145
Posttetanic potentiation, 20, 145, 425
Potassium
   as intracellular cation, 125
   extracellular, 290
Potential
   basis functions for measurement of in space, 173–176
   current and force relations in, 178
   extracellular contours of, 183
   as function along distance, 199–201
   gradient, 175
   spatial functions of, 219–228
   transmembrane current and, 182
Potential fields
   of axons, 185–188
   closed, 200
   compound, 202–211
   dipole, *see* Dipole field
   monopole, *see* Monopole field

   in olfactory bulb, 211–234
   in prepyriform cortex, 245–249
   tripole, 187
Potential functions
   for core conductor, 180–185
   reference electrode for, 175
Potential measurement, basis functions for, 173–176
Prepyriform cortex, 164
   AEP in, 246–247, 332
   attention mechanism and, 422–427
   dipole generators in, 244
   EEG and, 148, 405, 409
   factor analysis of AEP parameters for, 410–413
   feedback inhibition in, 458
   geometry and topology of, 234–238
   LOT stimulation of, 238–239, 364
   molecular layer of, 236
   neurons in, 161
   observed fields of potential for, 238–245
   PON stimulation and, 373–374
   potential fields in, 211–249
   potential fields versus active states in, 245–249
   in sleep–wake cycle, 341
   superficial pyramidal cells of, 236
   topological analysis of, 321–326
   zero isopotential surface in, 243, 339
Presynaptic facilitation, 20
Presynaptic inhibition, 20, 30, 163, 304
Primary olfactory nerve, *see* PON
Primary sensory areas, as KII sets, 459
PSP (postsynaptic potential), 19–21
   amplitudes in, 143–144
   changes in, 96–97
   energy source for, 141–142
   excitatory and inhibitory, 140
   information in, 98
   ionic emf of, 163
   loop current and, 140–141
   as straight line, 103
   tetanic input and, 145
PSTH (poststimulus time histogram), 37–39
   AEP and, 246, 315, 335, 438
   feedback and, 286
   glomerular, 296
   measurement of, 316–317
   of prepyriform cortex, 246
   types, 295, 315, 335
Pulse(s), *see* Action potential
Pulse logic hypothesis, 457

Pulse mode, background activity in, 150–154
Pulse probability
  conditional of pulse train, 162–163, 165
  expectation density (autocorrelation), 153
  in KI set, 162–163
Pulse probability density, 155–156
  time and amplitude in, 156–157
Pulse probability sigmoid curves, 158–159, 161, 164
Pulse probability wave, 49
  experimental, 159
  oscillation of, 162
Pulse-to-wave conversion
  dendrites and, 17
  in KI sets, 163–165
  nonlinearity in, 20, 143, 144
  at synapse, 12
  time variance in, 20, 145
Pulse trains, 151–154
  EEG and, 154
  Poisson process in, 151–152
  pulse probabilities in, 162–165
  tetanizing, 333
Pulse transmission, transfer functions for, 80–86
Pulse–wave relationships, 154–159, 250
  in cortex and olfactory bulb, 334–337

R

Ranvier, nodes of, 130, 137, 190, 196
Realizability, experimental, 47–49
Receptor field, 252, 456–458
Regression, nonlinear, 103–106
Resistance, electrical, 63, 87
Response, defined, 52
Rheobase, 60
Rhythmic potentials, 449–452
Root locus
  AEP measurements and, 392
  EEG amplitudes and, 370–378
  as describing functions, 348
  equilibrium states and, 355–366
  experimental and theoretical, 355–366
  families of, 386
  as function of feedback gain, 278–284
  for reduced KII set, 319

S

Saltatory conduction, 137
Schwann cells, of peripheral nerves, 10
Sensory and motor events, unit activity correlated
  with, 455–461
Septum, 210–211
Sherringtonian paradigm, 9
Shock, as driving energy, 60
Short-axis cylinder cell, 238
Sigmoid curve, pulse probability, 159, 164, 400–401
Signal, neural, 47, 402
Signal processing, by neural mass action, 427–429
Single feedback loops
  amplitude-dependent gain and stability in, 42–45, 284–285
  with fixed gain, 270, 341
  general properties of, 270–285
  reduction from KI level, 285–305
  reduction from KII level, 305–321
  reduction from KIII level, 305–309
Single neurons
  input–output relations of, 19–21
  potential fields of, 172–193
Single-shock input, to neural system, 60
Single-shock stimulation
  in prepyriform cortex, 239–241
  of primary olfactory nerve (PON), 219
Sleep, 341, 403, 413
Sodium
  as extracellular cation, 125
  spike amplitude versus concentration gradient for, 137
Sodium inactivation, 132
Sodium permeability model, 129–134
Solid angle, dipole moment and, 173
Soma, 11
  dendrites as low resistance shunt for, 90
  isopotentiality of, 145
  spherical, 192
Source–sink distributions, 197–202
  conversion of activity density function to, 250
Spatial distribution, of active states, 251–260
Spectrum
  AEP, 112, 117, 395
  EEG, 150
Spinal cord, in Sherringtonian paradigm, 9, 28
Spinal motorneuron, 18, 29, 35, 97, 142
Spontaneous activity, as background activity, 146, 150
Spontaneous variation of AEPs, 375, 390, 390, 409–410, 420
Stability properties,
  of K sets, 42–45, 284–285

Stability properties, *(continued)*
  of KI sets, 299–304
  of KII sets, 378–381
  of neurons, 22–24
Stability theory, Lyapunov, 348
Stable limit cycle domain, 23, 379–380
Stable nonzero equilibrium, 23, 46, 343
Stable states, multiple, 42–45, 343
Stable zero equilibrium, 23, 46, 343
  of neuron, 23
State variables
  in neural masses, 34–36
  in neuron, 13–15
  operations between, 16–19, 37–38
Steady state, excitatory feedback gain in, 299
Steady state spatial inhomogeneities, 6
Stellate neurons, 199
Stimulus, defined, 52
Stimulus–response pair, 52
Strength–duration curve, 60
Superior colliculus, 203, 288
Superior olivary nucleus, 203–205
Surface element, of brain, 7
Synapse, 11
  pulse–to–wave conversion, 12
Synaptic conductance change, 142, 423
Synaptic delay, 91–94
Synaptic divergence, 252
  evaluation of, 260–264
Synaptic inputs, excitatory and inhibitory, 19
Synaptic interaction, in neural mass models, 5
Synaptic noise, 145
  as random time series, 146–147, 449
Synaptic vesicles, 91
Synchronization, mechanisms of, 386, 389–390, 432–433, 449–450, 454–455

T

Temporal dispersion, at axon, 12
Tetanic input, postsynaptic potentials and, 145
Tetanic stimulation, LOT and, 330, 365, 425–426
Tetanizing pulse train, open-loop condition and, 333
Thalamic tetanization, 424–426
Theoretical chemistry, neural activity and, 6
Threshold, of neural activity, 22, 138, 160, 399
Time, functions of, 52
Tractile divergence, 252

Transfer function, 69
Transmarginal inhibition, 452
Transmembrane conductance
  change of, 141
  curve for, 136
Transmembrane current, 179–180
  depolarizing, 138
  sign reversal in, 200
Transmembrane current density, 135, 181, 186
Transmembrane potential difference, 16
  AEP and, 233, 249, 269
  active state and 16–19
  conductances in, 127–128, 141
Trigger zone, wave-to-pulse conversion, 21, 95, 145
Tripole field of potential, 187
Tufted cells, *see* Mitral-tufted cells

U

Undercutting, cortical, 331, 341, 373, 411–412, 449
Unit activity, correlation of with sensory and motor events, 455–461
Unit cluster, 49, 146, 193
Unit train, *see* Pulse

V

Vector, field, neural signal as, 433
Velocity
  axon conduction, 81
  distribution, 82
  spread of bulbar AEP, 227, 230
  spread of prepyriform AEP, 239–241

W

Wave activity
  behavioral correlates of, in KII sets, 402–427
  induced versus intrinsic, 386, 432
Wave mode
  notation for, 194
  spatial analysis of potentials in, 194
Wave packet
  defined, 433–434
  selective attention and, 445–446
Wave–pulse relations, 154–159, 250
Wave-to-pulse conversion, 21

feedback loops and, 275
in KI sets, 159–162
linear function for, 101–106
nonlinearity in, 21, 58, 145
time-invariant, 159–161
time-varying, 21, 58, 101–103, 139, 144
Wedensky theory of inhibition, 452
Wilson–Cowan model, 397–401

Z

Zero isopotential surface, in prepyriform cortex, 243
Zeros, in Laplace transform, 69–70, 109, 116, 278
  functional properties, 119, 314, 427
Zhabotinsky reaction, 6

A 5
B 6
C 7
D 8
E 9
F 0
G 1
H 2
I 3
J 4